Recent Development of Electrospinning for Drug Delivery

Recent Development of Electrospinning for Drug Delivery

Special Issue Editors
Romána Zelkó
Dimitrios A. Lamprou
István Sebe

MDPI • Basel • Beijing • Wuhan • Barcelona • Belgrade

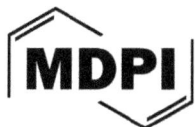

Special Issue Editors
Romána Zelkó
Semmelweis University
Hungary

Dimitrios A. Lamprou
Queen's University Belfast
UK

István Sebe
Semmelweis University
Hungary

Editorial Office
MDPI
St. Alban-Anlage 66
4052 Basel, Switzerland

This is a reprint of articles from the Special Issue published online in the open access journal *Pharmaceutics* (ISSN 1999-4923) from 2019 to 2020 (available at: https://www.mdpi.com/journal/pharmaceutics/special_issues/electrospinning_drug_delivery).

For citation purposes, cite each article independently as indicated on the article page online and as indicated below:

LastName, A.A.; LastName, B.B.; LastName, C.C. Article Title. *Journal Name* **Year**, *Article Number*, Page Range.

ISBN 978-3-03928-140-4 (Pbk)
ISBN 978-3-03928-141-1 (PDF)

Cover image courtesy of István Sebe.

© 2020 by the authors. Articles in this book are Open Access and distributed under the Creative Commons Attribution (CC BY) license, which allows users to download, copy and build upon published articles, as long as the author and publisher are properly credited, which ensures maximum dissemination and a wider impact of our publications.

The book as a whole is distributed by MDPI under the terms and conditions of the Creative Commons license CC BY-NC-ND.

Contents

About the Special Issue Editors vii

Romána Zelkó, Dimitrios A. Lamprou and István Sebe
Recent Development of Electrospinning for Drug Delivery
Reprinted from: *Pharmaceutics* 2020, 12, 5, doi:10.3390/pharmaceutics12010005 1

Panna Vass, Edit Hirsch, Rita Kóczián, Balázs Démuth, Attila Farkas, Csaba Fehér, Edina Szabó, Áron Németh, Sune K. Andersen, Tamás Vigh, Geert Verreck, István Csontos, György Marosi and Zsombor K. Nagy
Scaled-Up Production and Tableting of Grindable Electrospun Fibers Containing a Protein-Type Drug
Reprinted from: *Pharmaceutics* 2019, 11, 329, doi:10.3390/pharmaceutics11070329 6

Enni Hakkarainen, Arle Kõrkjas, Ivo Laidmäe, Andres Lust, Kristian Semjonov, Karin Kogermann, Heikki J. Nieminen, Ari Salmi, Ossi Korhonen, Edward Haeggström and Jyrki Heinämäki
Comparison of Traditional and Ultrasound-Enhanced Electrospinning in Fabricating Nanofibrous Drug Delivery Systems
Reprinted from: *Pharmaceutics* 2019, 11, 495, doi:10.3390/pharmaceutics11100495 18

Špela Zupančič, Katja Škrlec, Petra Kocbek, Julijana Kristl and Aleš Berlec
Effects of Electrospinning on the Viability of Ten Species of Lactic Acid Bacteria in Poly(Ethylene Oxide) Nanofibers
Reprinted from: *Pharmaceutics* 2019, 11, 483, doi:10.3390/pharmaceutics11090483 28

Silvia Pisani, Rossella Dorati, Enrica Chiesa, Ida Genta, Tiziana Modena, Giovanna Bruni, Pietro Grisoli and Bice Conti
Release Profile of Gentamicin Sulfate from Polylactide-*co*-Polycaprolactone Electrospun Nanofiber Matrices
Reprinted from: *Pharmaceutics* 2019, 11, 161, doi:10.3390/pharmaceutics11040161 42

Liis Preem, Frederik Bock, Mariliis Hinnu, Marta Putriņš, Kadi Sagor, Tanel Tenson, Andres Meos, Jesper Østergaard and Karin Kogermann
Monitoring of Antimicrobial Drug Chloramphenicol Release from Electrospun Nano- and Microfiber Mats Using UV Imaging and Bacterial Bioreporters
Reprinted from: *Pharmaceutics* 2019, 11, 487, doi:10.3390/pharmaceutics11090487 56

Urve Paaver, Jyrki Heinämäki, Ivan Kassamakov, Tuomo Ylitalo, Edward Hæggström, Ivo Laidmäe and Karin Kogermann
Quasi-Dynamic Dissolution of Electrospun Polymeric Nanofibers Loaded with Piroxicam
Reprinted from: *Pharmaceutics* 2019, 11, 491, doi:10.3390/pharmaceutics11100491 75

Emese Sipos, Nóra Kósa, Adrienn Kazsoki, Zoltán-István Szabó and Romána Zelkó
Formulation and Characterization of Aceclofenac-Loaded Nanofiber Based Orally Dissolving Webs
Reprinted from: *Pharmaceutics* 2019, 11, 417, doi:10.3390/pharmaceutics11080417 87

Khan Viet Nguyen, Ivo Laidmäe, Karin Kogermann, Andres Lust, Andres Meos, Duc Viet Ho, Ain Raal, Jyrki Heinämäki and Hoai Thi Nguyen
Preformulation Study of Electrospun Haemanthamine-Loaded Amphiphilic Nanofibers Intended for a Solid Template for Self-Assembled Liposomes
Reprinted from: *Pharmaceutics* 2019, 11, 499, doi:10.3390/pharmaceutics11100499 98

Amanda Cherwin, Shelby Namen, Justyna Rapacz, Grace Kusik, Alexa Anderson, Yale Wang, Matey Kaltchev, Rebecca Schroeder, Kellen O'Connell, Sydney Stephens, Junhong Chen and Wujie Zhang
Design of a Novel Oxygen Therapeutic Using Polymeric Hydrogel Microcapsules Mimicking Red Blood Cells
Reprinted from: *Pharmaceutics* **2019**, *11*, 583, doi:10.3390/pharmaceutics11110583 . . . . **111**

Mirja Palo, Sophie Rönkönharju, Kairi Tiirik, Laura Viidik, Niklas Sandler and Karin Kogermann
Bi-Layered Polymer Carriers with Surface Modification by Electrospinning for Potential Wound Care Applications
Reprinted from: *Pharmaceutics* **2019**, *11*, 678, doi:10.3390/pharmaceutics11120678 . . . . **119**

Irem Unalan, Stefan J. Endlein, Benedikt Slavik, Andrea Buettner, Wolfgang H. Goldmann, Rainer Detsch and Aldo R. Boccaccini
Evaluation of Electrospun Poly(ε-Caprolactone)/Gelatin Nanofiber Mats Containing Clove Essential Oil for Antibacterial Wound Dressing
Reprinted from: *Pharmaceutics* **2019**, *11*, 570, doi:10.3390/pharmaceutics11110570 . . . . **140**

Charu Dwivedi, Himanshu Pandey, Avinash C. Pandey, Sandip Patil, Pramod W. Ramteke, Peter Laux, Andreas Luch and Ajay Vikram Singh
In Vivo Biocompatibility of Electrospun Biodegradable Dual Carrier (Antibiotic + Growth Factor) in a Mouse Model—Implications for Rapid Wound Healing
Reprinted from: *Pharmaceutics* **2019**, *11*, 180, doi:10.3390/pharmaceutics11040180 . . . . **156**

Bishweshwar Pant, Mira Park and Soo-Jin Park
Drug Delivery Applications of Core-Sheath Nanofibers Prepared by Coaxial Electrospinning: A Review
Reprinted from: *Pharmaceutics* **2019**, *11*, 305, doi:10.3390/pharmaceutics11070305 . . . . **175**

About the Special Issue Editors

Romána Zelkó is a full-time professor at the Faculty of Pharmacy of the Semmelweis University, Budapest. Her research work focuses on polymeric delivery systems, the physical ageing of polymers, and the microstructural characterization of dosage forms associated with their functionality-related characteristics. She is the author of several scientific (over 200 journal papers, six patents) and expert works. She is a member of editorial boards of internationally recognized journals, and a peer reviewer for several scientific journals with impact factor ranking. Her expertise covers the planning, development and solid-state characterization of different dosage forms, as well as the regulatory aspects of medicines.

Dimitrios A. Lamprou has authored over 75 articles, over 200 conference abstracts, and over 90 Oral/Invited presentations, and has secured over 2 million GBP in research funding. His research and academic leadership have been recognized in a range of awards, including the Royal Pharmaceutical Society (RPS) Science Award and the Scottish Universities Life Sciences Alliance (SULSA) Leaders Scheme Award. His group is applying nano- and microfabrication techniques in pharmaceutical and medical device manufacturing. More specifically, his areas of interest include additive manufacturing (3D printing and bioprinting), electrospinning (melt and solution), and microfluidics (particle formulations and chip manufacturing).

István Sebe obtained a PhD in pharmaceutical sciences at Semmelweis University in 2018. His research focuses on the development of innovative drug delivery systems based on electrostatic fiber formation techniques. The results of his work so far have been presented at several national and international conferences and have been published in several international scientific journals. In 2016, he was awarded the prize for the most innovative PhD work at Semmelweis University. In 2018, he was awarded the Albert Szent-Györgyi Young Investigator Award by the New York Hungarian Scientific Society. He is one of the founding and board members of the Hungarian Medical Microbiology Association, and since 2017 he has been a board member of the Hungarian Pharmaceutical Society—Pharmaceutical Industry Organization. In addition to his research, he coordinates industrial drug product development projects.

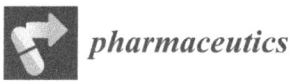

Editorial

Recent Development of Electrospinning for Drug Delivery

Romána Zelkó [1],*, Dimitrios A. Lamprou [2],* and István Sebe [1]

1. University Pharmacy Department of Pharmacy Administration, Semmelweis University, 7–9 Hőgyes Street, H-1092 Budapest, Hungary; istvan.sebe@gmail.com
2. School of Pharmacy, Queen's University Belfast, 97 Lisburn Road, Belfast BT9 7BL, UK
* Correspondence: zelko.romana@pharma.semmelweis-univ.hu (R.Z.); D.Lamprou@qub.ac.uk (D.A.L.)

Received: 17 December 2019; Accepted: 18 December 2019; Published: 19 December 2019

Electrospinning is one of the most widely used techniques for the fabrication of nano/microparticles and nano/microfibers, induced by a high voltage applied to the drug-loaded solution. The modification of environmental conditions, solution properties or operation parameters results in different fiber properties, thus enabling the fine-tuning of functionality-related characteristics of the final product. The latter includes the alteration of the rate and extent of the solubility of drugs, hence the rapid or prolonged onset of absorption.

This Special Issue serves to highlight and capture the contemporary progress of electrospinning techniques, with particular attention to their further pharmaceutical application as conventional and novel drug delivery systems or for tissue regeneration purposes. It comprises a series of 12 research articles and one review, illustrating the versatile researches and teams from 13 different countries, making profound contributions to the field.

Palo et al. investigated a combined technique for the fabrication of bi-layered carriers from a blend of polyvinyl alcohol (PVA) and sodium alginate (SA). The bi-layered carriers were prepared by solvent casting in combination with two surface modification approaches, electrospinning or three-dimensional (3D) printing. An initial inkjet printing trial for the incorporation of bioactive substances for drug delivery purposes was performed. The solvent cast (SC) film served as a robust base layer. The bi-layered carriers with electrospun nanofibers (NFs) as the surface layer showed improved physical durability and decreased adhesiveness compared to the SC film and bi-layered carriers with a patterned three-dimensional (3D) printed layer. The bi-layered carriers presented favorable properties for dermal use with minimal tissue damage. In addition, electrospun NFs on SC films (bi-layered SC/NF carrier) provided the best physical structure for cell adhesion, and proliferation as the highest cell viability was measured compared to the SC film and the carrier with a patterned 3D printed layer (bi-layered SC/3D carrier) [1].

Cherwin et al. developed a novel oxygen therapeutic made from a pectin-based hydrogel microcapsule carrier mimicking red blood cells. The study focused on three main criteria for developing the oxygen therapeutic to mimic red blood cells: Size (5–10 μm), morphology (biconcave shape), and functionality (encapsulation of oxygen carriers; e.g., hemoglobin (Hb)). The hydrogel carriers were generated via the electrospraying of the pectin-based solution into an oligochitosan crosslinking solution using an electrospinning setup. The pectin-based solution was investigated first to develop the simplest possible formulation for electrospray. The production process of the hydrogel microcapsules was also optimized. The microcapsule with the desired morphology and size was successfully prepared under the optimized condition. The encapsulation of Hb into the microcapsule did not adversely affect the microcapsule preparation process, and the encapsulation efficiency remained high (99.99%). The produced hydrogel microcapsule system offers a promising alternative for creating a novel oxygen therapeutic [2].

Unalan et al. prepared antibacterial poly(ε-caprolactone) (PCL)-gelatin (GEL) electrospun nanofiber mats containing clove essential oil (CLV) using glacial acetic acid (GAA) solvent. The addition of CLV increased the fiber diameter from 241 ± 96 nm to 305 ± 82 nm. Along with the increase of the CLV content of nanofibers, the wettability of PCL-GEL nanofiber mats was also increased. Fourier-transform infrared spectroscopy (FTIR) analysis confirmed the presence of CLV, and the actual content of CLV was determined by gas chromatography–mass spectrometry (GC-MS). It was confirmed that the CLV-loaded PCL-GEL nanofiber mats did not have cytotoxic effects on normal human dermal fibroblast (NHDF) cells, while the fibers exhibited antibacterial activity against *Staphylococcus aureus* and *Escherichia coli*. Consequently, PCL-GEL/CLV nanofiber mats can be potential candidates for antibiotic-free wound healing applications [3].

Viet Nguyen et al. developed novel amphiphilic electrospun nanofibers (NFs) loaded with haemanthamine (HAE), phosphatidylcholine (PC), and polyvinylpyrrolidone (PVP), intended for a stabilizing platform of self-assembled liposomes of the active agent. The NFs were fabricated with a solvent-based electrospinning method. The HAE-loaded fibers showed a nanoscale size ranging from 197 nm to 534 nm. The liposomes with a diameter between 63 nm and 401 nm were spontaneously formed as the NFs were exposed to water. HAE dispersed inside liposomes showed a tri-modal dissolution behavior. Amphiphilic NFs loaded with HAE are an alternative approach for the formulation of a liposomal drug delivery system and stabilization of the liposomes of the chemically instable and poorly water-soluble alkaloid [4].

Hakkarainen et al. investigated nozzleless ultrasound-enhanced electrospinning (USES) as a means to generate nanofibrous drug delivery systems (DDSs) for pharmaceutical and biomedical applications. Traditional electrospinning (TES) equipped with a conventional spinneret was used as a reference method. High-molecular polyethylene oxide (PEO) and chitosan were used as carrier polymers and theophylline anhydrate as a water-soluble model drug. The nanofibers were electrospun with the diluted mixture (7:3) of aqueous acetic acid (90% *v/v*) and formic acid solution (90% *v/v*) (with a total solid content of 3% *w/v*). The fiber diameter and morphology of the nanofibrous DDSs were modulated by varying ultrasonic parameters in the USES process (i.e., frequency, pulse repetition frequency, and cycles per pulse). The authors found that the USES technology produced nanofibers with a higher fiber diameter (402 ± 127 nm) than TES (77 ± 21 nm). An increase in burst count in USES increased the fiber diameter (555 ± 265 nm) and the variation in fiber size. The slight-to-moderate changes in a solid state (crystallinity) were detected in comparison to the nanofibers generated by TES and USES. In conclusion, USES provides a promising alternative for aqueous-based fabrication of nanofibrous DDSs for various pharmaceutical and biomedical applications [5].

Paaver et al. investigated and monitored the wetting and dissolution properties of Piroxicam (PRX)-loaded polymeric nanofibers in situ and determined the solid-state of the drug during dissolution. Hydroxypropyl methylcellulose (HPMC) and polydextrose (PD) were used as carrier polymers for electrospinning (ES). The initial-stage dissolution of the nanofibers was monitored in situ with three-dimensional white light microscopic interferometry (SWLI) and high-resolution optical microscopy. They confirmed that PRX recrystallizes in a microcrystalline form immediately after wetting of nanofibers, which could lead to enhanced dissolution of the drug. Initiation of crystal formation was detected by SWLI, indicating that PRX was partially released from the nanofibers, and the solid-state form of PRX changed from amorphous to crystalline. The amount, shape, and size of the PRX crystals depended on the carrier polymer used in the nanofibers and the pH of the dissolution media. The PRX-loaded nanofibers exhibited a quasi-dynamic dissolution via recrystallization. SWLI enabled a rapid, non-contacting, and non-destructive method for in situ monitoring of the early-stage dissolution of nanofibers and regional mapping of crystalline changes during wetting [6].

Preem et al. tested and compared different drug release model systems for electrospun chloramphenicol (CAM)-loaded nanofiber (polycaprolactone (PCL)) and microfiber (PCL in combination with polyethylene oxide) mats with different drug release profiles. The CAM release and its antibacterial effects in disc diffusion assay were assessed by bacterial bioreporters. The release into buffer solution showed larger differences in the drug release rate between differently designed mats compared to the hydrogel release tests. The UV imaging method provided an insight into the interactions with an agarose hydrogel mimicking wound tissue, thus providing information about early drug release from the mat. Bacterial bioreporters showed clear correlations between the drug release into gel and antibacterial activity of the electrospun CAM-loaded mats [7].

Zupančič et al. investigated the effect of electrospinning on the viability of bacteria incorporated into nanofibers. The morphology, zeta potential, hydrophobicity, average cell mass, and growth characteristics of nine different species of *Lactobacillus* and one of *Lactococcus* were characterized. The electrospinning of polymer solutions containing ~10 log colony forming units (CFU)/mL of lactic acid bacteria enabled the successful incorporation of all bacterial species tested, from the smallest (0.74 µm; *Lactococcus lactis*) to the largest (10.82 µm; *Lactobacillus delbrueckii* ssp. bulgaricus), into poly(ethylene oxide) nanofibers with an average diameter of ~100 nm. All of these lactobacilli were viable after incorporation into nanofibers, with 0 to 3 log CFU/mg loss in viability, depending on the species. Viability correlated with the hydrophobicity and extreme length of lactic acid bacteria, whereas a horizontal or vertical electrospinning set-up did not have any role. Therefore, electrospinning represents a promising method for the incorporation of lactic acid bacteria into solid delivery systems, while drying the bacterial dispersion at the same time [8].

Sipos et al. formulated aceclofenac-loaded poly(vinyl-pyrrolidone)-based nanofibers by electrospinning to obtain drug-loaded orally disintegrating webs to enhance the solubility and dissolution rate of the poorly soluble anti-inflammatory active that belongs to the Biopharmaceutical Classification System (BCS) Class-II. Triethanolamine-containing ternary composite of aceclofenac-poly(vinylpyrrolidone) nanofibers was formulated to exert the synergistic effect on the drug-dissolution improvement. The nanofibrous formulations had diameters in the range of a few hundred nanometers. FT-IR spectra and DSC thermograms indicated the amorphization of aceclofenac, which resulted in a rapid release of the active substance. The characteristics of the selected ternary fiber composition (10 mg/g aceclofenac, 1% w/w triethanolamine, 15% w/w PVPK90) were found to be suitable for obtaining orally dissolving webs of fast dissolution and potential oral absorption [9].

Vass et al. developed a processable, electrospun formulation of a model biopharmaceutical drug, β-galactosidase. They demonstrated that higher production rates of drug-loaded fibers could be achieved by using high-speed electrospinning compared to traditional electrospinning techniques. An aqueous solution of 7.6 w/w% polyvinyl alcohol, 0.6 w/w% polyethylene oxide, 9.9 w/w% mannitol, and 5.4 w/w% β-galactosidase was successfully electrospun with a 30 mL/h feeding rate, which is about 30 times higher than the feeding rate usually attained with single-needle electrospinning. According to X-ray diffraction measurements, each component was in an amorphous state in the fibers, except the mannitol, which was crystalline (δ-polymorph). The presence of crystalline mannitol and the low water content enabled appropriate grinding of the fibrous sample without secondary drying. The ground powder was mixed with commonly used tabletting excipients and was successfully directly compressed. β-galactosidase remained stable in the course of the whole processing and after one year of storage at room temperature in the tablets. The results demonstrate that high-speed electrospinning is a viable alternative to traditional biopharmaceutical drying methods, especially for heat-sensitive molecules, and further processing of electrospun fibers to tablets can be successfully achieved [10].

Dwivedi et al. designed a nanocomposite carrier using Poly(D,L-lactide-*co*-glycolide) (PLGA)/gelatin polymer solutions for the simultaneous release of recombinant human epidermal growth factor (rhEGF) and gentamicin sulfate at the wound site to hasten the process of diabetic wound healing and inactivation of bacterial growth. The bacterial inhibition percentage and detailed in vivo biocompatibility for wound healing efficiency was performed on diabetic C57BL6 mice with dorsal wounds. The scaffolds exhibited excellent wound healing and continuous proliferation of cells for 12 days, thus providing a promising means for the rapid healing of diabetic wounds and ulcers [11].

Pisani et al. studied electrospun nanofibers as antibiotic release devices for preventing bacteria biofilm formation after surgical operation. In their work gentamicin sulfate (GS) was loaded into polylactide-*co*-polycaprolactone (PLA-PCL) electrospun nanofibers; quantification and in vitro drug release profiles in static and dynamic conditions were investigated. The kinetics of the GS release from nanofibers was studied using mathematical models. A preliminary microbiological test was carried out towards *Staphylococcus aureus* and *Escherichia coli* bacteria. The prolonged effect of the antibiotic at the site of action can reduce administration frequency and improve patient compliance [12].

Pant et al. summarized that electrospinning has emerged as a potential technique for producing nanofibers. The use of electrospun nanofibers in drug delivery has increased rapidly over recent years due to their valuable properties, which include a large surface area, high porosity, small pore size, superior mechanical properties, and ease of surface modification. A drug-loaded nanofiber membrane can be prepared via electrospinning using a model drug and polymer solution; however, the release of the drug from the nanofiber membrane in a safe and controlled way is challenging as a result of the initial burst release. Employing a core-sheath design provides a promising solution for controlling the initial burst release. This paper summarizes the physical phenomena, the effects of various parameters in coaxial electrospinning, and the usefulness of core-sheath nanofibers in drug delivery. It also highlights the future challenges involved in utilizing core-sheath nanofibers for drug delivery applications [13].

All the articles presented in this Special Issue represent a small fraction of the great research interest in the field of nanofibrous system applications as drug delivery bases or for tissue engineering purposes. Their diverse and tunable features enable a wide variety of use, which opens a new dimension in the case of their feasible scaling-up.

Funding: This research received no external funding.

Conflicts of Interest: The authors declare no conflicts of interest.

References

1. Palo, M.; Rönkönharju, S.; Tiirik, K.; Viidik, L.; Sandler, N.; Kogermann, K. Bi-Layered Polymer Carriers with Surface Modification by Electrospinning for Potential Wound Care Applications. *Pharmaceutics* **2019**, *11*, 678. [CrossRef] [PubMed]
2. Cherwin, A.; Namen, S.; Rapacz, J.; Kusik, G.; Anderson, A.; Wang, Y.; Kaltchev, M.; Schroeder, R.; O'Connell, K.; Stephens, S.; et al. Design of a Novel Oxygen Therapeutic Using Polymeric Hydrogel Microcapsules Mimicking Red Blood Cells. *Pharmaceutics* **2019**, *11*, 583. [CrossRef] [PubMed]
3. Unalan, I.; Endlein, S.J.; Slavik, B.; Buettner, A.; Goldmann, W.H.; Detsch, R.; Boccaccini, A.R. Evaluation of Electrospun Poly(ε-Caprolactone)/Gelatin Nanofiber Mats Containing Clove Essential Oil for Antibacterial Wound Dressing. *Pharmaceutics* **2019**, *11*, 570. [CrossRef] [PubMed]
4. Viet Nguyen, K.; Laidmäe, I.; Kogermann, K.; Lust, A.; Meos, A.; Viet Ho, D.; Raal, A.; Heinämäki, J.; Thi Nguyen, H. Preformulation Study of Electrospun Haemanthamine-Loaded Amphiphilic Nanofibers Intended for a Solid Template for Self-Assembled Liposomes. *Pharmaceutics* **2019**, *11*, 499. [CrossRef] [PubMed]
5. Hakkarainen, E.; Kõrkjas, A.; Laidmäe, I.; Lust, A.; Semjonov, K.; Kogermann, K.; Nieminen, H.J.; Salmi, A.; Korhonen, O.; Haeggström, E.; et al. Comparison of Traditional and Ultrasound-Enhanced Electrospinning in Fabricating Nanofibrous Drug Delivery Systems. *Pharmaceutics* **2019**, *11*, 495. [CrossRef] [PubMed]
6. Paaver, U.; Heinämäki, J.; Kassamakov, I.; Ylitalo, T.; Hæggström, E.; Laidmäe, I.; Kogermann, K. Quasi-Dynamic Dissolution of Electrospun Polymeric Nanofibers Loaded with Piroxicam. *Pharmaceutics* **2019**, *11*, 491. [CrossRef] [PubMed]
7. Preem, L.; Bock, F.; Hinnu, M.; Putrinš, M.; Sagor, K.; Tenson, T.; Meos, A.; Østergaard, J.; Kogermann, K. Monitoring of Antimicrobial Drug Chloramphenicol Release from Electrospun Nano- and Microfiber Mats Using UV Imaging and Bacterial Bioreporters. *Pharmaceutics* **2019**, *11*, 487. [CrossRef] [PubMed]
8. Zupančič, Š.; Škrlec, K.; Kocbek, P.; Kristl, J.; Berlec, A. Effects of Electrospinning on the Viability of Ten Species of Lactic Acid Bacteria in Poly(Ethylene Oxide) Nanofibers. *Pharmaceutics* **2019**, *11*, 483. [CrossRef] [PubMed]

9. Sipos, E.; Kósa, N.; Kazsoki, A.; Szabó, Z.-I.; Zelkó, R. Formulation and Characterization of Aceclofenac-Loaded Nanofiber Based Orally Dissolving Webs. *Pharmaceutics* **2019**, *11*, 417. [CrossRef] [PubMed]
10. Vass, P.; Hirsch, E.; Kóczián, R.; Démuth, B.; Farkas, A.; Fehér, C.; Szabó, E.; Németh, Á.; Andersen, S.K.; Vigh, T.; et al. Scaled-Up Production and Tableting of Grindable Electrospun Fibers Containing a Protein-Type Drug. *Pharmaceutics* **2019**, *11*, 329. [CrossRef] [PubMed]
11. Dwivedi, C.; Pandey, H.; Pandey, A.C.; Patil, S.; Ramteke, P.W.; Laux, P.; Luch, A.; Singh, A.V. In Vivo Biocompatibility of Electrospun Biodegradable Dual Carrier (Antibiotic + Growth Factor) in a Mouse Model—Implications for Rapid Wound Healing. *Pharmaceutics* **2019**, *11*, 180. [CrossRef] [PubMed]
12. Pisani, S.; Dorati, R.; Chiesa, E.; Genta, I.; Modena, T.; Bruni, G.; Grisoli, P.; Conti, B. Release Profile of Gentamicin Sulfate from Polylactide-*co*-Polycaprolactone Electrospun Nanofiber Matrices. *Pharmaceutics* **2019**, *11*, 161. [CrossRef] [PubMed]
13. Pant, B.; Park, M.; Park, S.-J. Drug Delivery Applications of Core-Sheath Nanofibers Prepared by Coaxial Electrospinning: A Review. *Pharmaceutics* **2019**, *11*, 305. [CrossRef] [PubMed]

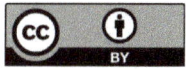

© 2019 by the authors. Licensee MDPI, Basel, Switzerland. This article is an open access article distributed under the terms and conditions of the Creative Commons Attribution (CC BY) license (http://creativecommons.org/licenses/by/4.0/).

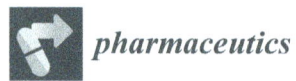

Article

Scaled-Up Production and Tableting of Grindable Electrospun Fibers Containing a Protein-Type Drug

Panna Vass [1], Edit Hirsch [1,*], Rita Kóczián [1], Balázs Démuth [1], Attila Farkas [1], Csaba Fehér [2], Edina Szabó [1], Áron Németh [2], Sune K. Andersen [3], Tamás Vigh [3], Geert Verreck [3], István Csontos [1], György Marosi [1] and Zsombor K. Nagy [1]

1. Department of Organic Chemistry and Technology, Budapest University of Technology and Economics (BME), Műegyetem rakpart 3, H-1111 Budapest, Hungary
2. Department of Applied Biotechnology and Food Science, Budapest University of Technology and Economics (BME), Műegyetem rakpart 3, H-1111 Budapest, Hungary
3. Oral Solids Development, Janssen R&D, Turnhoutseweg 30, 2340 Beerse, Belgium
* Correspondence: ehirsch@oct.bme.hu; Tel.: +36-1463-2254

Received: 29 May 2019; Accepted: 9 July 2019; Published: 11 July 2019

Abstract: The aims of this work were to develop a processable, electrospun formulation of a model biopharmaceutical drug, β-galactosidase, and to demonstrate that higher production rates of biopharmaceutical-containing fibers can be achieved by using high-speed electrospinning compared to traditional electrospinning techniques. An aqueous solution of 7.6 w/w% polyvinyl alcohol, 0.6 w/w% polyethylene oxide, 9.9 w/w% mannitol, and 5.4 w/w% β-galactosidase was successfully electrospun with a 30 mL/h feeding rate, which is about 30 times higher than the feeding rate usually attained with single-needle electrospinning. According to X-ray diffraction measurements, polyvinyl alcohol, polyethylene oxide, and β-galactosidase were in an amorphous state in the fibers, whereas mannitol was crystalline (δ-polymorph). The presence of crystalline mannitol and the low water content enabled appropriate grinding of the fibrous sample without secondary drying. The ground powder was mixed with excipients commonly used during the preparation of pharmaceutical tablets and was successfully compressed into tablets. β-galactosidase remained stable during each of the processing steps (electrospinning, grinding, and tableting) and after one year of storage at room temperature in the tablets. The obtained results demonstrate that high-speed electrospinning is a viable alternative to traditional biopharmaceutical drying methods, especially for heat sensitive molecules, and tablet formulation is achievable from the electrospun material prepared this way.

Keywords: electrospinning; scale-up; processability; biopharmaceuticals; oral dosage form; grinding

1. Introduction

Biotechnology-based medicinal products have exhibited spectacular growth over the past decade and are presently one of the most rapidly expanding segments of the pharmaceutical industry [1]. A significant challenge is maintaining the activity of biopharmaceuticals, like proteins and other biologics, during storage, shipping, and upon administration. In liquid dosage forms, biopharmaceuticals often show instability due to being prone to physical and chemical degradation [2]. Therefore, retaining the initial activity of biopharmaceuticals during product development is a cornerstone in their commercialization. The elimination of water from the formulations not only improves the stability of the biopharmaceuticals, but has additional benefits, like reduced transportation costs and easier handling and storage [3]. However, biopharmaceuticals are usually very sensitive to water removal due to their structural complexity. This poses a great challenge to finding a cost-effective drying method that is capable of dehydrating the molecule without inducing degradation, and which can produce a powder suitable for oral downstream processing (e.g., tableting).

Currently, the most widely used drying technologies employed to obtain solid biopharmaceuticals are freeze drying and spray drying, despite their disadvantages. Besides being a highly energy- and time-intensive batch process, freeze drying exposes biopharmaceuticals to freezing stresses that can cause degradation. On the contrary, spray drying can be operated continuously and is more economical, but the high drying temperature applied during the process can induce inactivation of heat-sensitive biomolecules [4,5]. Electrospinning (ES) is a novel and efficient continuous drying technology providing rapid and gentle drying at an ambient temperature. ES is a fiber production method based on the effect of a high voltage on highly viscous polymer solutions. The technology generates a dried product by elongation (due to the electrostatic forces) of the liquid feed into ultra-fine (generally < 10 μm [6]) jets, resulting in a large surface area that enables near-instantaneous drying at room temperature. Over the past years, a large number of papers have been published about the application of electrospinning for the solid formulation of various biopharmaceuticals, such as enzymes, peptides, proteins (e.g., monoclonal antibodies), oligonucleotides, and probiotics [7–15], showing the high interest in the application of ES for biopharmaceuticals. In order for ES to be applied for industrial use, it is necessary to scale-up the technology to achieve adequate production rates and develop downstream processing steps, e.g., milling for conversion of the produced fibers into powders suitable for powder filling (oral capsules and parenteral applications) and tableting (oral dosage forms).

The laboratory-scale electrospinning device with a single needle has a rather low (0.01–2 g dry product per hour) productivity [14]. The scale-up of the technology is challenging, but a device has already been developed that uses high-speed electrospinning and is compatible with the requirements of the pharmaceutical industry [16]. With this method, productivity can be significantly increased by combining electrostatic [17] and high-speed rotational [18] jet generation and fiber elongation (Figure 1).

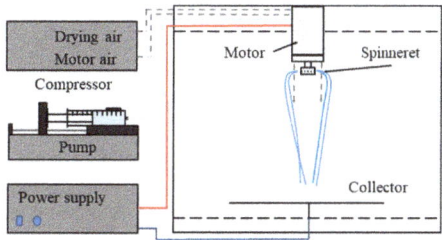

Figure 1. Schematic representation of high-speed electrospinning.

Another great challenge in addition to process scalability is achieving appropriate downstream processability of the electrospun fibers [19,20]. In this respect, the friability/grindability of the fibers and the properties (e.g., flowability) of the ground fibrous powder are also critical. A recent study by Hirsch et al. [21] evaluated the effect of various sugars and sugar alcohols on fiber friability in placebo fibers based on polyvinyl alcohol (PVA) and polyethylene oxide (PEO). They found mannitol to be the best friability increasing excipient due to its high crystallinity and the low moisture content in the fibrous samples. Mannitol-containing PVA- and PEO-based fibers were grindable directly after electrospinning, and there was no need for post-drying of the samples.

According to the authors' best knowledge, there has been no attempt to develop grindable, and thus downstream processable, electrospun formulations of biopharmaceuticals. Therefore, the aim of this work was twofold: to develop grindable fibers containing a model biopharmaceutical produced by high-speed electrospinning and to produce a stable, solid oral formulation from the ground fibrous powder. Oral administration of biopharmaceuticals has many advantages, especially when targeted delivery to the colon is needed. The advantages include a high local concentration of the therapeutic agent, smaller dose, and reduced risk of drug interactions, besides limited or no systemic exposure to the biopharmaceutical, which is usually associated with toxicity and serious adverse effects, including immunogenetic responses and hypersensitivity reactions [11].

The model biopharmaceutical in the present work was a protein-type drug, β-galactosidase (lactase), which is an enzyme widely used as a drug for the treatment of lactose intolerance. It is estimated that about 70% of adults worldwide are not able to digest lactose due to the insufficient production of β-galactosidase in the colon, which brings on gastrointestinal symptoms when dairy products are consumed [22]. Structurally, β-galactosidase is a multidomain monomeric glycoprotein, which has been shown to inactivate during spray drying without excipients, due to surface denaturation [23]. Aggregation of the enzyme has also been observed during the storage of a freeze-dried formulation of β-galactosidase [24]. An earlier study demonstrated that the enzyme remained stable during electrospinning and storage [15].

2. Materials and Methods

2.1. Materials

Polyvinyl alcohol (PVA, M_w: 130,000, 86.7–88.7 mol% hydrolysis) purchased from Sigma-Aldrich (Merck, Darmstadt, Germany) and polyethylene oxide (PEO, M_w: 2 M) supplied by Colorcon (Dartford, UK) were used as polymer matrices. Mannitol (Mannogem EZ, SPI Pharma, Wilmington, DE, USA) was used as a grindable additive during electrospinning. Powder of β-galactosidase (opti-lactase A-100) from *Aspergillus oryzae* was kindly provided by Optiferm GmbH (Oy-Mittelberg, Germany; min. 100,000 FCC Unit/g). O-nitrophenyl-β-D-galactopyranoside (ONPG) was obtained from Carbosynth (Compton, UK). Microcrystalline cellulose (MCC) (Vivapur 200) was purchased from JRS Pharma (Rosenberg, Germany). Crospovidone was obtained from BASF (Ludwigshafen, Germany). Mannitol (Pearlitol 400DC) used as a tableting excipient was a kind gift from Roquette Pharma (Lestrem, France). The water used was from a Millipore Milli-Q ultrapure water system.

2.2. Scaled-Up Electrospinning of β-Galactosidase

The scaled-up electrospinning experiments were performed using a lab-scale high-speed electrostatic spinning (HSES) setup (Figure 1) consisting of a circular-shaped, stainless steel spinneret connected to a high-speed motor [16]. The rotational speed of the spinneret equipped with orifices (number of orifices: 8, diameter of the orifices: 330 μm, diameter of the spinneret 34 mm), combined with the effect of the electrical field, allowed increased productivity. PVA and PEO were added to purified water and the mixture was dissolved under heating (40 °C) and stirring (600 rpm). After complete dissolution, the solution was cooled down to room temperature and mannitol and β-galactosidase were added to the mixture, which was stirred (600 rpm) without heating until complete dissolution. The enzyme-containing polymer solution was fed with an SEP-10 S Plus syringe pump (Viltechmeda Ltd., Vilnius, Lithuania) with a 30 mL/h feeding rate. The rotational speed of the spinneret was fixed at 8000 rpm. The applied voltage was 37 kV during the experiments using a high-voltage power supply (Unitronik Ltd., Nagykanizsa, Hungary). A vertical drying air flow (2 bar) and the electrostatic forces directed the fibers to the grounded metal collector covered with aluminum foil, which was placed at a fixed distance (35 cm) from the spinneret. The experiments were performed at room temperature (25 °C).

2.3. Scanning Electron Microscopy

The morphology of the electrospun samples was studied by a JEOL 6380LVa-(JEOL, Tokyo, Japan) type scanning electron microscope in a high vacuum. Conductive double-sided carbon adhesive tape was used to fix the samples, which were subsequently sputtered by gold using ion sputtering (JEOL 1200, JEOL, Tokyo, Japan). A 15 kV accelerating voltage and 10 mm working distance were used during the measurements.

2.4. Determination of Residual Water Content

The residual water content of the samples was measured right after the electrospinning process using a Sartorius MA40 moisture balance (Göttingen, Germany). The residual water content was determined based on the moisture loss of approximately 0.1 g sample after 10 min at 105 °C.

2.5. Grinding/Milling of the Electrospun Material

To assess the friability of the produced fibers, the electrospun enzyme-containing material was pushed through a sieve with a 0.8 mm hole size to make it suitable for blending with excipients. This kind of milling is conceptually similar to oscillatory or conical milling (both methods produce powder by pushing the material through a sieve) with respect to the achieved powder properties.

2.6. Modulated Differential Scanning Calorimetry (DSC)

Modulated differential scanning calorimetry (DSC) measurements were carried out using a DSC3+ (Mettler Toledo AG, Switzerland) DSC machine in TOPEM® mode (sample weight was 5–15 mg, pierced pan, nitrogen flush, 50 mL/min). The instrument applies stochastic temperature modulation superimposed on the underlying heating rate. A 1 °C/min overall heating rate and 1 °C pulse height (which means that the temperature was modulated by ±0.5 °C) were used during the measurements. The pulse width (the frequency of the modulation) was fluctuating randomly between 15 and 30 s. The temperature was increased from 0 °C to 200 °C.

2.7. X-ray Powder Diffraction (XRPD)

A PANalytical X'pert Pro MDP X-ray diffractometer (Almelo, The Netherlands) using Cu-Kα radiation (1.506 Å) and an Ni filter was used to study the X-ray powder diffraction patterns of the samples. The applied voltage and the current were 40 kV and 30 mA, respectively. The reference and the fibrous samples were analyzed between 2 θ angles of 4° and 42°, in reflection mode with a step size of 0.0167°.

2.8. FTIR Measurement

Fourier-transform infrared (FTIR) spectra were collected using a Bruker Tensor 37-type FTIR spectrometer equipped with a DTGS detector (Bruker Corporation, Billerica, MA, USA). The samples were ground with KBr and cold-pressed (200 bars) into discs. The measurement was carried out in transmission mode, at a scanning range of 400–4000 cm^{-1} with a resolution of 4 cm^{-1}.

2.9. Raman Mapping

For Raman mapping, the ground fibrous sample was compressed slightly to gain a flat surface of the material. Spectrum collection was carried out using a Labram-type Raman instrument (Horiba Jobin–Yvon, Kyoto, Japan) coupled with an external 532 nm Nd:YAG laser source and Olympus BX-40 optical microscope. A 100× objective (laser spot size: ~2 µm) was employed in the high-resolution measurements. Raman photons were dispersed with a 950 groove/mm grating monochromator, directing them to the CCD detector. The spectral range of 390–1500 cm^{-1} with a 1 cm^{-1} resolution was measured. A 1 µm step size in both directions was used and the collected map consisted of 31 × 31 points. The spectrum acquisition length was 30 s and it was accumulated two times in each mapping point. The classical least squares (CLS) method using the spectra of the reference substances was applied to evaluate the data.

2.10. Tablet Preparation

Standard convex-shaped tablets were prepared from powder composed of the ground enzyme-loaded electrospun material mixed with different excipients (MCC, mannitol, crospovidone) on a CPR-6 eccentric tablet press (Dott Bonapace, Limbiate, Italy) equipped with 14 mm concave punches using manual powder filling.

2.11. Determination of Enzyme Activity

The activity of β-galactosidase was determined with ONPG as the substrate. ONPG is a colorless substance, which is cleaved by β-galactosidase to galactose (colorless) and o-nitrophenol (ONP, yellow, if pH ≥ 9) (Figure 2). The amount of ONP can be measured spectrophotometrically (at 420 nm, based on a previously created calibration (data not shown)). A total of 1.5 mL of a 6 M ONPG solution in 0.1 M acetate buffer (pH = 4.8) was pipetted to 0.1 mL of 10^{-3} g/L aqueous enzyme solution, preincubated to 55 °C. After running the reaction for 10 min at 55 °C, it was stopped by adding 1 mL of 1 M Na_2CO_3 solution to the reaction mixture. The solution was left to cool to room temperature and the absorbance of the sample was measured using a UV/V is spectrophotometer (Pharmacia Ultraspec III, Cambridge, UK). A stable enzyme formulation (over the course of the experiments) was measured in parallel to each fibrous enzyme-containing sample to serve as a reference. Experiments were conducted in quadruplicate.

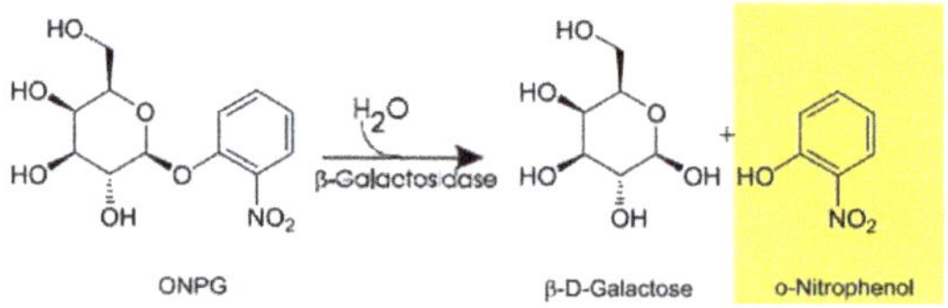

Figure 2. Enzymatic hydrolysis of O-nitrophenyl-β-D-galactopyranoside (ONPG) by β-galactosidase [20].

2.12. Storage Stability Test

For storage stability testing, the reference enzyme formulation and the prepared enzyme-loaded tablets were kept in locked glass vials at 4 °C and 25 °C. The activity of β-galactosidase in the tablets was measured after 1, 3, 6, and 12 months of storage.

3. Results and Discussion

3.1. High-Speed Electrospinning of β-Galactosidase

The broadly applied single-needle electrospinning is not capable of the mass production of fibers, and therefore, its productivity is far from the needs of commercial pharmaceutical manufacturing. In this research, HSES was used to increase the throughput of the technology. Based on the results of our previous study [21] on placebo systems, a matrix solution composed of 7.65 *w/w*% PVA, 0.57 *w/w*% PEO, and 15.30 *w/w*% mannitol was selected for the experiments with β-galactosidase to achieve a grindable fibrous product.

The placebo system was supplemented with β-galactosidase powder so that the enzyme would be 20 *w/w*% of the solid product (Table 1).

Table 1. Composition of the PVA-based electrospinning solutions of β-galactosidase.

Material	Amount (g)		Concentration (w/w%)		Ratio of Components in the Solid Product (%)	
	Original	Optimized	Original	Optimized	Original	Optimized
PVA 130,000	1.000	1.000	7.2	7.6	26.0	32.5
PEO 2M	0.075	0.075	0.5	0.6	2.0	2.4
Mannitol	2.000	1.300	14.4	9.9	52.0	42.3
β-galactosidase	0.770	0.700	5.6	5.4	20.0	22.8
Water	10.00	10.00	72.2	76.5	-	-

Even though it was possible to obtain enzyme-containing fibers by electrospinning of this solution, the high solid content caused premature drying of the material, which resulted in blocking of the spinneret and it needed to be cleaned regularly during the electrospinning process. To address this problem, the amount of mannitol in the system was reduced so that, together with β-galactosidase, their amount would equal the amount of mannitol in the placebo system (Table 1). Electrospinning could be performed seamlessly using the optimized solution composition, which suggests that decreasing the amount of mannitol in the matrix leads to a better processability. However, in our earlier study, it was shown that when the sugar alcohol content in the fibers was decreased below a critical concentration, fiber grindability deteriorated [21]. Due to this, the mannitol amount was not decreased further in the present work.

The feeding rate used in the electrospinning experiment with the optimized composition was 30 mL/h, which is about 30 times higher than what is achievable with single-needle electrospinning for aqueous solutions [21]. The obtained fibrous mat was easily removable from the aluminum foil used on the collector (Figure S1). The product was examined by means of SEM. The fibrous nature of the produced β-galactosidase-containing sample can be seen in Figure 3A. Bead-free fibers were obtained with diameters around 1–5 μm, but submicronic fibers were also observable.

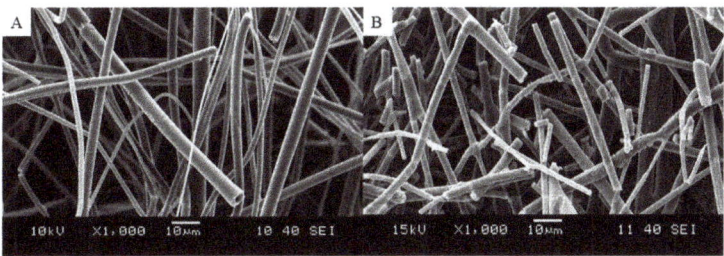

Figure 3. Scanning electron microscope images of β-galactosidase containing polyvinyl alcohol (PVA)-based fibers after electrospinning (**A**) and grinding (**B**) (at 1000-fold magnification).

3.2. Processing of the β-Galactosidase-Containing Fibers

Processability of the formed fibers (e.g., milling, powder properties, etc.) is critical in the development of solid pharmaceutical products. The produced enzyme-containing fibers collected in the form of a fibrous mat were not suitable for conventional tablet production. Therefore, the collected mat needed to be ground to a powder before further processing. Grindability of the fibrous mats from the two matrix compositions containing β-galactosidase was evaluated right after electrospinning by pushing the material through a sieve with a pestle. The friability of the enzyme-containing fibers was sufficient without secondary drying, and the grinding of the mat resulted in a fibrous powder (Figure S1). It was noticed, however, that the fibers with the optimized matrix composition were slightly less friable than the fibers with the original composition. This suggests that less mannitol in the fibers results in decreased grindability, which is in line with our previous findings [21]. Further examinations were only carried out on the fibers with an optimized composition.

The morphology of the enzyme-loaded fibrous powder was studied with SEM (Figure 3B). It can be seen that the fibrous structure of the electrospun material was preserved during the grinding process and the diameter of the fibers was unchanged. However, grinding reduced the length of the fibers, resulting in a powder with improved flowability compared to the original unground material.

3.3. Characterization of the Fibers

In order to reveal the physical state of the different materials in the fibers, DSC, XRPD, and Raman examinations were carried out. The reference PEO and PVA are semi-crystalline polymers (glass transition temperature of PVA could be detected at 46.1 °C), which was confirmed by the DSC (Figure 4) measurement. The reference β-galactosidase powder did not show any significant peak (except for water loss). The reference δ-mannitol had a sharp melting peak at 165.9 °C, even though other researchers detected two peaks (the first belonging to the melting of the δ polymorph, followed by the fast recrystallization to the more stable β polymorph, with a second melting peak) [25,26]. Similarly, the fibrous material had two endothermic peaks at 148.8 °C and 160.8 °C, which probably belong to mannitol. During the DSC run, a melting point depression was seen (165.9 °C → 148.8 °C) due to the submicronic mannitol crystals with a large specific surface [27], which was probably followed by recrystallization to a more stable form and the melting of it [25,26]. Based on these results, it can be concluded that all fiber components are amorphous except mannitol.

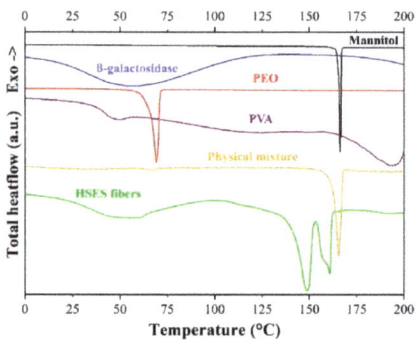

Figure 4. Differential scanning calorimetry (DSC) thermograms of δ-mannitol, β-galactosidase, polyethylene oxide (PEO), polyvinyl alcohol (PVA), the physical mixture of the fiber components, and the ground electrospun PVA + PEO + mannitol + β-galactosidase (high-speed electrostatic spinning (HSES) fibers).

In order to confirm the results obtained by DSC, XRPD measurements were performed. According to the diffractograms, only mannitol was crystalline in the fibers, showing the characteristic peaks of the δ-polymorph. This polymorph of mannitol has been shown to be the least stable at ambient conditions [28] and it can transform into the α- or β-polymorph [26], which can be found in the physical mixture of the electrospinning matrix and β-galactosidase (Figure 5). During drying (e.g., spray drying), the formation of α- and β-mannitol is expected [29]. However, in the fibers, δ-mannitol can be found, which might be ascribed to the even faster drying with ES (and therefore, no possibility for rearrangement into a stable form) or to the presence of the other substances.

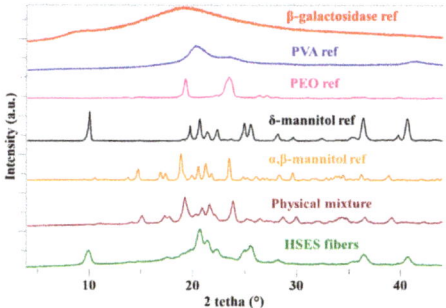

Figure 5. X-ray powder diffraction (XRPD) patterns of β-galactosidase; polyvinyl alcohol (PVA); polyethylene oxide (PEO); δ-mannitol; α, β-mannitol; the physical mixture of PVA, PEO, α, β-mannitol, and β-galactosidase; and the ground electrospun PVA + PEO + mannitol + β-galactosidase.

To evaluate the molecular interactions, FTIR spectroscopy was applied on the samples (Figure 6). PVA and mannitol molecules contain free hydroxyl groups (which can act as potential proton donors for hydrogen bonding) and β-galactosidase possesses numerous different groups that can act as potential proton donors or receptors. Therefore, hydrogen bonding might occur in the fibers. Characteristic absorption peaks of β-galactosidase are at 3298 cm^{-1} due to OH stretching and at 2939 cm^{-1} due to CH stretching. The absorption bands at 1651 cm^{-1} indicate the CONH vibration, and the 1541 cm^{-1} peak is the NH bending vibration of the β-galactosidase structure [30]. These peaks indicate the protein nature of β-galactosidase. PVA has a broad absorption band from OH at 3319 cm^{-1}, bands from stretching vibrations of CH$_2$/CH groups at 2941/2910 cm^{-1} and from C=O at 1736 cm^{-1} (characteristic of the carbonyl group of polyvinyl acetate), together with deformation bands of CH$_2$/CH at 1437/1375 cm^{-1}, and CO stretching vibrations at 1096 cm^{-1} and 1261 cm^{-1} [31]. Characteristic absorption bands of PEO include the band at 2893 cm^{-1} due to symmetric and antisymmetric CH stretching, and bands at 1468 cm^{-1} (asymmetric CH$_2$ bending) and 846 cm^{-1} (CH$_2$ rocking). The band in PEO at 1104 cm^{-1} indicates asymmetric COC stretching [32]. Mannitol showed the characteristic peaks of the OH group at 3289 cm^{-1} and the CH stretching at 2936 cm^{-1}. Multiple characteristic absorption bands of δ-mannitol can be observed in the 500–1500 cm^{-1} region, which can also be seen in the spectrum of the electrospun sample, indicating the presence of the crystalline δ polymorph in the fibers [25]. The characteristic bands of β-galactosidase, PVA, and PEO either disappeared or appeared shifted in the spectrum of the HSES fibers, indicating molecular interaction (presumably hydrogen bonding) between the components.

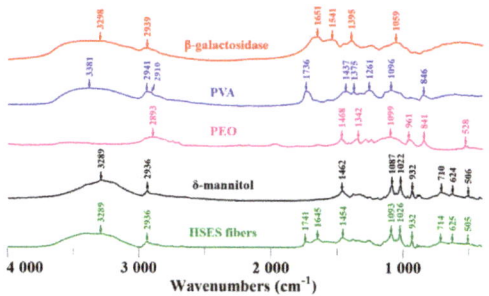

Figure 6. Fourier-transform infrared (FTIR) spectra of β-galactosidase, polyvinyl alcohol (PVA), polyethylene oxide (PEO), δ-mannitol, and the ground electrospun PVA + PEO + mannitol + β-galactosidase.

The local distribution of the components in the ground fibers was analyzed by Raman mapping. For accurate dosing, homogeneity of the enzyme in the formulation is required. According to the Raman chemical map (Figure 7A), β-galactosidase seems to be uniformly distributed in the ground fibers as very small differences in color are seen.

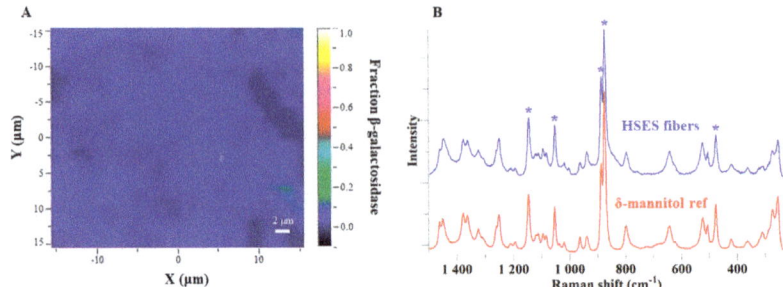

Figure 7. (**A**) Homogeneity study of β-galactosidase in the electrospun fibers by Raman mapping; (**B**) Raman spectra of the ground electrospun fibers and δ-mannitol (characteristic peaks marked with *).

The Raman mapping results also confirmed that the electrospun fibers mainly contained δ-mannitol. The characteristic peaks of the δ polymorph are shown in Figure 7B and these are in good agreement with data reported by others in the literature [33,34]. The ground electrospun fibers were reanalyzed by DSC, XRPD, and Raman after one year of storage at 4 °C. Even though the δ-polymorph is the least stable among the mannitol polymorphs, no recrystallization was observed in the fibers after this extended storage.

It has been previously shown that sugars and sugar alcohols can interact with water vapor and they have different water sorption capacities based on their physical state [35,36]. Amorphous sugars tend to absorb large amounts of water into their bulk structure, whereas crystalline sugars interact with water based on surface adsorption only. Water can act as a plasticizer in electrospun fibers and consequently, the water content of the electrospun materials influences their grindability significantly. It has been shown that a water content below 8% ensures acceptable grindability of sugar-containing fibers [21]. It was also shown that the physical state of excipients could impact the grindability, with crystalline mannitol eliminating the need for post-drying. The water content of the β-galactosidase-containing fibrous sample measured by the loss on drying (LOD) method was 6.0%. Presumably, this relatively low water content is due to the crystalline nature of mannitol in the fibers.

3.4. Tableting and Long-Term Stability Study of the Tablets

As the marketable final form of a lactase enzyme is preferably a tablet, the purpose of this study was not only to investigate the processability of enzyme-containing electrospun fibers, but also to produce tablets without losing the achieved advantages (i.e., activity preserved after processing). The fibrous powder was mixed with MCC, mannitol, and crospovidone, and the powder mixture was subsequently tableted (Figure S2). The main compression force was ~8 kN in this experiment. The composition of the produced tablets can be found in Table 2.

Table 2. Composition of the produced tablets.

Ingredients	Amount (mg)/Tablet	Amount (%)/Tablet
MCC 200	150	30
Mannitol	150	30
Crospovidone	50	10
Fibrous powder	150	30
Σ	500	100

Enzyme activity was measured after HSES, grinding, and tableting to assess the effect of the processing steps on β-galactosidase. The activity of a stable enzyme formulation was measured parallel to each sample to serve as a reference. The results are depicted in Figure 8. No significant difference can be seen between the activity of the reference enzyme and the electrospun and processed β-galactosidase, which suggests that the drying conditions with HSES are so gentle temperature wise that no degradation of this protein-type drug is seen.

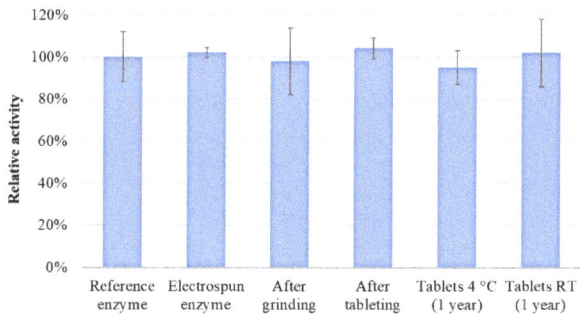

Figure 8. Enzyme activity of β-galactosidase in the fibers after high-speed electrostatic spinning (HSES), after grinding, after tableting, and the one-year stability result of the tablets (stored at 4 °C and room temperature).

Ensuring long-term stability of biopharmaceutical products is one of the main challenges in their pharmaceutical use and new formulations thus need to stabilize biopharmaceuticals to maintain their activity during storage. The storage stability of the electrospun and tableted β-galactosidase was compared with a reference enzyme formulation. The tablets of electrospun β-galactosidase were kept at 4 °C and room temperature and their activity were measured after 1 month, 3 months, 6 months, and 1 year. The periodic activity measurements showed that the enzyme remained stable in the tablets at both 4 °C and 25 °C, even after one year of storage (Figure 8). This result shows that the processable matrix containing PVA, PEO, and mannitol is suitable for stabilizing β-galactosidase in the long term.

4. Conclusions

The present work demonstrated that HSES is a feasible technology for producing biopharmaceutical-containing, processable fibers. A PVA-PEO-mannitol matrix was used to incorporate a model protein-type drug, β-galactosidase. A feeding rate of 30 mL/h was achieved in the experiments, which is 30 times higher than what is achievable for aqueous systems using single-needle ES. The produced fibrous mat was easily removed from the collector and it was found to be grindable without the need for a post-drying step, which simplifies downstream processing. All excipients were in an amorphous state in the fibers, except mannitol. The low water content and the crystalline mannitol in the fibrous sample could be the reason for the adequate grindability. The ground fibrous powder was mixed with tableting excipients and was successfully tableted. No decrease in enzyme activity was observed after either of the processing steps (electrospinning, grinding, and tableting). Besides, β-galactosidase remained stable in the tablets after one year of storage both at 4 °C and room temperature. In conclusion, the gentle drying by HSES and the processability of the applied matrix enabled the production of a final dosage form for the easy oral administration of this model protein without decreasing its activity.

Supplementary Materials: The following are available online at http://www.mdpi.com/1999-4923/11/7/329/s1, Figure S1. Electrospun sample removal from the collector and grinding process. Figure S2. Tablets prepared from ground fibrous enzyme-containing powder, MCC, mannitol, and crospovidone.

Author Contributions: P.V. designed and accomplished the electrospinning experiment. E.H. completed the SEM analysis. R.K. and C.F. performed the enzyme activity measurements. B.D. and P.V. evaluated the fiber grindability and produced tablets. A.F. performed the Raman mapping measurement. Z.K.N., Á.N., and I.C. evaluated the results. S.K.A., T.V., G.V., and G.M. contributed to the conception and design of the work. All authors were involved in the drafting and revision of the manuscript and are aligned on the final version to be published.

Funding: This work was supported by OTKA grants K-112644, PD-128241, KH-124541. Support of grant BME FIKP-BIO by EMMI is kindly acknowledged.

Conflicts of Interest: The authors declare no conflict of interest. Sune K. Andersen, Tamás Vigh, and Geert Verreck are employees of the Janssen R&D. The company had no role in the design of the study; in the collection, analyses, or interpretation of data; in the writing of the manuscript, and in the decision to publish the results.

References

1. Walsh, G. Biopharmaceutical benchmarks 2018. *Nat. Biotechnol.* **2018**, *36*, 1136–1145. [CrossRef] [PubMed]
2. Jameel, F.; Hershenson, S. *Formulation and Process Development Strategies for Manufacturing Biopharmaceuticals*; John Wiley and Sons: Hoboken, NJ, USA, 2010.
3. Langford, A.; Bhatnagar, B.; Walters, R.; Tchessalov, S.; Ohtake, S. Drying technologies for biopharmaceutical applications: Recent developments and future direction. *Dry. Technol.* **2018**, *36*, 677–684. [CrossRef]
4. Ameri, M.; Maa, Y.F. Spray drying of biopharmaceuticals: Stability and process considerations. *Dry. Technol.* **2006**, *24*, 763–768. [CrossRef]
5. Angkawinitwong, U.; Sharma, G.; Khaw, P.T.; Brocchini, S.; Williams, G.R. Solid-state protein formulations. *Ther. Deliv.* **2015**, *6*, 59–82. [CrossRef] [PubMed]
6. Cramariuc, B.; Cramariuc, R.; Scarlet, R.; Manea, L.R.; Lupu, I.G.; Cramariuc, O. Fiber diameter in electrospinning process. *J. Electrost.* **2013**, *71*, 189–198. [CrossRef]
7. Broeckx, G.; Vandenheuvel, D.; Claes, I.J.J.; Lebeer, S.; Kiekens, F. Drying techniques of probiotic bacteria as an important step towards the development of novel pharmabiotics. *Int. J. Pharm.* **2016**, *505*, 303–318. [CrossRef] [PubMed]
8. Jiang, H.; Wang, L.; Zhu, K. Coaxial electrospinning for encapsulation and controlled release of fragile water-soluble bioactive agents. *J. Control. Release* **2014**, *193*, 296–303. [CrossRef]
9. Zussman, E. Encapsulation of cells within electrospun fibers. *Polym. Adv. Technol.* **2011**, *22*, 366–371. [CrossRef]
10. Hu, X.; Liu, S.; Zhou, G.; Huang, Y.; Xie, Z.; Jing, X. Electrospinning of polymeric nanofibers for drug delivery applications. *J. Control. Release* **2014**, *185*, 12–21. [CrossRef]
11. Vass, P.; Démuth, B.; Hirsch, E.; Nagy, B.; Andersen, S.K.; Vigh, T.; Verreck, G.; Csontos, I.; Nagy, Z.K.; Marosi, G. Drying technology strategies for colon-targeted oral delivery of biopharmaceuticals. *J. Control. Release* **2019**, *296*, 162–178. [CrossRef]
12. Angkawinitwong, U.; Awwad, S.; Khaw, P.T.; Brocchini, S.; Williams, G.R. Electrospun formulations of bevacizumab for sustained release in the eye. *Acta Biomater.* **2017**, *64*, 126–136. [CrossRef] [PubMed]
13. Škrlec, K.; Zupančič, Š.; Prpar Mihevc, S.; Kocbek, P.; Kristl, J.; Berlec, A. Development of electrospun nanofibers that enable high loading and long-term viability of probiotics. *Eur. J. Pharm. Biopharm.* **2019**, *136*, 108–119. [CrossRef] [PubMed]
14. Nagy, Z.K.; Wagner, I.; Suhajda, A.; Tobak, T.; Harasztos, A.H.; Vigh, T.; Soti, P.L.; Pataki, H.; Molnar, K.; Marosi, G. Nanofibrous solid dosage form of living bacteria prepared by electrospinning. *Express Polym. Lett.* **2014**, *8*, 352–361. [CrossRef]
15. Wagner, I.; Nagy, Z.K.; Vass, P.; Fehér, C.; Barta, Z.; Vigh, T.; Sóti, P.L.; Harasztos, A.H.; Pataki, H.; Balogh, A.; et al. Stable formulation of protein-type drug in electrospun polymeric fiber followed by tableting and scaling-up experiments. *Polym. Adv. Technol.* **2015**, *26*, 1461–1467. [CrossRef]
16. Nagy, Z.K.; Balogh, A.; Demuth, B.; Pataki, H.; Vigh, T.; Szabo, B.; Molnar, K.; Schmidt, B.T.; Horak, P.; Marosi, G.; et al. High speed electrospinning for scaled-up production of amorphous solid dispersion of itraconazole. *Int. J. Pharm.* **2015**, *480*, 137–142. [CrossRef]
17. Lukas, D.; Sarkar, A.; Pokorny, P. Self-organization of jets in electrospinning from free liquid surface: A generalized approach. *J. Appl. Phys.* **2008**, *103*, 084309. [CrossRef]

18. Sebe, I.; Szabó, B.; Nagy, Z.K.; Szabó, D.; Zsidai, L.; Kocsis, B.; Zelkó, R. Polymer structure and antimicrobial activity of polyvinylpyrrolidone-based iodine nanofibers prepared with high-speed rotary spinning technique. *Int. J. Pharm.* **2013**, *458*, 99–103. [CrossRef]
19. Démuth, B.; Farkas, A.; Szabó, B.; Balogh, A.; Nagy, B.; Vágó, E.; Vigh, T.; Tinke, A.P.; Kazsu, Z.; Demeter, Á.; et al. Development and tableting of directly compressible powder from electrospun nanofibrous amorphous solid dispersion. *Adv. Powder Technol.* **2017**, *28*, 1554–1563. [CrossRef]
20. Szabo, E.; Demuth, B.; Nagy, B.; Molnar, K.; Farkas, A.; Szabo, B.; Balogh, A.; Hirsch, E.; Nagy, B.; Marosi, G.; et al. Scaled-up preparation of drug-loaded electrospun polymer fibres and investigation of their continuous processing to tablet form. *Express Polym. Lett.* **2018**, *12*, 436–451. [CrossRef]
21. Hirsch, E.; Vass, P.; Démuth, B.; Pethő, Z.; Bitay, E.; Andersen, S.K.; Vigh, T.; Verreck, G.; Molnár, K.; Nagy, Z.K.; et al. Electrospinning scale-up and formulation development of PVA nanofibers aiming oral delivery of biopharmaceuticals. *Express Polym. Lett.* **2019**, *13*, 590–603. [CrossRef]
22. Ugidos-Rodríguez, S.; Matallana-González, M.C.; Sánchez-Mata, M.C. Lactose malabsorption and intolerance: A review. *Food Funct.* **2018**, *9*, 4056–4068. [CrossRef] [PubMed]
23. Branchu, S.; Forbes, R.T.; York, P.; Petrén, S.; Nyqvist, H.; Camber, O. Hydroxypropyl-β-cyclodextrin inhibits spray-drying-induced inactivation of β-galactosidase. *J. Pharm. Sci.* **1999**, *88*, 905–911. [CrossRef] [PubMed]
24. Yoshioka, S.; Aso, Y.; Izutsu, K.I.; Terao, T. Aggregates Formed During Storage of Galactosidase in Solution and in the Freeze-Dried State. *Pharm. Res.* **1993**, *10*, 687–691. [CrossRef] [PubMed]
25. Burger, A.; Henck, J.-O.; Hetz, S.; Rollinger, J.M.; Weissnicht, A.A.; Stöttner, H. Energy/Temperature Diagram and Compression Behavior of the Polymorphs of d-Mannitol. *J. Pharm. Sci.* **2000**, *89*, 457–468. [CrossRef]
26. Hao, H.; Su, W.; Barrett, M.; Caron, V.; Healy, A.-M.; Glennon, B. A Calibration-Free Application of Raman Spectroscopy to the Monitoring of Mannitol Crystallization and Its Polymorphic Transformation. *Org. Process Res. Dev.* **2010**, *14*, 1209–1214. [CrossRef]
27. Sun, C.Q.; Wang, Y.; Tay, B.K.; Li, S.; Huang, H.; Zhang, Y.B. Correlation between the Melting Point of a Nanosolid and the Cohesive Energy of a Surface Atom. *J. Phys. Chem. B* **2002**, *106*, 10701–10705. [CrossRef]
28. Cares-Pacheco, M.G.; Vaca-Medina, G.; Calvet, R.; Espitalier, F.; Letourneau, J.J.; Rouilly, A.; Rodier, E. Physicochemical characterization of d-mannitol polymorphs: The challenging surface energy determination by inverse gas chromatography in the infinite dilution region. *Int. J. Pharm.* **2014**, *475*, 69–81. [CrossRef] [PubMed]
29. Lee, Y.Y.; Wu, J.X.; Yang, M.; Young, P.M.; van den Berg, F.; Rantanen, J. Particle size dependence of polymorphism in spray-dried mannitol. *Eur. J. Pharm. Sci.* **2011**, *44*, 41–48. [CrossRef]
30. Barth, A. Infrared spectroscopy of proteins. *Biochim. Biophys. Acta* **2007**, *1767*, 1073–1101. [CrossRef]
31. Sun, X.-Z.; Williams, G.R.; Hou, X.-X.; Zhu, L.-M. Electrospun curcumin-loaded fibers with potential biomedical applications. *Carbohydr. Polym.* **2013**, *94*, 147–153. [CrossRef]
32. Wen, S.J.; Richardson, T.J.; Ghantous, D.I.; Striebel, K.A.; Ross, P.N.; Cairns, E.J. FTIR characterization of PEO+LiN(CF3SO2)2 electrolytes. *J. Electroanal. Chem.* **1996**, *408*, 113–118. [CrossRef]
33. Cornel, J.; Kidambi, P.; Mazzotti, M. Precipitation and Transformation of the Three Polymorphs of d-Mannitol. *Ind. Eng. Chem. Res.* **2010**, *49*, 5854–5862. [CrossRef]
34. De Beer, T.R.M.; Allesø, M.; Goethals, F.; Coppens, A.; Vander Heyden, Y.; Lopez De Diego, H.; Rantanen, J.; Verpoort, F.; Vervaet, C.; Remon, J.P.; et al. Implementation of a Process Analytical Technology System in a Freeze-Drying Process Using Raman Spectroscopy for In-Line Process Monitoring. *Anal. Chem.* **2007**, *79*, 7992–8003. [CrossRef] [PubMed]
35. Hancock, B.C.; Shamblin, S.L. Water vapour sorption by pharmaceutical sugars. *Pharm. Sci. Technol. Today* **1998**, *1*, 345–351. [CrossRef]
36. Burnett, D.J.; Thielmann, F.; Booth, J. Determining the critical relative humidity for moisture-induced phase transitions. *Int. J. Pharm.* **2004**, *287*, 123–133. [CrossRef] [PubMed]

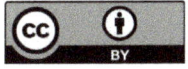 © 2019 by the authors. Licensee MDPI, Basel, Switzerland. This article is an open access article distributed under the terms and conditions of the Creative Commons Attribution (CC BY) license (http://creativecommons.org/licenses/by/4.0/).

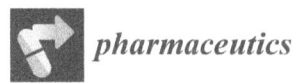

Article

Comparison of Traditional and Ultrasound-Enhanced Electrospinning in Fabricating Nanofibrous Drug Delivery Systems

Enni Hakkarainen [1,†], Arle Kõrkjas [2,†], Ivo Laidmäe [2,3], Andres Lust [2], Kristian Semjonov [2], Karin Kogermann [2], Heikki J. Nieminen [4,5], Ari Salmi [4], Ossi Korhonen [1], Edward Haeggström [4] and Jyrki Heinämäki [2,*]

1. School of Pharmacy, University of Eastern Finland, 70210 Kuopio, Finland; hakkarainen.enni@gmail.com (E.H.); ossi.korhonen@uef.fi (O.K.)
2. Institute of Pharmacy, Faculty of Medicine, University of Tartu, 50411 Tartu, Estonia; arle.korkjas@ut.ee (A.K.); ivo.laidmae@ut.ee (I.L.); andres.lust@ut.ee (A.L.); kristian.semjonov@ut.ee (K.S.); kkogermann@gmail.com (K.K.)
3. Department of Immunology, Institute of Biomedicine and Translational Medicine, University of Tartu, 50411 Tartu, Estonia
4. Electronics Research Laboratory, Department of Physics, University of Helsinki, 00014 Helsinki, Finland; heikki.j.nieminen@aalto.fi (H.J.N.); ari.salmi@helsinki.fi (A.S.); edward.haeggstrom@helsinki.fi (E.H.)
5. Medical Ultrasonics Laboratory, Department of Neuroscience and Biomedical Engineering, Aalto University, 02150 Espoo, Finland
* Correspondence: jyrki.heinamaki@ut.ee; Tel.: +372-7375281
† These authors contributed equally to this work.

Received: 31 August 2019; Accepted: 23 September 2019; Published: 26 September 2019

Abstract: We investigated nozzleless ultrasound-enhanced electrospinning (USES) as means to generate nanofibrous drug delivery systems (DDSs) for pharmaceutical and biomedical applications. Traditional electrospinning (TES) equipped with a conventional spinneret was used as a reference method. High-molecular polyethylene oxide (PEO) and chitosan were used as carrier polymers and theophylline anhydrate as a water-soluble model drug. The nanofibers were electrospun with the diluted mixture (7:3) of aqueous acetic acid (90% v/v) and formic acid solution (90% v/v) (with a total solid content of 3% w/v). The fiber diameter and morphology of the nanofibrous DDSs were modulated by varying ultrasonic parameters in the USES process (i.e., frequency, pulse repetition frequency and cycles per pulse). We found that the USES technology produced nanofibers with higher fiber diameter (402 ± 127 nm) than TES (77 ± 21 nm). An increase of a burst count in USES increased the fiber diameter (555 ± 265 nm) and the variation in fiber size. The slight-to-moderate changes in a solid state (crystallinity) were detected when compared the nanofibers generated by TES and USES. In conclusion, USES provides a promising alternative for aqueous-based fabrication of nanofibrous DDSs for pharmaceutical and biomedical applications.

Keywords: nanotechnology; nanofibers; traditional electrospinning; ultrasound-enhanced electrospinning; drug delivery system

1. Introduction

Electrospinning (ES) is a method for fabricating polymeric nanofibrous constructs, which have potential applications in pharmaceutical and biomedical fields. Nanofibers are typically tenth-to-hundred nanometers thick, they feature large outer surface, substantial surface- area-to-volume ratio, and high porosity (nanomats). This makes these fibers interesting for drug delivery and tissue engineering applications [1–3]. To date, nanofibers have found use, e.g., in formulation of poorly water-soluble drugs, fabrication of novel drug delivery systems (DDSs), supporting wound healing as wound dressings or artificial skin substitutes, and as scaffolds in tissue engineering [3–5].

ES has been applied as a manufacturing method in the clothing, electronics and optical industries, and during the past twenty years it has gained increasing interest in the pharmaceutical and biomedical industries. In traditional ES (TES), a polymer solution is first translated via a capillary tube to a spinneret and then spun towards a grounded collector plate or roll using a high-voltage electron field between the spinneret and collector [6,7]. The major limitations associated with the use of a simple single-fluid TES are blockage of a spinneret (nozzle) system, hazards related to the use of organic solvents (including residual solvent in the nanofibers), and long processing times. More recently, modified two-fluid and tri-fluid coaxial ES methods have been introduced to advance ES of even complicated nanostructures [8]. The clogging phenomena associated with ES can be eliminated by using such modified coaxial ES and concentric needle spinneret [8]. The morphology and diameter of TES nanofibers depend on the intrinsic properties of the solution, the type of polymer, conformation of the polymer chain, the viscosity, elasticity, electric conductivity, as well as the polarity and surface tension of the solvent [1–4]. In recent years, interest has been focused on developing nozzleless ES technologies to avoid the above-mentioned challenges related to TES.

Ultrasound-enhanced ES (USES) provides an orifice-free ES technique that employs ultrasound (US) to create nanofibers [9]. In this technique, high-intensity focused US bursts generate a liquid protrusion with a Taylor cone from the surface of an electrospinning solution (Figure 1). When the drug-polymer solution is charged with high negative voltage, a nanofiber jet is generated from the tip of the protrusion and this jet is led to an electrically grounded collector residing at a constant distance from the fountain [10]. The USES have some advantages over TES: the blockage of a spinneret system and the inclusion of hazardous organic solvents can be avoided with USES. In a USES setup, there is no nozzle that may clog and the evaporation of solvent is more efficient than in a TES setup. With USES, the evaporation of solvent is advanced by using a high-intensity focused US. A travelling US wave generates acoustic streaming inside the solution and induces thermal effect (heating) on the surface of the liquid, thus advancing the evaporation of the solvent. The generation of a liquid protrusion with a Taylor cone can be modified by changing US frequency, pulse repetition frequency and cycles per pulse [9,10].

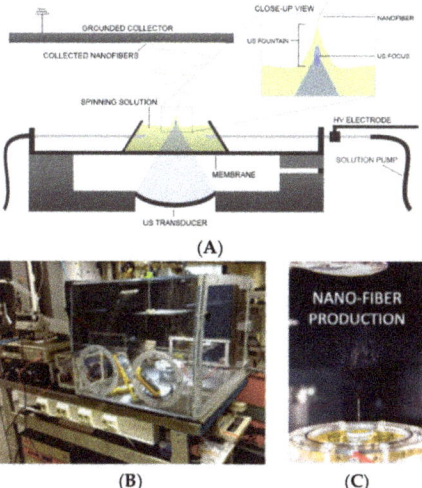

Figure 1. (**A**) Schematic diagram of the ultrasound-enhanced electrospinning (USES) setup, (**B**) photograph of the USES system and process environment (including a humidity cabinet), and (**C**) close-up photograph on the formation of nanofibers in a USES process.

In the present study, we compared the TES and USES techniques as means to fabricate drug-loaded polymeric nanofibers and we investigated the physicochemical and pharmaceutical properties of the produced nanofibers/nanofibrous DDSs. The influence of these two nanofabrication processes on the fiber formation, geometric fiber properties, surface morphology and physical solid-state properties of nanoconstructs were investigated. Special attention was paid to the formation and physical characterization of the drug-loaded nanofibers generated by the USES method.

2. Materials and Methods

2.1. Materials

Theophylline anhydrate (CAS No. 58-55-9; chemical purity ≥ 99%; Sigma-Aldrich Inc., Saint Louis, MO, U.S.A) was used as a water-soluble model drug. Polyethylene oxide, PEO (CAS No. 25322-68-3; Product No. 189456; average molecular weight 900,000 Da) and chitosan (CAS No. 9012-76-4; Product No. 448877; medium molecular weight grade) (Sigma-Aldrich Inc., Saint Louis, MO, U.S.A) were investigated as carrier polymers in both TES and USES nanofabrication. The diluted mixture (7:3) of aqueous acetic acid (CAS No. 64-19-7; chemical purity 99.9%) (90% v/v) and formic acid (CAS No. 64-18-6; chemical purity ≥ 98%; Ph. Eur., Strasbourg, France) solution (90% v/v) (with a total solid content of 3% w/v) was used as a solvent system for ES.

2.2. Fabrication of Nanoconstructs

The composition of the electrospun nanofibers is shown in Table 1. The nanofibers were generated in a TES (ESR-200Rseries, eS-robot®, NanoNC, Seoul, Korea) and in a custom-made in-house USES method. The USES method is described in detail in [8]. In brief, the USES setup features a vessel containing a spinning solution, a US generator and a transducer, a membrane system between the bottom of the vessel and the US transducer, a high-voltage electrode, and a grounded collector plate.

Table 1. Composition (% w/w) of nanofibers generated by traditional electrospinning (TES) (I) and ultrasound-enhanced electrospinning (USES) (II–IV.)

Formulation/Ingredient	I	II	III	IV
Chitosan	43.5	43.5	34.8	40
Polyethylene oxide (PEO)	43.5	43.5	52.2	60
Theophylline	13.0	13.0	13.0	0

To modulate the fiber diameter, specific US parameters (frequency, pulse repetition frequency and cycles per pulse) were exploited in an ES process. Table 2 lists the process parameters applied to fabricate TES and USES nanofibers.

Table 2. Process parameters applied in the traditional electrospinning (TES) (I) and ultrasound-enhanced electrospinning (USES) (II–IV) of nanofibers.

Formulation/Parameter	I	II	III	IV
Voltage (kV)	11.5–14.0	16.0	16.0	14.0–16.0
Voltage of collector (kV)	NA	−5.0	−5.0	−5.0
Distance (cm)	15.0	17.0	17.0	17.0
Pumping rate (mL/h)	0.3	0.8	0.6	0.6
Amplitude (mV)	NA	250	240	200–240
Frequency (MHz)	NA	2.06	2.06	2.06
Burst count (Cycles)	NA	1000	1000	1000
Burst rate (Hz)	NA	70	70	70
Humidity (RH%)	18	19	24	30

NA = not applicable.

2.3. Characterization of Nanofibers

The nanofibrous samples were stored in a zip-lock plastic bag in ambient room temperature (22 ± 2 °C) prior to characterization. Scanning electron microscopy, SEM (Zeiss EVO MA15, Jena, Germany) and optical microscopy were applied to study fiber size distribution and morphology of nanofibers. The samples were coated with a platinum layer (6 nm) prior to imaging with SEM. Three SEM images of each sample were taken using three different magnifications (400×, 2000–2500× and 10,000×). ImageJ software Version 1.51K was used to measure the diameter of nanofibers. Statistical evaluation (*t*-test) was made using Microsoft Excel 2016 (Microsoft Corp., Albuquerque, NM, USA).

Physical solid-state and thermal properties were investigated by means of Fourier Transform Infrared (FTIR) spectroscopy (IRPrestige 21, Shimadzu corporation, Kyoto, Japan) with a single reflection attenuated total reflection (ATR) crystal (Specac Ltd., Orpington, UK), X-ray diffraction, XRD (Bruker D8 Advance diffractometer, Bruker AXS GmbH, Karlsruhe, Germany), and differential scanning calorimetry, DSC (DSC 4000, Perkin Elmer Ltd., Shelton, CT, USA). XRD and FTIR spectroscopy results were normalized and scaled. In all DSC experiments, the sample size was 3–6 mg. The samples were first cooled down and kept at 0 °C for three minutes, and then heated to 350 °C at a rate of 10 °C/min. The samples were then cooled to 0 °C (10 °C/min) and then heated to 350 °C (10 °C/min). The DSC thermogram for PEO was obtained by heating the sample from 30 °C to 170 °C with a heating rate of 10 °C/min. For solid-state characterization, the corresponding binary or ternary physical mixtures (PMs) were prepared manually with a mortar and pestle, and they were used as reference samples for the nanofibrous samples.

3. Results and Discussion

3.1. Topographical and Fiber Size Comparison of Nanoconstructs

Figure 2 illustrates the topography (surface morphology) of the polymeric nanofibrous constructs generated by TES (A, B) and USES (C, D). Figure 3 shows the comparison of the average diameter of individual nanofibers produced by TES and USES. With all fiber compositions tested, TES produced thinner and more uniform-by-size polymeric nanofibers in comparison with those generated by the nozzle-free USES technique. The diameter of nanofibers produced by TES was 77 ± 21 nm, and the diameter of the corresponding nanofibers generated by USES were 402 ± 127 nm (with a burst count of 400 cycles) and 555 ± 265 nm (with a burst count of 700 cycles). Statistically significant difference ($p < 0.001$) was shown between the fiber diameter of nanofibers obtained with TES and the nanofibers generated with USES. This difference in fiber size could be explained by the fact that the USES is a multivariate process involving an open vessel and more critical process parameters (including US parameters) to be controlled than in the TES. The sensitivity of the polymer solution to US and the variations in distance between the surface of the ES solution and the collector plate could be potential reasons for these differences. In aqueous polymer solution ES, the process and ambient parameters such as conductivity, applied voltage, relative humidity, and the distance between a nozzle tip and collector plate could affect the diameter of nanofibers (i.e., increasing the level of these parameters leads to generation of thinner fibers) [4]. However, in fabricating nanofibers for pharmaceutical and biomedical applications, having nanofibers as small as possible is not of intrinsic value in itself and is not necessarily an ultimate goal. For example, in wound healing and many tissue engineering applications, a fiber size close to the micron-scale is considered beneficial in terms of cell adhesion and proliferation [11].

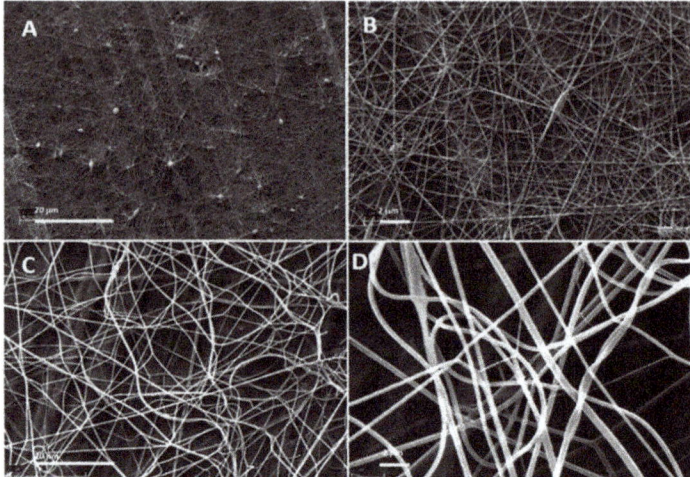

Figure 2. Scanning electron microscopy (SEM) images of traditional electrospun (TES) and ultrasound-enhanced electrospun (USES) nanofibers. (**A,B**) TES nanofibers (magnification 2500× and 10,000×); (**C,D**) USES nanofibers (2500× and 10,000×).

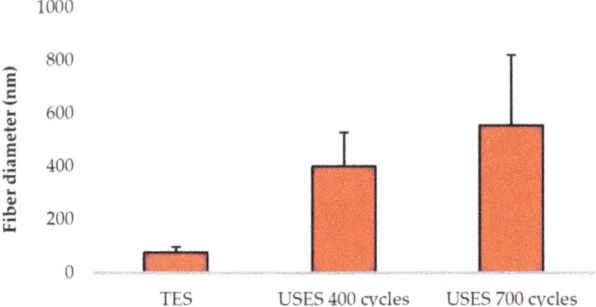

Figure 3. Average diameter (mean ± SD) of traditional electrospun (TES) and ultrasound-enhanced electrospun (USES) nanofibers. The fiber size analysis is based on three SEM images, and the total number of analyzed individual nanofibers was $n = 100$ (with USES 700 cycles $n = 53$). The number of cycles in the USES process (US signal) refers to pulse duration.

With USES, the fiber diameter can be modulated by changing the burst count (cycles per US pulse = duty factor). As seen in Figure 3, changing a burst count from 400 to 700 cycles generated nanofibers with the average diameter of 402 nm and 555 nm, respectively (the other critical US parameters, i.e., frequency and pulse repetition frequency, were kept constant). The statistical analysis showed that the diameters of USES nanofibers generated with the two burst count cycles were different ($p < 0.001$). In the TES, solutions with high conductivity and high surface tension require high voltages and the change in applied voltage (electric field) has only a minor effect on fiber diameter of the nanofibers [4]. Therefore, the process flexibility of USES (i.e., the dynamic modulation of fiber size) is an advantage over TES. The use of higher voltages in the TES increases also the risk of "bead" formation (= defects) in the nanofibrous mats due to the instability of a Taylor cone [4]. As seen in Figure 2, the USES nanofibrous constructs can be generated without signs of "beads" in the final nanofibrous mat. This is advantageous since the formation of "beads" is considered to be a sign of improper ES process.

3.2. Characterization of Nanoconstructs

3.2.1. X-Ray Diffraction

The carrier polymer PEO has two typical diffraction peaks (2θ) at 19° and 23° [12]. As seen in Figure 4, both characteristic diffraction peaks of PEO are visible in the XRD patterns of the PEO powder and in the PM, thus revealing the semi-crystalline nature of PEO. According to the literature, crystalline theophylline gives several characteristic reflections at diffraction angles (2θ) at 7.2°, 12.6°, 14.3°, 24.1°, 25.6°, 26.4° and 29.4° [13]. The major reflection (2θ) is located at 12.6°. Crystalline chitosan has also two characteristic reflections (2θ) at approximately 10° and 20° [14].

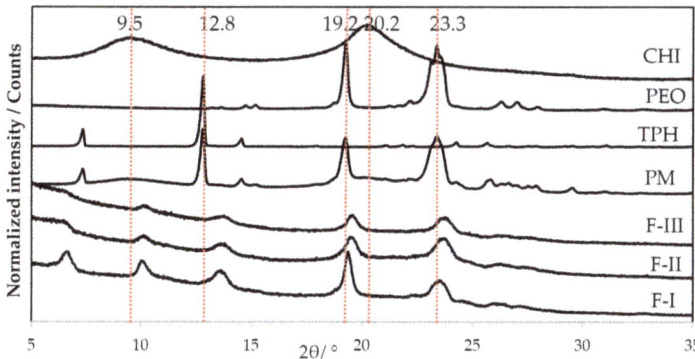

Figure 4. Normalized X-ray diffraction (XRD) patterns of pure materials, physical mixture (PM) of drug and carrier materials, and nanofibers generated with traditional electrospinning, TES (formulation F-I), and ultrasound-enhanced electrospinning, USES (F-II, F-III). Key: CHI = Chitosan, PEO = Polyethylene oxide, TPH = Theophylline anhydrate form II.

The XRD patterns for the nanofibers produced by TES and USES appear nearly identical, and the characteristic diffraction peaks for the three pure materials can be distinguished (Figure 4). Both carrier polymers PEO and chitosan preserved their semi-crystallinity and crystallinity, respectively. We found differences between the diffraction patterns of nanofibrous samples fabricated by these two methods. As seen in Figure 4, nanofibers produced with TES displayed a slightly shifted diffraction peak at 6.6° 2θ which suggests a solid-state change in theophylline. We also found that this reflection and the characteristic peak of theophylline (at 7.2° 2θ) are absent in the XRD patterns of nanofibers generated by USES. Moreover, the other characteristic reflection (2θ) of theophylline at 12.8° 2θ is not distinguished in the XRD patterns of nanofibers (a new reflection shows less intensity and it is shifted to 13.5° 2θ). Therefore, it is evident that solid-state (crystallinity) changes in theophylline have taken place during the TES and USES nanofabrication. It is possible that in addition to an amorphous form, theophylline monohydrate or metastable theophylline or even the mixture of different forms may appear during or immediately after ES. Furthermore, all diffraction peaks in the XRD pattern of the nanofibers generated by USES appear weaker and less sharp than the corresponding reflections of the XRD pattern for the nanofibers produced by TES (Figure 4). This can be seen with the diffraction reflection (2θ) 19.2° which originates from PEO. With nanofibers generated by USES, the diffraction reflections (2θ) characteristic to semi-crystalline PEO at 19.2° and 23.3° are seen as slightly weaker than those in the XRD pattern of PM (Figure 4). These differences in the XRD patterns reveal that there is a difference in the crystallinity of nanofibers fabricated with the different methods. Application of high-intensity focused US in the USES process affects the solid-state properties of the nanofibers resulting in more amorphous (less ordered) nanostructures than those obtained with TES.

3.2.2. Differential Scanning Calorimetry

The thermal behavior (DSC thermograms) of the pure materials, PM, and nanofibers produced by TES and USES are shown in 5 and 6. As seen in Figure 5, the melting endotherms for PEO and theophylline are at 70 °C and at 270 °C, respectively. The characteristic melting endotherm of PEO is seen in the DSC thermograms of PM (Figure 5) and in the thermograms of nanofibers generated by TES and USES (Figure 6). Chitosan as a pure material exhibited a broad endothermic event at 40–120 °C (due to water evaporation) and an exothermic event at 300 °C (chemical degradation) [15]. The melting of theophylline cannot be seen in the DSC thermograms of PMs and nanofibers due to the melting of polymer at lower temperatures and subsequent dissolution of theophylline in the molten polymer (PEO, chitosan). Hence, the DSC results cannot reveal whether theophylline exists in a crystalline form or an amorphous form in the nanofibers generated by TES or USES. However, the XRD patterns shown previously confirmed the solid-state of the drug (crystalline form rather than amorphous form) in the nanofibers generated by USES.

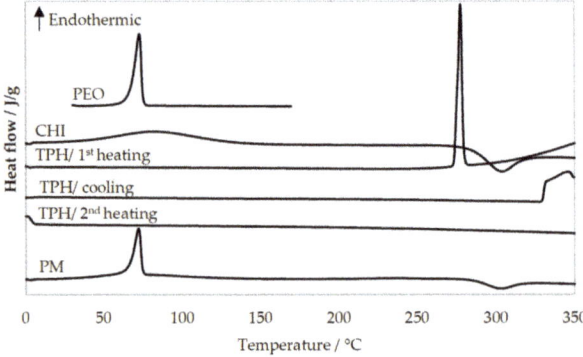

Figure 5. Differential scanning calorimetry (DSC) thermograms of pure materials and physical mixture (PM) of drug and carrier materials. For PEO, CHI, and PM, only the first heating is presented. Key: CHI = Chitosan, PEO = Polyethylene oxide, TPH = Theophylline.

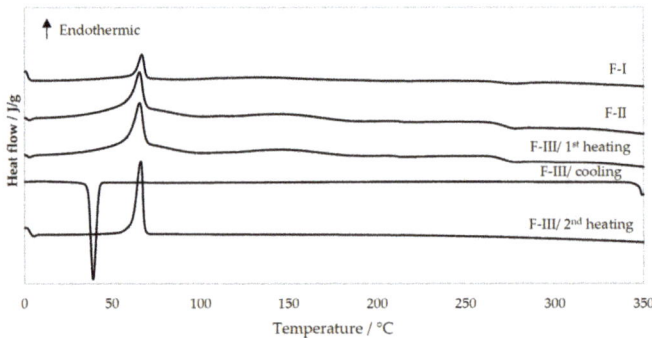

Figure 6. Differential scanning calorimetry (DSC) thermograms of nanofibers generated with traditional electrospinning, TES (formulation F-I) and ultrasound-enhanced electrospinning, USES (F-II, F-III). For F-I and F-II only the first heating is presented. Key: CHI = Chitosan, PEO = Polyethylene oxide, TPH = Theophylline.

The DSC profiles of drug-loaded nanofibers generated by TES or USES were nearly identical suggesting that applying focused high-intensity US in the USES process does not significantly affect the solid-state properties of the nanofibers (Figure 6). As shown in Figure 6, the lower peak height of a characteristic melting endotherm for PEO at 70 °C indicates lower enthalpy of transition (ΔH) with the nanofibers produced by TES than that of the fibers produced by USES. In the DSC thermograms of nanofibers generated by both TES and USES, a small exothermic event at 270 °C is seen, which is probably caused by the chemical decomposition of chitosan.

In the cooling phase, only the crystallization of PEO is observed in the DSC thermogram of the F-III nanofibers generated by USES (Figure 6). During re-heating of the sample (F-III), the thermal event (melting endotherm) of PEO is seen. Chitosan decomposed during the first heating but the fate of theophylline is not clear. No visible thermal events nor signals were detected in the DSC thermogram of pure theophylline after the first heating and no decomposition during heating nor any solidification during the cooling (Figure 5). The relatively small amount of theophylline (13%) in the PM and nanofibers may explain why the melting of theophylline is not recognized in the DSC thermograms of PM or nanofibers, but it cannot account for the lack of thermic events during the cooling phase or in the second heating of pure theophylline. Crystallization of theophylline during the DSC cooling phase has been reported previously [13,16].

3.2.3. Fourier Transform Infrared (FTIR) Spectroscopy

Figure 7 shows FTIR spectra for the pure materials, a physical mixture (PM) and the nanofibers produced by TES and USES. No significant changes in chemical structure of the materials were found in the nanofibers generated with TES or the USES nanofabrication process. The characteristic peaks for theophylline were identified in both TES (F-I) and USES (F-II, III) nanofibrous constructs. The FTIR spectra were close to identical for both types of nanofibers. A characteristic peak of PEO at 2875 cm^{-1} presents the stretching of C–H [17]. It can be observed in all FTIR spectra except in the spectrum for chitosan and theophylline (Figure 7). The characteristic absorption peaks of the theophylline spectrum at 1665–1550 cm^{-1} are derived from C–C and C–N bonds [18]. We found small and characteristic absorption peaks for chitosan (as a pure material) and a peak with a higher intensity for the PM in the same spectral region (Figure 7). This specific peak (1658 cm^{-1}) is partially visible in the FTIR spectra of the nanofibers produced by TES (F-I) and USES (F-II, III). The intensity of the characteristic peak of theophylline at 1658 cm^{-1} for nanofibrous samples (F-II, F-III), however, is smaller than that observed in the FTIR spectra of PM or pure theophylline powder.

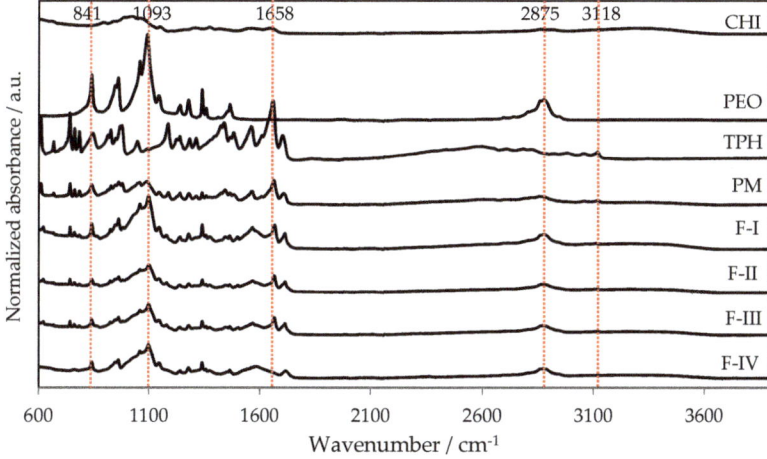

Figure 7. Normalized FTIR spectra for pure materials, the physical mixture (PM) of drug and carrier materials, and nanofibers generated with traditional electrospinning, TES (formulation F-I) and ultrasound-enhanced electrospinning, USES (F-II, F-III and F-IV). Key: CHI = Chitosan, PEO = Polyethylene oxide, TPH = Theophylline.

4. Conclusions

We compared traditional electrospinning (TES) and nozzleless ultrasound-enhanced electrospinning (USES) as methods to fabricate nanofibrous polymeric drug delivery systems (DDSs). The physicochemical and pharmaceutical properties of the nanofibrous DDSs were studied. Both methods can be applied for aqueous-based fabrication of non-woven DDSs using PEO and chitosan as carrier polymers. With USES, the evaporation of solvent is advanced by using a high-intensity focused US enabling acoustic streaming and thermal effect inside the solution. Therefore, USES is associated with more pronounced process-induced solid-state changes of the materials compared to those induced by TES. Nanofibers generated by USES are amorphous, whereas the nanofibers produced by TES are less prone to being amorphous. The controlled phase transformation of higher-energy amorphous form is especially poorly applicable for water-soluble drugs. Further research is needed to discover all potential strengths and limitations of USES in fabricating nanofibrous DDSs.

Author Contributions: Conceptualization, E.H. (Enni Hakkarainen), I.L., K.K., J.H. and E.H. (Edward Haeggström); methodology, E.H. (Enni Hakkarainen), A.K., I.L., H.J.N., A.S., A.L. and K.K.; investigation, E.H. (Enni Hakkarainen), A.K., A.L., K.S. and I.L.; resources, J.H., K.K. and E.H. (Edward Haeggström); writing—original draft preparation, E.H. (Enni Hakkarainen); writing—review and editing, A.K., J.H., K.K., I.L., A.L., H.J.N., A.S., K.S., O.K. and E.H. (Edward Haeggström); visualization, E.H. (Enni Hakkarainen), A.K. and H.J.N.; supervision, I.L., K.K., J.H., O.K. and E.H. (Edward Haeggström); project administration, J.H., K.K., O.K. and E.H. (Edward Haeggström); funding acquisition, J.H., K.K., O.K. and E.H. (Edward Haeggström).

Funding: This work was funded by the Erasmus Programme Student Mobility (E. Hakkarainen) and the Finnish (Acouspin) and Estonian national research grant projects (IUT 34-18 and PUT 1088).

Acknowledgments: J. Aruväli is kindly acknowledged for performing XRD analyses.

Conflicts of Interest: The authors declare no conflicts of interest.

References

1. Agarwal, S.; Wendorff, J.H.; Greiner, A. Use of electrospinning technique for biomedical applications. *Polymer* **2008**, *49*, 5603–5621. [CrossRef]
2. Bhardwaj, N.; Kundu, S.; Bhardwaj, N.; Kundu, S.C. Electrospinning: A fascinating fiber fabrication technique. *Biotechnol. Adv.* **2010**, *28*, 325–347. [CrossRef] [PubMed]
3. Sebe, I.; Szabó, P.; Kállai-Szabó, B.; Zelkó, R. Incorporating small molecules or biologics into nanofibers for optimized drug release: A Review. *Int. J. Pharm.* **2015**, *494*, 516–530. [CrossRef] [PubMed]
4. Pelipenko, J.; Kocbek, P.; Kristl, J. Critical attributes of nanofibers: Preparation, drug loading, and tissue regeneration. *Int. J. Pharm.* **2015**, *484*, 57–74. [CrossRef] [PubMed]
5. Pant, B.; Park, M.; Park, S.-J. Drug delivery applications of core-sheath nanofibers prepared by coaxial electrospinning: a review. *Pharmaceutics* **2019**, *11*, 305. [CrossRef] [PubMed]
6. Huang, Z.; Zhang, Y.; Kotaki, M.; Ramakrishna, S. A review on polymer nanofibers by electrospinning and their applications in nanocomposites. *Compos. Sci. Technol.* **2003**, *63*, 2223–2253. [CrossRef]
7. Naraghi, M.; Chasiotis, I.; Kahn, H.; Wen, Y.; Dzenis, Y. Novel method for mechanical characterization of polymeric nanofibers. *Rev. Sci. Instrum.* **2007**, *78*, 085108. [CrossRef] [PubMed]
8. Wang, M.; Hai, T.; Fang, Z.; Yu, D.-G.; Yang, Y.; Bligh, S.W.A. The relationships between the working fluids, process characteristics and products from the modified coaxial electrospinning of zein. *Polymers* **2019**, *11*, 1287. [CrossRef] [PubMed]
9. Nieminen, H.J.; Laidmäe, I.; Salmi, A.; Rauhala, T.; Paulin, T.; Heinämäki, J.; Haeggström, E. Ultrasound-enhanced electrospinning. *Sci. Rep.* **2018**, *8*. [CrossRef] [PubMed]
10. Laidmäe, I.; Nieminen, H.; Salmi, A.; Paulin, T.; Rauhala, T.; Falk, K.; Yliruusi, J.; Heinämäki, J.; Haeggström, E.; Veski, P. Device and method to produce nanofibers and constructs thereof. World Intellectual Property Organization Patent No. WO2016151191A1, 29 September 2016. Available online: https://patents.google.com/patent/WO2016151191A1/en (accessed on 5 July 2019).
11. Badami, A.S.; Kreke, M.R.; Thompson, M.S.; Riffle, J.S.; Goldstein, A.S. Effect of fiber diameter on spreading, proliferation, and differentiation of osteoblastic cells on electrospun poly (lactic acid) substrates. *Biomaterials* **2006**, *27*, 596–606. [CrossRef] [PubMed]

12. Chrissopoulou, K.; Andrikopoulos, K.S.; Fotiadou, S.; Bollas, S.; Karageorgaki, C.; Christofilos, D.; Voyiatzis, G.A.; Anastasiadis, S.H. Crystallinity and chain conformation in PEO/layered silicate nanocomposites. *Macromolecules* **2011**, *44*, 9710–9722. [CrossRef]
13. Szterner, P.; Legendre, B.; Sghaier, M. Thermodynamic properties of polymorphic forms of theophylline. Part I: DSC, TG, X-ray study. *J. Therm. Anal. Calorim.* **2009**, *99*, 325–335. [CrossRef]
14. Mukhopadhyay, P.; Maity, S.; Chakraborty, S.; Rudra, R.; Ghodadara, H.; Solanki, M.; Chakraborti, A.S.; Prajapati, A.K.; Kundu, P.P. Oral delivery of quercetin to diabetic animals using novel pH responsive carboxypropionylated chitosan/ alginate microparticles. *RSC Adv.* **2016**, *6*, 73210–73221. [CrossRef]
15. Zhang, M.; Li, X.H.; Gong, Y.D.; Zhao, N.M.; Zhang, X.F. Properties and biocompatibility of chitosan films modified by blending with PEGs. *Biomaterials* **2002**, *23*, 2641–2648. [CrossRef]
16. Schnitzler, E.; Kobelnik, M.; Sotelo, G.F.C.; Bannach, G.; Ionashiro, M. Thermoanalytical study of purine derivatives compounds. *Ecl. Quím.* **2004**, *29*, 71–78. [CrossRef]
17. Surov, O.V.; Voronova, M.I.; Afineevskii, A.V.; Zakharov, A.G. Polyethylene oxide films reinforced by cellulose nanocrystals: Microstructure-properties relationship. *Carbohydr. Polym.* **2018**, *181*, 489–498. [CrossRef] [PubMed]
18. Nafisi, S.; Shamloo, D.S.; Mohajerani, N.; Omidi, A.A. Comparative study of caffeine and theophylline binding to Mg(II) and Ca(II) ions: Studied by FTIR and UV spectroscopic methods. *J. Mol. Struct.* **2002**, *608*, 1–7. [CrossRef]

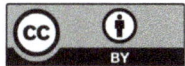

© 2019 by the authors. Licensee MDPI, Basel, Switzerland. This article is an open access article distributed under the terms and conditions of the Creative Commons Attribution (CC BY) license (http://creativecommons.org/licenses/by/4.0/).

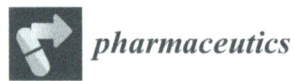

Article

Effects of Electrospinning on the Viability of Ten Species of Lactic Acid Bacteria in Poly(Ethylene Oxide) Nanofibers

Špela Zupančič [1,†], Katja Škrlec [2,†], Petra Kocbek [1], Julijana Kristl [1,*] and Aleš Berlec [1,2,*]

1. Faculty of Pharmacy, University of Ljubljana, Aškerčeva 7, SI-1000 Ljubljana, Slovenia; spela.zupancic@ffa.uni-lj.si (Š.Z.); petra.kocbek@ffa.uni-lj.si (P.K.)
2. Department of Biotechnology, Jožef Stefan Institute, Jamova 39, SI-1000 Ljubljana, Slovenia; katja.luzarskrlec@gmail.com
* Correspondence: julijana.kristl@ffa.uni-lj.si (J.K.); ales.berlec@ijs.si (A.B.); Tel.: + 386-1-476-9500 (J.K.); + 386-1-477-3754 (A.B.)
† These authors contributed equally.

Received: 30 August 2019; Accepted: 15 September 2019; Published: 18 September 2019

Abstract: Lactic acid bacteria can have beneficial health effects and be used for the treatment of various diseases. However, there remains the challenge of encapsulating probiotics into delivery systems with a high viability and encapsulation efficacy. The electrospinning of bacteria is a novel and little-studied method, and further investigation of its promising potential is needed. Here, the morphology, zeta potential, hydrophobicity, average cell mass, and growth characteristics of nine different species of *Lactobacillus* and one of *Lactococcus* are characterized. The electrospinning of polymer solutions containing ~10 log colony forming units (CFU)/mL lactic acid bacteria enabled the successful incorporation of all bacterial species tested, from the smallest (0.74 µm; *Lactococcus lactis*) to the largest (10.82 µm; *Lactobacillus delbrueckii* ssp. *bulgaricus*), into poly(ethylene oxide) nanofibers with an average diameter of ~100 nm. All of these lactobacilli were viable after incorporation into nanofibers, with 0 to 3 log CFU/mg loss in viability, depending on the species. Viability correlated with the hydrophobicity and extreme length of lactic acid bacteria, whereas a horizonal or vertical electrospinning set-up did not have any role. Therefore, electrospinning represents a promising method for the incorporation of lactic acid bacteria into solid delivery systems, while drying the bacterial dispersion at the same time.

Keywords: nanotechnology; biotechnology; probiotics; *Lactobacillus*; *Lactococcus*; electrospinning; nanofibers; drying; local delivery; viability

1. Introduction

Probiotics are living microbes that have beneficial health effects when administered to a host in a sufficient quantity. They most often belong to the very diverse genus of *Lactobacillus*, which includes a large number of species with a "generally recognized as safe" or "qualified presumption of safety" status [1,2]. In 2015, 175 genomes of lactobacilli were included in a comparative taxonomic study [2]. These are non-spore-forming rods or coccobacilli that are characterized by low genomic guanine and cytosine contents, the production of lactic acid, and complex nutritional requirements. They are aero-tolerant or anaerobic, aciduric, or acidophilic [1]. *Lactobacillus* spp. are particularly important in human nutrition and are also considered to be important cell factories in biotechnology, for the production of valuable chemicals. They have also been tested in several clinical trials to evaluate their efficiency for the treatment of a wide spectrum of diseases [1,3].

Lactobacillus probiotics are usually administered orally for the treatment of intestinal diseases, such as acute gastroenteritis [4], necrotizing enterocolitis [5], antibiotic-associated diarrhea [6], and inflammatory bowel disease [7], among others. Moreover, these probiotics have also shown promising potential for the treatment of extra-intestinal diseases, including urinary tract infections, periodontal disease, and bacterial vaginosis [8,9]. However, for such diseases, topical administration of the lactobacilli would appear advisable, to promote their higher efficiency.

For example, the vagina is densely colonized by microbiota (10^7–10^8 colony-forming units [CFU]/g vaginal fluid) [10,11]. Among the distinct ecological environments of the human body, the vaginal microbiota is the least diverse [12], where bacteria from the genus *Lactobacillus* predominate in the majority of healthy women (> 70%) [10,11]. A healthy vaginal microbiota includes from four to 12 different species [13], and the species that dominate individual microbiota include *Lactobacillus crispatus*, *Lactobacillus jensenii*, *Lactobacillus gasseri*, and *Lactobacillus iners* [11,14]. Their use for re-establishing the dominance of lactobacilli in vaginal dysbiosis (e.g., bacterial vaginosis and vaginal candidiasis) is therefore rational, and might even be the most justified among the different applications of these probiotics.

For successful treatments, probiotics need to be incorporated into patient-friendly delivery systems with large numbers of incorporated probiotics, which need to remain stable and survive for prolonged periods during storage [8]. Liquid and semi-solid dosage forms (e.g., hydrogels [15,16]) can have shorter residence times at the local site [10] and issues regarding probiotic stability compared to solid dosage forms. For preparations of these forms, different encapsulation and drying techniques have been used, including microencapsulation, emulsification, coacervation, spray drying, and lyophilization [17,18]. The main drawbacks of these techniques are the use of organic solvents and high temperatures [17]. Electrospinning represents a promising method for the incorporation of probiotics into nanofibers, allowing drying of the bacteria and preparation of a solid delivery system in a single step [19], and thereby offering considerable advantages over techniques such as microencapsulation and lyophilization.

Electrospinning is an established technique used to produce fibers with small diameters, in the range of several nanometers to micrometers, which are often called nanofibers. The manufacturing process is based on the drying of a thin liquid jet that is formed from a drop of polymer solution in a strong electric field [20]. The use of nanofibers has been suggested for several biomedical applications, including wound dressing, drug delivery, and tissue engineering [20]. Of these, drug delivery is the most promising, whereby its advantages include high drug loading, a high incorporation efficiency, the simultaneous delivery of diverse therapeutics, an increased surface area, a good mechanical resistance, an enhanced distribution at mucosal surfaces, ease of operation, and cost effectiveness [20–22].

To date, there have only been a few studies on the electrospinning of probiotics [23–28]. *Bifidobacterium animalis* subsp. *lactis* Bb12 has been incorporated into poly(vinyl alcohol) nanofibers [24]. Among the lactobacilli, *Lactobacillus acidophilus* was incorporated into poly(vinyl alcohol) and poly(vinyl pyrrolidone) nanofibers [25], and into agrowaste-based nanofibers [23]. *Lb. gasseri* was incorporated into poly(vinyl alcohol) nanofibers [28] and *Lb. rhamnosus* into poly(vinyl alcohol) and sodium alginate-based nanofibers [27]. Recently, we optimized the incorporation of *Lactobacillus plantarum* into poly(ethylene oxide) (PEO) nanofibers, and confirmed that their viability can be improved by the addition of lyoprotectants, such as trehalose [26].

Lactobacilli-containing nanofibers represent an innovative delivery system that would be particularly appropriate for topical administration. Due to scarce data on the influence of electrospinning on the viability of different *Lactobacillus* species, in the present study, we incorporated nine different species from the genus *Lactobacillus* and one from the genus *Lactococcus* into PEO nanofibers and assessed their viabilities following their incorporation, as a single study. To explain the higher susceptibilities of some strains to electrospinning, the morphology, zeta potential, hydrophobicity, average mass of bacterial cells, and growth characteristics of these 10 strains were also characterized.

2. Materials and Methods

2.1. Materials

Poly(ethylene oxide) (Mw, 900 kDa) and chloramphenicol were obtained from Sigma Aldrich (Steinheim, Germany). Phosphate-buffered saline (pH 7.4; osmolality: 280–315 mOsm/kg) was sourced from Gibco (Life Technologies, Carlsbad, CA, USA). De Man, Rogosa and Sharpe (MRS) and M-17 media for culturing the *Lactobacillus* spp. and *L. lactis*, respectively, were obtained from Merck (Darmstadt, Germany). Water, buffers, and growth media were sterilized by autoclaving at 2 bar and 121 °C for 20 min.

2.2. Bacterial Strains and Culturing Conditions

The *Lactobacillus* strains were grown at 37 °C in MRS medium without aeration. *L. lactis* MG1363 was grown at 30 °C in M-17 medium supplemented with 0.5% glucose (GM-17), without aeration (Table 1). For long-term storage, the bacterial strains were kept frozen at −80 °C in their corresponding growth medium with 20% (v/v) glycerol. For each experiment, fresh bacteria cultures were cultivated. Frozen cultures were first transferred onto an appropriate growth medium agar plate and incubated for 2 days at 37 °C (*Lactobacillus* spp.) or 30 °C (*L. lactis*). A single bacteria colony was picked, inoculated into 10 mL of the appropriate medium, and incubated at 37 °C or 30 °C for 24 h. Overnight cultures were diluted in fresh medium (1:100, v/v) and grown until a stationary growth phase was reached (as determined from the growth curves; see below). The cultures were centrifuged at 5000× g for 10 min (Sorvall Lynx 4000; ThermoFisher Scientific, Waltham, MA, USA). The cells were then washed twice with phosphate-buffered saline and resuspended in an appropriate volume of water.

Table 1. Bacterial strains used in this study, and some of their properties.

Strain	Source	Fermentation Type	Genome Size [bp]	Reference
Lactobacillus sp.				
Lb. acidophilus ATCC 4356	Infant feces	Homofermentative	1956.699	[29]
Lb. delbrueckii ssp. *bulgaricus* ATCC 11842	Yoghurt	Homofermentative	1864.998	[30]
Lb. casei ATCC 393	Cheese	Facultative heterofermentative	2924.929	[31]
Lb. gasseri ATCC 33323	Human isolate	Homofermentative	1894.360	[32]
Lb. paracasei ATCC 25302	Milk product	Facultative heterofermentative	2991.737	NCBI
Lb. plantarum ATCC 8014	n/a	Facultative heterofermentative	3254.764	NCBI
Lb. reuteri ATCC 55730	Breast milk	Heterofermentative	2036.000	[33]
Lb. rhamnosus ATCC 53103	Human intestine	Homofermentative	3005.051	[34]
Lb. salivarius ATCC 11741	Infant feces	Homofermentative	1956.699	NCBI
Lactococcus sp.				
Lactococcus lactis ssp. *cremoris* MG1363	Cheese	Homofermentative	2529.478	[35]

n/a: not available, NCBI: National Center for Biotechnology Information, ATCC: American Type Culture Collection.

2.3. Characterization of Bacterial Strains

2.3.1. Determination of Cell Surface Charge of the Bacteria

The cell-surface net charge of the bacteria (as represented by the zeta potential) was determined by laser Doppler micro-electrophoresis (Zetasizer Nano ZS; Malvern Instruments, Malvern, UK). Bacteria dispersions in 0.9% (m/v) NaCl with a concentration of 10.3 log CFU/mL were 200-fold diluted with deionized water, put into plastic cuvettes, and covered with the Zeta Dip Cell. The measurements of zeta potential were performed at 25 °C using an He-Ne laser, with a wavelength of 633 nm and the backscatter detector at the scattering angle of 173°. The electrophoretic mobilities measured for the bacterial cells in the applied electric field were employed to automatically calculate their zeta potential using the Smoluchowski approximation of the Henry equation. At least three measurements were performed for each bacterial strain.

2.3.2. Determination of Cell Surface Hydrophobicity of the Bacteria

The hydrophobicity of the bacteria was determined according to the method of Perez et al. [36], with some modifications. Cultures of the strains were harvested in the stationary phase by centrifugation at 12,000× g for 5 min at 4 °C, washed twice with 50 mM K_2HPO_4 (pH 6.5) buffer, and finally resuspended in the same buffer. The cell suspensions were adjusted to an absorbance at 560 nm (A_{560}) of 0.5. Three milliliters of bacterial suspensions was added to 0.6 mL n-hexadecane, vortexed for 120 s, and left for 30 min at room temperature, to allow separation of the two phases. The aqueous phase was carefully removed and A_{560} was measured using a spectrophotometer (Lambda Bio+; Perkin Elmer, Weltham, MA, USA). The decrease in the absorbance of the aqueous phase was taken as the measure of the cell surface hydrophobicity (H%), which was calculated as in Equation (1):

$$H\% = [(A_0-A)/A_0] \times 100 \qquad (1)$$

where A_0 and A are the absorbances before and after extraction with n-hexadecane, respectively.

2.3.3. Determination of Mass of the Bacterial Cells

Bacterial dispersions in water with known numbers of cells and known dispersion volumes were frozen at −80 °C for 24 h, and then lyophilized (Beta 1-8K; Martin Christ, Osterode am Harz, Germany). The first drying phase (T_{shelf} = −5 °C; P = 0.63 mbar) was performed for 24 h, and the second drying phase (T_{shelf} = 20 °C) for 1 h. The lyophilizates obtained were weighed.

2.3.4. Growth Curves of *Lactobacillus* spp. and *L. lactis*

Overnight cultures of *Lactobacillus* spp. and *L. lactis* MG1363 were diluted (1:100) in 200 μL fresh MRS or GM-17 growth medium, respectively, in 96-well microplates. The plates were sealed with sealing film and incubated in a microplate reader (Sunrise; Tecan, Salzburg, Austria) at 37 °C (or 30 °C for *L. lactis*) for 24 h. A_{595} was measured every 2 min. The plates were shaken for 10 s before each measurement. Each culture was grown in quadruplicate. The growth rates and lag phases of the growth curves were analyzed using the DMFit 3.5 software and the model of Baranyi and Roberts [37].

2.4. Preparation of Polymer Solutions with the Bacteria

Overnight cultures of bacteria were diluted (1:100) in 500 mL fresh medium and grown to an optical density at 600 nm (OD_{600}) of 2.50 to 3.00. The cultures were centrifuged at 5000× *g* for 10 min, and washed twice with phosphate-buffered saline. To obtain 4% (*w/v*) PEO bacterial dispersions, the cells were dispersed in an appropriate volume of deionized water. PEO was added to the bacterial dispersions with 10.6 ± 0.8 log CFU/mL in deionized water, and stirred at room temperature for 4 h.

2.5. Rheological Characterization of Polymer Solutions with the Bacteria

Rotational and oscillatory tests of PEO solutions with the bacteria were performed using a rheometer (Physica MCR 301; Anton Paar, Graz, Austria) with a cone-plate measuring system (CP50-2; cone radius, 24.981 mm; cone angle, 2.001°) at a constant temperature of 25.0 ± 0.1 °C, as previously described [27,28]. The zero-gap was set to 0.209 mm. The shear rate during the rotational tests ranged from 1 /s to 100 /s, and the viscosity (η) was calculated as $\eta = \tau_c/\dot{\gamma}$, where τ_c is the shear stress and $\dot{\gamma}$ is the shear rate. The relative viscosity was calculated as the viscosity of the PEO solutions with bacteria, divided by the viscosity of the PEO solution, at a shear rate of 1 /s. Oscillatory tests were performed at a frequency from 0.2 /s to 100 /s, and an amplitude of 1%, which was within the linear viscoelastic region determined in prior amplitude-sweep experiments, to define the phase shift angle (δ). The storage (*G'*) and loss modulus (*G"*) were calculated as in Equations (2) and (3), respectively:

$$G' = (\tau_a/\gamma_a) \times \cos\delta \qquad (2)$$

$$G'' = (\tau_a/\gamma_a) \times \sin\delta \qquad (3)$$

where τ_a is the shear stress and γ_a is the deformation. The damping factor was calculated as $\tan\delta = G''/G'$.

2.6. Preparation of Bacteria-Loaded Nanofibers by Electrospinning

The bacterial dispersions in 4% (m/v) PEO solutions were transferred into a 5 mL syringe fitted with a metallic needle of a 1 mm inner diameter and located horizontally on a syringe pump (model R-99E; RazelTM, Linari Engineering, Valpiana, Italy). The electrode of a high-voltage power supply (model HVG-P60-R-EU; Linari Engineering, Valpiana, Italy) was clamped onto the metallic needle, and the collector was grounded and covered with a piece of aluminum foil. The process was set to a flow rate of 0.4 mL/h, voltage of 15 kV, and nozzle-to-collector distance of 15 cm. Additionally, PEO solution with *Lb. delbrueckii* ssp. *bulgaricus* was electrospun in a vertical electrospinning set-up employing the same equipment and conditions as used for the horizontal electrospinning.

2.7. Characterization of Nanofibers Loaded with the Bacteria

2.7.1. Morphology of the Bacterial Cells and Nanofibers

Three microliters of each bacterial dispersion was pipetted onto a metal stub and air dried, and the nanofiber mats were attached to metal stubs with double-sided conductive tape. The samples were not coated prior to the imaging under scanning electron microscopy (Supra 35 VP; Carl Zeiss, Oberkochen, Jena, Germany), which was operated at an acceleration voltage of 1 kV, with a secondary detector. The length and width of at least 30 randomly selected bacteria and the diameters of 50 randomly selected nanofibers (as parts not containing any bacteria) were measured using the ImageJ 1.51j8 software (National Institutes of Health, Bethesda, MD, USA).

2.7.2. Viability of the Bacteria

The viability of the bacterial cells in the PEO solutions was determined prior to the electrospinning and after their incorporation into the nanofibers. The number of viable suspended bacteria in a known volume of bacterial dispersion was determined using the drop plate method [38]. Eight ten-fold serial dilutions of bacterial cells in PEO solutions were prepared using 50 mM phosphate buffer at pH 7.4, with each dilution in a final volume of 1 mL. Ten microliters of each dilution was pipetted onto agar plates as five replicates, and after incubation, the dilution that contained 3 to 30 colonies per single drop was counted, and replicates were averaged. These data were expressed as CFU/mL and were converted into log CFU/mL. The viability of the bacteria incorporated into the nanofibers was determined by dissolving a known mass of nanofibers in 50 mM phosphate buffer, with a pH of 7.4. Bacterial diluting and counting were performed as described above; here, the data were expressed as CFU/mg nanofibers, and were converted to log CFU/mg. The experimental bacteria loading was compared to the theoretical bacteria loading. The theoretical bacteria loading (CFU/mg) was calculated as the number of bacterial cells in the polymer solution (CFU) per dry weight of polymer and bacterial cells, in 1 mL dispersion. The dry weight of PEO was assumed to be 4 mg, while the dry weight of 1×10^{10} bacterial cells was determined as described in Section 2.3.3, and is shown in Table 2.

2.8. Statistics

The effects of hydrophobicity on the viability of the bacteria were analyzed by applying Mann–Whitney nonparametric tests (*, $p < 0.05$), using the GraphPad Prism 5.00 software. All of the data are presented as means ± standard deviation (SD).

3. Results

3.1. Physical Characteristics of the Lactobacillus spp. and L. lactis

The physical properties of the lactic acid bacteria (e.g., size, charge, and hydrophobicity) were hypothesized to affect their viability after incorporation into the nanofibers. Despite the wealth of information on lactic acid bacteria available, studies that compare physical properties and growth characteristics of multiple lactic acid bacteria are scarce; these were therefore determined in the present study for the selected pool of lactobacilli and *L. lactis* (Table 2, Figure 1). The lactobacilli differed little in terms of their average cell width. Two species had average cell lengths >2 µm, namely *Lb. gasseri* (4.68 µm) and *Lb. delbrueckii* ssp. *bulgaricus* (10.82 µm). The zeta potentials of the different species were comparable, at around −10 mV. The exceptions here were *Lactobacillus casei* and *Lactobacillus rhamnosus*, with zeta potentials of ~0 mV, and *Lactobacillus paracasei*, with the lowest zeta potential (−23.9 mV). There were considerable differences in the cell hydrophobicities, allowing division of the bacterial species into two groups: bacteria with a lower hydrophobicity (<40%; hydrophilic) and bacteria with a higher hydrophobicity (>70%; hydrophobic). Differences in mass (dry weight) of the bacteria might be attributed to the production of exopolysaccharides that differ among these different species. Exopolysaccharides can remain attached to bacteria, despite the washing step. The highest mass was determined for *Lb. rhamnosus* ATCC 53103 and *Lb. delbrueckii* ssp. *bulgaricus* ATCC 11842, which are known producers of exopolysaccharides [39,40].

Table 2. Selected physical characteristics of the bacterial species used in this study.

Bacteria Species	Average Cell Width [µm]	Average Cell Length [µm]	Zeta Potential [mV]	Hydrophobicity [%]	Mass of 1×10^{10} Bacterial Cells [mg]
Lb. acidophilus	0.56 ± 0.04	1.28 ± 0.26	−9.1 ± 5.0	78.6 ± 1.0	0.65
Lb. delbrueckii ssp. *bulgaricus*	0.51 ± 0.07	10.82 ± 3.31	−9.4 ± 5.5	28.5 ± 3.9	9.14
Lb. casei	0.58 ± 0.06	1.54 ± 0.36	−0.4 ± 5.5	11.3 ± 0.5	4.22
Lb. gasseri	0.65 ± 0.07	4.68 ± 1.43	−7.9 ± 4.6	92.5 ± 2.1	5.59
Lb. paracasei	0.68 ± 0.09	2.05 ± 0.49	−23.9 ± 4.4	36.4 ± 4.8	2.13
Lb. plantarum	0.52 ± 0.04	1.33 ± 0.29	−12.7 ± 4.0	74.2 ± 2.3	0.54
Lb. reuteri	0.72 ± 0.08	1.43 ± 0.37	−13.7 ± 5.7	71.9 ± 5.8	1.04
Lb. rhamnosus	0.64 ± 0.08	2.16 ± 0.51	−3.9 ± 4.4	31.5 ± 7.7	16.31
Lb. salivarius	0.70 ± 0.07	1.39 ± 0.31	−11.7 ± 4.6	90.1 ± 1.3	1.92
L. lactis	0.53 ± 0.05	0.74 ± 0.18	−12.8 ± 5.5	24.2 ± 6.3	0.48

3.2. Growth Characteristics of the Lactobacillus spp. and L. lactis

Apart from their physical properties, the bacteria also differed in their growth characteristics when cultured under the same conditions (Figure 1). *Lactobacillus salivarius* was the fastest growing *Lactobacillus* spp., with a growth rate of ~0.3 /h. *Lb. plantarum* and *Lactobacillus reuteri* had a growth rate of ~0.2 /h, while the majority of strains grew at growth rates of 0.1 /h to 0.2 /h. The slowest growers were *Lb. delbrueckii* ssp. *bulgaricus* and *Lb. casei*, with growth rates just above 0.05 /h. These last two and *Lb. paracasei* also had the longest lag times (>5 h), while the rest of the bacteria had lag times of <3 h.

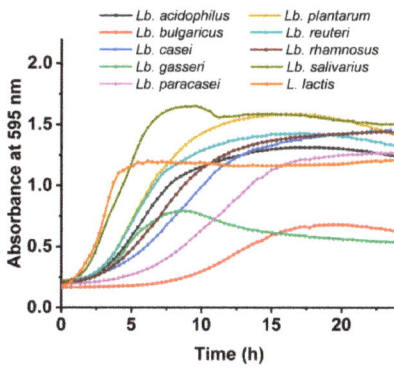

Figure 1. Representative growth curves of the *Lactobacillus* spp. and *L. lactis*.

3.3. Viscosity of Polymer Solutions with the Dispersed Bacteria

The dispersions of the bacteria in 4% (*m/v*) PEO solution increased the viscosity in comparison to 4% (*m/v*) PEO solution without the bacteria (Figure 2). The viscosity at the low shear rate (1 /s) of the PEO solution was 1.36 Pas. PEO solutions with *Lb. rhamnosus* and *Lb. salivarius* had the highest viscosities, with 2.8-fold and 2.5-fold increases, respectively, compared to the PEO solution without these bacteria. Conversely, *Lb. casei* and *Lb. plantarum* had the lowest viscosities among these bacterial dispersions, with only a 1.3-fold increase (Figure 2a). The PEO solutions and all of the PEO solutions with dispersed bacteria showed shear-thinning behavior, which was similar for all of the samples tested, with the exception of the PEO solution with *Lb. rhamnosus*, where the viscosity decreased more rapidly through an increase in the shear rate (Figure 2b). For all of the dispersions tested, the loss modulus dominated over the storage modulus (Figure 2c), and consequently, the damping factor (tan δ), as the ratio between the loss and storage modulus was >1 at all of the tested angular frequencies (Figure 2d). Therefore, in these viscoelastic dispersions, the viscous portion prevailed over the elastic one. All of these dispersions were comparable, with the exception of the PEO solution with *Lb. rhamnosus*, where the storage modulus was a lot higher (Figure 2c) and the damping factor was lower (Figure 2d). This might be attributed to the production of exopolysaccharides and the pronounced growth of *Lb. rhamnosus* as chains, as seen in Figure 3. Viscosity did not correlate with zeta potential or bacterial hydrophobicity.

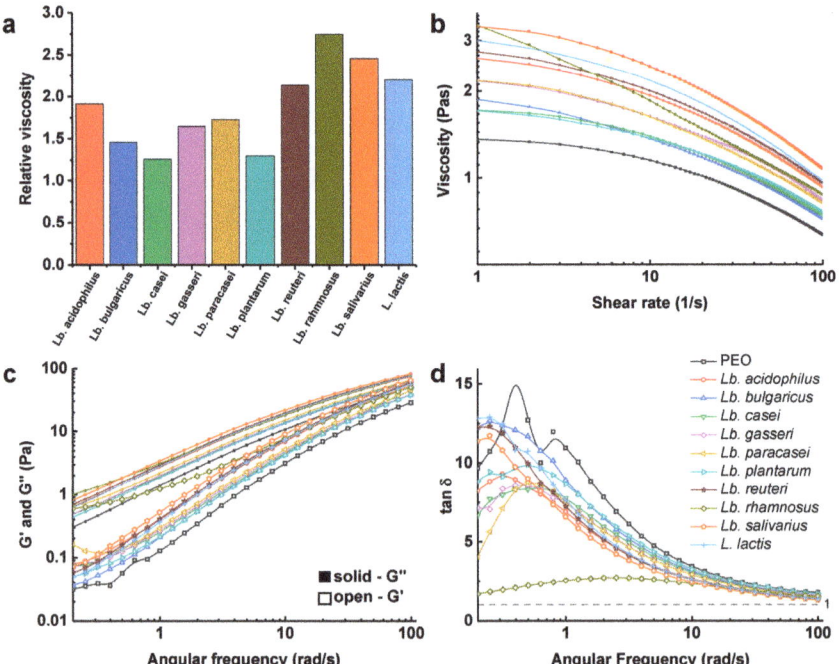

Figure 2. Rheological characterization of 4% (*m/v*) poly(ethylene oxide) (PEO) solutions without bacteria and with the dispersed *Lactobacillus* spp. or *L. lactis*. (**a**) Relative viscosity, as the ratio of the viscosity of the PEO dispersions with bacteria to that of the PEO solution, at a 1 /s shear rate. (**b**) Viscosity of the dispersions as a function of the shear rate. (**c**) Storage (G′) and loss (G″) moduli, and (**d**) tan δ as a function of the angular frequency.

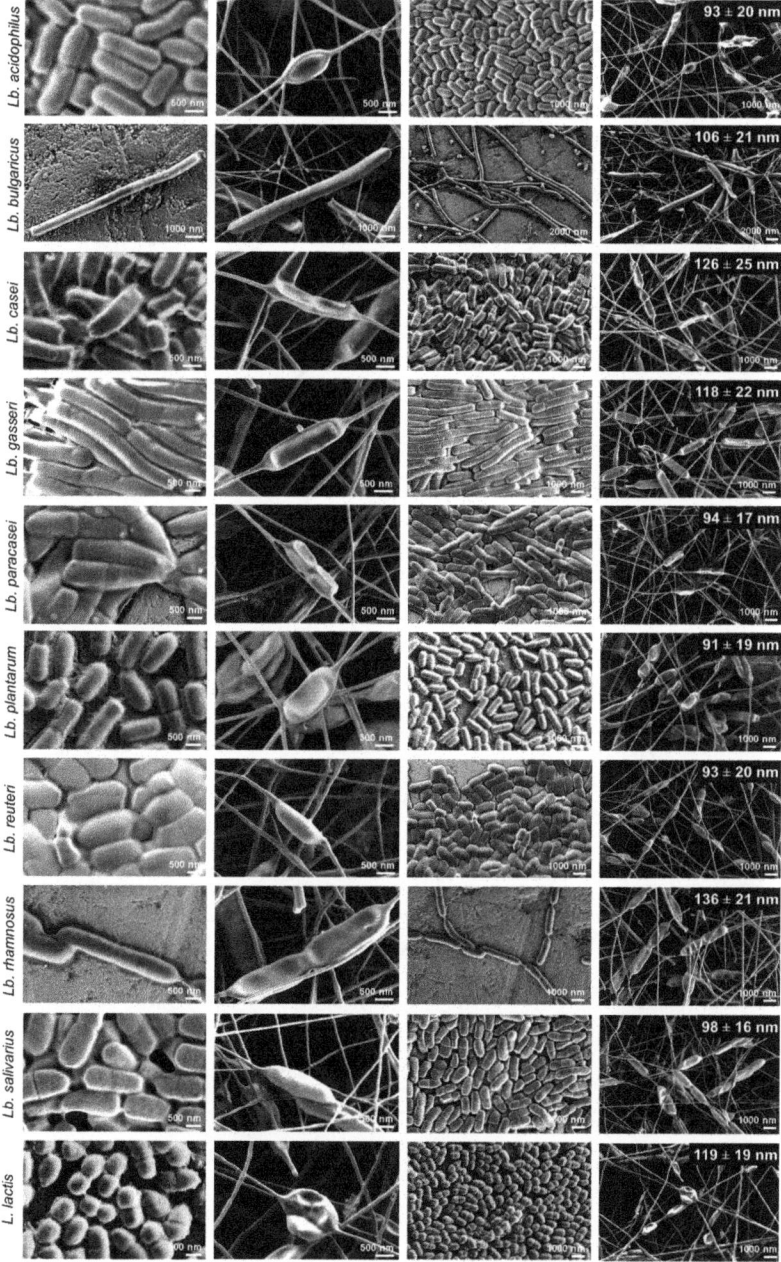

Figure 3. Scanning electron microscopy images of the lactic acid bacteria air dried from the water dispersion (columns 1, 3; under high and low magnification, respectively) and bacteria-loaded nanofibers (columns 2, 4; under high and low magnification, respectively). The numbers given in column 4 indicate the average nanofiber diameters.

3.4. Morphology of Nanofibers with the Bacteria

Under scanning electron microscopy, the thin nanofibers with a thickness of ~100 nm showed local thickenings in the shape of the bacteria, which confirmed the effective incorporation of all of these bacterial species into nanofibers (Figure 3). During SEM analysis, we did not observe any bacteria, which were not incorporated into nanofibers. The nanofiber polymer coating of the bacterial cells was thin, homogenous, and showed no cracks. Single or dividing cells were oriented along the nanofibers and evenly distributed over the nanofiber mats. These mostly retained their shape, compared to the bacteria before the incorporation; however, in some cases, the flattening of cells was seen (Figure 3). The diameters of the nanofibers with the incorporated bacteria in regions without the bacteria varied slightly among these different strains (Table 3). However, these differences did not correlate with the viscosities of the bacterial/PEO dispersions.

Table 3. Growth rates and lag times of the *Lactobacillus* spp. and *L. lactis* determined from their growth curves.

Bacterial Species	Growth Rate [/h]	Lag Time [h]
Lb. acidophilus	0.158 ± 0.005	2.31 ± 0.09
Lb. bulgaricus	0.066 ± 0.001	8.14 ± 0.15
Lb. casei	0.116 ± 0.002	3.41 ± 0.07
Lb. gasseri	0.118 ± 0.004	1.60 ± 0.15
Lb. paracasei	0.102 ± 0.010	5.50 ± 0.23
Lb. plantarum	0.199 ± 0.002	2.52 ± 0.21
Lb. reuteri	0.193 ± 0.009	1.82 ± 0.51
Lb. rhamnosus	0.125 ± 0.001	1.92 ± 0.34
Lb. salivarius	0.297 ± 0.028	1.11 ± 0.08
L. lactis	0.326 ± 0.013	0.84 ± 0.07

3.5. Viability of the Different Lactic Acid Bacteria after Electrospinning

All of the bacterial species were viable following their incorporation into the nanofibers. For five species (*Lb. acidophilus*, *Lb. gasseri*, *Lb. reuteri*, *Lb. salivarius*, and *L. lactis*), the survival decreased by <1 log unit, indicating a high viability. Four species (*Lb. casei*, *Lb. paracasei*, *Lb. plantarum*, and *Lb. rhamnosus*) showed a decreased survival of between 1 and 2 log units. The worst survival was for *Lb. delbrueckii* ssp. *bulgaricus*, with more than a 2 log decrease in viability (Table 4).

Table 4. Viability of the lactic acid bacteria in PEO solution before and after their incorporation into nanofibers.

Bacterial Species	Theoretical Bacteria Loading (log CFU/mg)	Experimental Bacteria Loading (log CFU/mg)	Decrease in Viability (log CFU/mg)
Lb. acidophilus	9.89 ± 0.18	9.18 ± 0.21	0.71
Lb. bulgaricus	8.74 ± 0.15	5.91 ± 0.15	2.83
Lb. casei	8.85 ± 0.21	7.33 ± 0.19	1.52
Lb. gasseri	9.30 ± 0.18	9.20 ± 0.11	0.09
Lb. paracasei	9.53 ± 0.12	8.02 ± 0.18	1.51
Lb. plantarum	9.99 ± 0.06	8.70 ± 0.38	1.29
Lb. reuteri	9.76 ± 0.13	9.32 ± 0.04	0.44
Lb. rhamnosus	8.55 ± 0.13	7.41 ± 0.16	1.14
Lb. salivarius	9.21 ± 0.06	6.75 ± 0.07	0.73
L. lactis	9.06 ± 0.14	8.19 ± 0.33	0.87

Interestingly, the loss of viability correlated with the hydrophobicity of the bacterial cells. The hydrophilic bacteria showed significantly higher decreases in viability than the hydrophobic bacteria (Figure 4). This suggests that hydrophobic molecules at the bacterial surface (e.g., including exopolysaccharides) offer better protection for the bacteria during their incorporation into nanofibers. There were no correlations between the loss of viability and viscosity of dispersion or zeta potential of cells.

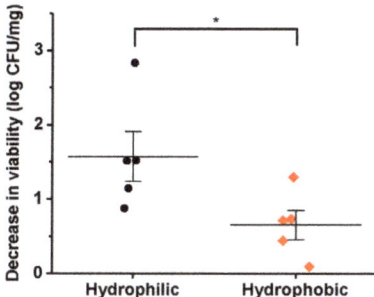

Figure 4. Bacterial cells with a lower hydrophobicity (< 40%, hydrophilic, black circles) showed larger decreases in viability after incorporation into nanofibers, in comparison to bacterial cells with a higher hydrophobicity (> 70%, hydrophobic, red diamonds). The horizontal lines indicate the means. *, $p < 0.05$ (Mann–Whitney tests).

In general, the width or length of the cells did not correlate with the viability of the bacteria. However, for *Lb. delbrueckii* ssp. *bulgaricus* in particular, the loss of viability might also be correlated with the bacterial cell size, as these bacteria had by far the longest cells and by far the highest decrease in viability. To exclude any influence of the direction of the electrospinning and possible losses of bacteria during the electrospinning due to the gravitational force, horizontal electrospinning was replaced with vertical electrospinning. The survivals here were not significantly different (Figure 5), which suggests that the direction of electrospinning has no major role in the bacterial viability.

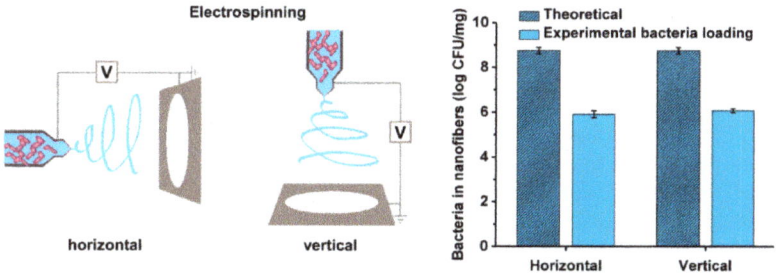

Figure 5. Theoretical and experimental loading of *Lb. delbrueckii* ssp. *bulgaricus* in nanofibers using either horizontal or vertical electrospinning.

4. Discussion

The scope of the use of probiotics can be widened by the introduction of novel delivery systems. The incorporation of probiotics into nanofibers is an emerging approach for the delivery of probiotics to body sites that require their controlled and/or sustained release. We and others have recently demonstrated the effective incorporation of lactic acid bacteria into nanofibers, and have shown that these incorporated bacteria retain their viability. However, previous studies have been limited to just five species of lactic acid bacteria: *Lb. acidophilus*, *Lb. gasseri* *Lb. plantarum*, *Lb. rhamnosus*, and *Bifidobacterium animalis* [19,23–28]. Different species of lactic acid bacteria can differ considerably in their properties and therapeutic effects, and therefore, it is crucial to strengthen our knowledge of the behavior of the different lactic acid bacteria during electrospinning.

We effectively incorporated nine taxonomically different species of the genus *Lactobacillus* and one species of the genus *Lactococcus* into PEO nanofibers, and have thus considerably increased our knowledge of the number of lactic acid bacteria that can be delivered using electrospun nanofibers. The dispersions of these bacteria in 4% (*m/v*) PEO solution had different rheological properties. A higher viscosity was attributed to the production of exopolysaccharides or to the pronounced chain growth phenotype. Although the bacteria in the PEO solution affected the viscosity, there was no need to change the process parameters during the electrospinning of the previously optimized electrospinning of PEO solutions without the bacteria, which enabled the production of smooth PEO nanofibers in a continuous process [26]. The previously reported mean diameter of PEO nanofibers without the incorporated bacteria was 135 ± 25 nm [26], which was similar to *Lb. rhamnosus*-loaded nanofibers here, whereas the other nanofibes were a little smaller, with the lowest mean diameter of 91 ± 19 nm for *Lb. plantarum*-loaded nanofibers. In line with previous studies, the addition of the bacteria to the PEO solutions did not only changed the viscosity, but also the dispersion conductivity. A prominent influence of conductivity over viscosity might lead to the decreased nanofiber diameters seen for the bacteria-loaded nanofibers [19,26].

While observing the bacteria-loaded nanofibers using scanning electron microscopy, we could clearly distinguish incorporated cells in nanofibers. Thus, electrospinning provided complete incorporation of the bacteria, even for the strain with the largest cells among those studied here (i.e., *Lb. delbrueckii* ssp. *bulgaricus*; cell length, 10.82 μm). As observed previously [26], although the morphology of the bacterial cells in the nanofibers was similar to their morphology obtained after air-drying the bacterial dispersions, some of the cells were flattened due to their drying and dehydration, or to the mechanical stress they had undergone [41].

All of these species of lactic acid bacteria that were incorporated survived the electrospinning; however, the theoretical and experimental bacterial loading differed. The electrospinning process results in a high incorporation efficiency of drugs [42] or bacteria [19] and here, the difference between both loadings was probably due to the decrease of bacterial viability. There were no correlations between the growth characteristics, viscosity of the dispersion, or zeta potential of the lactic acid bacteria and their survival. On the other hand, the decrease in viability of the bacteria in the nanofibers correlated with the hydrophobicities of the cells. Hydrophobicity depends on the surface structures of the bacterial cells, such as lipoteichoic acid, S-layer proteins, outer membrane proteins and lipids, surface fibrils, and various fimbriae or core oligosaccharides [43]. Considerable differences among the surface properties of lactic acid bacteria were also seen in our previous study [44]. We hypothesize that the hydrophobic surface offers better protection from the hydrophilic solution in which the bacteria are dispersed.

Another possible predictor of bacterial viability in these nanofibers is their extreme morphology. *Lb. delbrueckii* ssp. *bulgaricus* had by far the largest cells and the lowest viability, as the only species with a >2 log unit decrease in viability. This might be a consequence of the large bacteria surface per cell. The viability was not affected by the direction of electrospinning, which thus excluded gravitational effects.

To summarize, while the electrospinning process is feasible regardless of the species of lactic acid bacteria used, the prediction of viability is challenging and will require the testing of individual strains.

5. Conclusions

In the present study, we incorporated a range of safe lactic acid bacteria into PEO-based nanofibers, several of which are confirmed probiotics. All of the lactic acid bacteria remained viable after their incorporation into the nanofibers using an electrospinning procedure appropriate for PEO solutions, without the need for additional optimization. However, the survival of these lactic acid bacteria differed across two log units, and despite the determination of the physical and growth characteristics and the viscosities of the bacterial dispersions, no clear relationships were seen between the survival and the parameters measured. This suggests that the prediction of bacterial survival during the electrospinning process is challenging, and that the formulation of each particular bacterial strain will need to be optimized separately. The exceptions are the cell hydrophobicity and the extreme morphological characteristics of the bacteria (e.g., greatest size for *Lb. delbrueckii* ssp. *bulgaricus*), which offer some indications in terms of bacterial survival after their incorporation into nanofibers. The developed nanofiber-based delivery systems could be useful for the delivery of lactic acid bacteria to mucosal surfaces, such as oral, nasal, or vaginal surfaces.

Author Contributions: Conceptualization, methodology, investigation, K.Š. and Š.Z.; writing—original draft preparation, A.B., K.Š. and Š.Z.; writing—review and editing, A.B., J.K., K.Š., P.K. and Š.Z.; visualization, A.B. and Š.Z.; supervision, project administration, resources, funding acquisition, A.B. and J.K.

Funding: This research was funded by the Slovenian Research Agency, grant numbers P4-0127, P1-0189 and J1-9194.

Acknowledgments: We thank Christopher Berrie for critical reading of the manuscript.

Conflicts of Interest: The authors declare that they have no conflict of interest. The funders had no role in the design of the study; in the collection, analyses, or interpretation of data; in the writing of the manuscript; or in the decision to publish the results.

References

1. Salvetti, E.; Torriani, S.; Felis, G.E. The Genus Lactobacillus: A Taxonomic Update. *Probiotics Antimicrob. Proteins* **2012**, *4*, 217–226. [CrossRef] [PubMed]
2. Sun, Z.; Harris, H.M.; McCann, A.; Guo, C.; Argimon, S.; Zhang, W.; Yang, X.; Jeffery, I.B.; Cooney, J.C.; Kagawa, T.F.; et al. Expanding the biotechnology potential of lactobacilli through comparative genomics of 213 strains and associated genera. *Nat. Commun.* **2015**, *6*, 8322. [CrossRef] [PubMed]
3. Bosma, E.F.; Forster, J.; Nielsen, A.T. Lactobacilli and pediococci as versatile cell factories - Evaluation of strain properties and genetic tools. *Biotechnol. Adv.* **2017**, *35*, 419–442. [CrossRef] [PubMed]
4. Guarino, A.; Guandalini, S.; Lo Vecchio, A. Probiotics for Prevention and Treatment of Diarrhea. *J. Clin. Gastroenterol.* **2015**, *49* (Suppl. 1), S37–S45. [CrossRef]
5. AlFaleh, K.; Anabrees, J. Probiotics for prevention of necrotizing enterocolitis in preterm infants. *Cochrane Database Syst. Rev.* **2014**. [CrossRef] [PubMed]
6. Cai, J.; Zhao, C.; Du, Y.; Zhang, Y.; Zhao, M.; Zhao, Q. Comparative efficacy and tolerability of probiotics for antibiotic-associated diarrhea: Systematic review with network meta-analysis. *United Eur. Gastroenterol. J.* **2018**, *6*, 169–180. [CrossRef] [PubMed]
7. Ganji-Arjenaki, M.; Rafieian-Kopaei, M. Probiotics are a good choice in remission of inflammatory bowel diseases: A meta analysis and systematic review. *J. Cell. Physiol.* **2018**, *233*, 2091–2103. [CrossRef] [PubMed]
8. Rupa, P.; Mine, Y. Recent advances in the role of probiotics in human inflammation and gut health. *J. Agric. Food Chem.* **2012**, *60*, 8249–8256. [CrossRef] [PubMed]
9. Matsubara, V.H.; Bandara, H.M.; Ishikawa, K.H.; Mayer, M.P.; Samaranayake, L.P. The role of probiotic bacteria in managing periodontal disease: A systematic review. *Expert Rev. Anti. Infect. Ther.* **2016**, *14*, 643–655. [CrossRef]
10. Borges, S.; Barbosa, J.; Teixeira, P. Drug Delivery Systems for Vaginal Infections. *Front. Clin. Drug Res.* **2016**, *2*, 233.
11. Petrova, M.I.; Lievens, E.; Malik, S.; Imholz, N.; Lebeer, S. Lactobacillus species as biomarkers and agents that can promote various aspects of vaginal health. *Front. Physiol.* **2015**, *6*, 81. [CrossRef] [PubMed]
12. Belkaid, Y.; Naik, S. Compartmentalized and systemic control of tissue immunity by commensals. *Nat. Immunol.* **2013**, *14*, 646. [CrossRef] [PubMed]
13. Sycuro, L.K.; Fredricks, D.N. *Microbiota of the Genitourinary Tract*. The Human Microbiota: How Microbial Communities Affect. Health and Disease; John Wiley Sons: Hoboken, NJ, USA, 2013; pp. 167–210.
14. Ravel, J.; Gajer, P.; Abdo, Z.; Schneider, G.M.; Koenig, S.S.; McCulle, S.L.; Karlebach, S.; Gorle, R.; Russell, J.; Tacket, C.O.; et al. Vaginal microbiome of reproductive-age women. *Proc. Natl. Acad. Sci. USA* **2011**, *108*, 4680–4687. [CrossRef] [PubMed]
15. Gao, S.; Tang, G.; Hua, D.; Xiong, R.; Han, J.; Jiang, S.; Zhang, Q.; Huang, C. Stimuli-responsive bio-based polymeric systems and their applications. *J. Mater. Chem. B* **2019**, *7*, 709–729. [CrossRef]

16. Ding, Q.; Xu, X.; Yue, Y.; Mei, C.; Huang, C.; Jiang, S.; Wu, Q.; Han, J. Nanocellulose-Mediated Electroconductive Self-Healing Hydrogels with High Strength, Plasticity, Viscoelasticity, Stretchability, and Biocompatibility toward Multifunctional Applications. *ACS App. Mater. Inter.* **2018**, *10*, 27987–28002. [CrossRef] [PubMed]
17. Ghorani, B.; Tucker, N. Fundamentals of electrospinning as a novel delivery vehicle for bioactive compounds in food nanotechnology. *Food Hydrocolloid* **2015**, *51*, 227–240. [CrossRef]
18. Mirtič, J.; Rijavec, T.; Zupančič, S.; Zvonar Pobirk, A.; Lapanje, A.; Kristl, J. Development of probiotic-loaded microcapsules for local delivery: Physical properties, cell release and growth. *Eur. J. Pharm. Sci.* **2018**, *121*, 178–187. [CrossRef] [PubMed]
19. Zupancčič, Š.; Rijavec, T.; Lapanje, A.; Petelin, M.; Kristl, J.; Kocbek, P. Nanofibers with Incorporated Autochthonous Bacteria as Potential Probiotics for Local Treatment of Periodontal Disease. *Biomacromolecules* **2018**, *19*, 4299–4306. [CrossRef]
20. Hu, X.; Liu, S.; Zhou, G.; Huang, Y.; Xie, Z.; Jing, X. Electrospinning of polymeric nanofibers for drug delivery applications. *J. Control. Release* **2014**, *185*, 12–21. [CrossRef]
21. Chou, S.F.; Carson, D.; Woodrow, K.A. Current strategies for sustaining drug release from electrospun nanofibers. *J. Control. Release* **2015**, *220*, 584–591. [CrossRef]
22. Zupančič, Š. Core-shell nanofibers as drug delivery systems. *Acta Pharm.* **2019**, *69*, 131–153. [CrossRef] [PubMed]
23. Fung, W.Y.; Yuen, K.H.; Liong, M.T. Agrowaste-based nanofibers as a probiotic encapsulant: Fabrication and characterization. *J. Agric. Food Chem.* **2011**, *59*, 8140–8147. [CrossRef] [PubMed]
24. Lopez-Rubio, A.; Sanchez, E.; Wilkanowicz, S.; Sanz, Y.; Lagaron, J.M. Electrospinning as a useful technique for the encapsulation of living bifidobacteria in food hydrocolloids. *Food Hydrocolloid* **2012**, *28*, 159–167. [CrossRef]
25. Nagy, Z.K.; Wagner, I.; Suhajda, A.; Tobak, T.; Harasztos, A.H.; Vigh, T.; Soti, P.L.; Pataki, H.; Molnar, K.; Marosi, G. Nanofibrous solid dosage form of living bacteria prepared by electrospinning. *Express Polym. Lett.* **2014**, *8*, 352–361. [CrossRef]
26. Skrlec, K.; Zupancic, S.; Prpar Mihevc, S.; Kocbek, P.; Kristl, J.; Berlec, A. Development of electrospun nanofibers that enable high loading and long-term viability of probiotics. *Eur. J. Pharm. Biopharm.* **2019**, *136*, 108–119. [CrossRef] [PubMed]
27. Ceylan, Z.; Meral, R.; Karakaş, C.Y.; Dertli, E.; Yilmaz, M.T. A novel strategy for probiotic bacteria: Ensuring microbial stability of fish fillets using characterized probiotic bacteria-loaded nanofibers. *Innov. Food Sci. Emerg. Technol.* **2018**, *48*, 212–218. [CrossRef]
28. Amna, T.; Hassan, M.S.; Pandeya, D.R.; Khil, M.S.; Hwang, I.H. Classy non-wovens based on animate L. gasseri-inanimate poly(vinyl alcohol): Upstream application in food engineering. *Appl. Microbiol. Biotechnol.* **2013**, *97*, 4523–4531. [CrossRef] [PubMed]
29. Palomino, M.M.; Allievi, M.C.; Fina Martin, J.; Waehner, P.M.; Prado Acosta, M.; Sanchez Rivas, C.; Ruzal, S.M. Draft Genome Sequence of the Probiotic Strain Lactobacillus acidophilus ATCC 4356. *Genome Announc.* **2015**, *3*. [CrossRef] [PubMed]
30. van de Guchte, M.; Penaud, S.; Grimaldi, C.; Barbe, V.; Bryson, K.; Nicolas, P.; Robert, C.; Oztas, S.; Mangenot, S.; Couloux, A.; et al. The complete genome sequence of Lactobacillus bulgaricus reveals extensive and ongoing reductive evolution. *Proc. Natl. Acad. Sci. USA* **2006**, *103*, 9274–9279. [CrossRef] [PubMed]
31. Toh, H.; Oshima, K.; Nakano, A.; Takahata, M.; Murakami, M.; Takaki, T.; Nishiyama, H.; Igimi, S.; Hattori, M.; Morita, H. Genomic adaptation of the Lactobacillus casei group. *PLoS ONE* **2013**, *8*, e75073. [CrossRef] [PubMed]
32. Azcarate-Peril, M.A.; Altermann, E.; Goh, Y.J.; Tallon, R.; Sanozky-Dawes, R.B.; Pfeiler, E.A.; O'Flaherty, S.; Buck, B.L.; Dobson, A.; Duong, T.; et al. Analysis of the genome sequence of Lactobacillus gasseri ATCC 33323 reveals the molecular basis of an autochthonous intestinal organism. *Appl. Environ. Microbiol.* **2008**, *74*, 4610–4625. [CrossRef] [PubMed]
33. Saulnier, D.M.; Santos, F.; Roos, S.; Mistretta, T.A.; Spinler, J.K.; Molenaar, D.; Teusink, B.; Versalovic, J. Exploring metabolic pathway reconstruction and genome-wide expression profiling in Lactobacillus reuteri to define functional probiotic features. *PLoS ONE* **2011**, *6*, e18783. [CrossRef] [PubMed]

34. Morita, H.; Toh, H.; Oshima, K.; Murakami, M.; Taylor, T.D.; Igimi, S.; Hattori, M. Complete genome sequence of the probiotic Lactobacillus rhamnosus ATCC 53103. *J. Bacteriol.* **2009**, *191*, 7630–7631. [CrossRef] [PubMed]
35. Linares, D.M.; Kok, J.; Poolman, B. Genome sequences of Lactococcus lactis MG1363 (revised) and NZ9000 and comparative physiological studies. *J. Bacteriol.* **2010**, *192*, 5806–5812. [CrossRef] [PubMed]
36. Perez, P.F.; Minnaard, Y.; Disalvo, E.A.; De Antoni, G.L. Surface properties of bifidobacterial strains of human origin. *Appl. Environ. Microbiol.* **1998**, *64*, 21–26. [PubMed]
37. Baranyi, J.; Roberts, T.A. A dynamic approach to predicting bacterial growth in food. *Int. J. Food Microbiol.* **1994**, *23*, 277–294. [CrossRef]
38. Herigstad, B.; Hamilton, M.; Heersink, J. How to optimize the drop plate method for enumerating bacteria. *J. Microbiol. Methods* **2001**, *44*, 121–129. [CrossRef]
39. Lebeer, S.; Verhoeven, T.L.; Francius, G.; Schoofs, G.; Lambrichts, I.; Dufrene, Y.; Vanderleyden, J.; De Keersmaecker, S.C. Identification of a Gene Cluster for the Biosynthesis of a Long, Galactose-Rich Exopolysaccharide in Lactobacillus rhamnosus GG and Functional Analysis of the Priming Glycosyltransferase. *Appl. Environ. Microbiol.* **2009**, *75*, 3554–3563. [CrossRef]
40. Zeidan, A.A.; Poulsen, V.K.; Janzen, T.; Buldo, P.; Derkx, P.M.F.; Oregaard, G.; Neves, A.R. Polysaccharide production by lactic acid bacteria: From genes to industrial applications. *FEMS Microbiol. Rev.* **2017**, *41*, S168–S200. [CrossRef]
41. Reznik, S.N.; Yarin, A.L.; Zussman, E.; Bercovici, L. Evolution of a compound droplet attached to a core-shell nozzle under the action of a strong electric field. *Phys. Fluids* **2006**, *18*, 062101. [CrossRef]
42. Kajdič, S.; Vrečer, F.; Kocbek, P. Preparation of poloxamer-based nanofibers for enhanced dissolution of carvedilol. *Eur. J. Pharm. Sci.* **2018**, *117*, 331–340. [CrossRef] [PubMed]
43. Krasowska, A.; Sigler, K. How microorganisms use hydrophobicity and what does this mean for human needs? *Front. Cell Infect. Microbiol.* **2014**, *4*, 112. [CrossRef] [PubMed]
44. Zadravec, P.; Štrukelj, B.; Berlec, A. Improvement of LysM-mediated surface display of designed ankyrin repeat proteins (DARPins) in recombinant and nonrecombinant strains of Lactococcus lactis and Lactobacillus Species. *Appl. Environ. Microbiol.* **2015**, *81*, 2098–2106. [CrossRef] [PubMed]

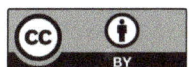

© 2019 by the authors. Licensee MDPI, Basel, Switzerland. This article is an open access article distributed under the terms and conditions of the Creative Commons Attribution (CC BY) license (http://creativecommons.org/licenses/by/4.0/).

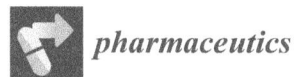

Article

Release Profile of Gentamicin Sulfate from Polylactide-*co*-Polycaprolactone Electrospun Nanofiber Matrices

Silvia Pisani [1], Rossella Dorati [1,2,*], Enrica Chiesa [1], Ida Genta [1], Tiziana Modena [1,2], Giovanna Bruni [3], Pietro Grisoli [1] and Bice Conti [1,2]

1. Department of Drug Sciences, University of Pavia, Viale Taramelli 12/14, 27100 Pavia, Italy; silvia.pisani01@universitadipavia.it (S.P.); enrica.chiesa01@universitadipavia.it (E.C.); ida.genta@unipv.it (I.G.); tiziana.modena@unipv.it (T.M.); pietro.grisoli@unipv.it (P.G.); bice.conti@unipv.it (B.C.)
2. Polymerix S.r.l., Via Taramelli 24, 27100 Pavia, Italy
3. Department of Chemistry, University of Pavia, Viale Taramelli 12/14, 27100 Pavia, Italy; giovanna.bruni@unipv.it
* Correspondence: rossella.dorati@unipv.it; Tel.: +39-0382-987393

Received: 10 March 2019; Accepted: 30 March 2019; Published: 3 April 2019

Abstract: The advent and growth of resistance phenomena to antibiotics has reached critical levels, invalidating the action of a majority of antibiotic drugs currently used in the clinical field. Several innovative techniques, such as the nanotechnology, can be applied for creating innovative drug delivery systems designed to modify drug release itself and/or drug administration route; moreover, they have proved suitable for overcoming the phenomenon of antibiotic resistance. Electrospun nanofibers, due to their useful structural properties, are showing promising results as antibiotic release devices for preventing bacteria biofilm formation after surgical operation and for limiting resistance phenomena. In this work gentamicin sulfate (GS) was loaded into polylactide-*co*-polycaprolactone (PLA-PCL) electrospun nanofibers; quantification and in vitro drug release profiles in static and dynamic conditions were investigated; GS kinetic release from nanofibers was studied using mathematical models. A preliminary microbiological test was carried out towards *Staphylococcus aureus* and *Escherichia coli* bacteria.

Keywords: electrospinning; gentamicin sulfate; polylactide-*co*-polycaprolactone; drug release kinetics

---

1. Introduction

Electrospinning is a straightforward method of producing polymeric matrices made of ultrafine entangled polymeric fibers with micro- to nano-meter range diameters and controlled surface morphology. The ultrafine fibers are generated by application of a strong electric field on a polymer solution or melt; fibers are stretched and collected on a metallic surface (plate or mandrel). During fiber formation, solvent must evaporate in order to achieve dry and homogeneous fibers. Electrospinning process parameters have been extensively studied and reviewed in the literature in the recent years [1,2].

In these years, the electrospinning technique raised tremendous interest in the pharmaceutical field, as an emerging processing technique of drug delivery systems. Different kinds of drug delivery systems have been investigated to improve the therapeutic effect and to reduce the toxicity of conventional dosage forms. Nanoscale formulations, such as liposomes, polymeric micelles, complexes, and nanofibers, attracted special attention during the last decade. Compared with other formulations, electrospinning affords great flexibility in selecting and combining materials and drugs. Drug molecule encapsulation into electrospun polymer nanofibers, promotes intimate drug to polymer contact, also modifying drug apparent solubility [3–11]. As far as electrospun materials are concerned, the ability of reaching high encapsulation efficiencies, simultaneous delivery of diverse drugs, and drug release modification are recognized as significant advantages. Moreover, the electrospinning process itself has notable advantages, such as ease of operation, cost-effectiveness, reproducibility, and easy up-scalability [1,12,13]. The use of electrospun nanofibers as drug carriers is promising in diverse pathologies, such as postoperative local chemotherapy administration wound dressing [14,15].

Several studies can be found in the literature concerning drug release from drug loaded electrospun matrices, either reporting drug release behavior or drug release kinetic evaluation. The latter is an important parameter to be investigated since drug release kinetic gives an indication of drug release mechanism. While a zero-order kinetic with constant release rate is preferred, drug release from polymeric drug delivery systems, such as electrospun nanofibers, in many cases shows initial burst release followed by a more controlled release of the drug over a longer duration.

The behavior depends on the drug dispersion state in the polymer fibers (i.e., molecular dispersion (obtained starting from drug/polymer solution) or solid dispersion (obtained starting from a drug suspension into polymer solution)). Therefore, in order to attain successful encapsulation of a drug into the electrospun nanofibers, the physicochemical properties of polymers, as well as their interaction with the drug molecules, must be precisely considered, as they significantly affect drug-encapsulation efficiency, drug distribution inside the fibers, and, ultimately, drug release from the nanofibers.

Various carrier materials, including natural and synthetic (biodegradable and non-degradable) polymers and a blend of both, were used and are being studied for electrospinning. The drugs investigated for electrospinning belong to different therapeutic classes, such as anticancer drugs, antibiotics and anti-infective, proteins, cardiovascular, DNA, and RNA [9,16–25].

The aim of this work was to prepare electrospun matrices loaded with GS and to in vitro evaluate the drug kinetic profile and its microbiologic activity. In vitro release profiles were attained through conventional static in vitro release test, and through an innovative dynamic bioreactor system that was tested in this work and compared to the conventional in vitro drug release test. The data were elaborated by kinetic release equation models [26]. The GS-loaded electrospun matrices could be used for local controlled drug delivery for treating infected skin and gum or during bone surgery in order to prevent or arrest infection.

Rationale for GS local administration resides in its poor oral bioavailability, and the high occurrence of side effects, such as ototoxicity and toxicity in the kidney, when the drug is administered by intravenous or intramuscular routes, which are the preferential administration routes for Gentamicin. Moreover, topical administration of GS is required with infected burns, excoriations, acne, and impetigo, and in these cases local delivery through a polymer nano-fibrous matrix promoting controlled drug release and prolonged therapeutic effect could be of interest.

2. Materials

Copolymer poly-L-lactide-poly-ε-caprolactone (PLA-PCL) 70:30 molar ratio (Resomer LC 703 S – M_w 160,000 Da), freely soluble in methylene chloride (MC), soluble in N,N-dimethylformamide (DMF), was obtained from Evonik Industries (Evonik Nutrition and Care GmbH, 64275 Damstadt, Germany). Analytical grade MC and DMF were supplied by Carlo Erba, with no further purification. Gentamicin sulfate, GS (Gentamicin C_1, $C_{21}H_{43}N_5O_7$, M_w 477.6 g/mol, Gentamicin C_2, $C_{20}H_{41}N_5O_7$, M_w 463.6 g/mol, Gentamicin C_{1a}, $C_{19}H_{39}N_5O_7$, M_w 449.5 g/mol), water solubility 100 mg/mL, insoluble in MC, slightly soluble in DMF (1% w/w), and ninhydrin (NH), M_w 178,14 g/mol; purity grade ≥ 95% were from Sigma Aldrich, Milano, Italy.

3. Methods

3.1. Preparation of Polymeric Electrospun Fibers Loaded with GS

GS powder (3.3% w/w) was first dissolved in DMF and then it was added to PLA-PCL solution (20% w/w, solubilized in MC) and maintained under magnetic stirring at 300 rpm for 2 h, until formation of creaming homogeneous yellowish system. The final PLA-PCL/GS solution, whose composition was 1% w/w GS and 14% w/w PLA-PCL, was sonicated to eliminate air bubbles.

The polymer solubility in MC:DMF 70:30 ratio was previously evaluated. The process parameter, set up in a previous work of the research group, were as follows: flow rate 1 mL/h, voltage 20 k/V, needle Gauge 18 [27]. A metallic plate collector covered with aluminum foil was used for avoiding any fiber damage during recovering; syringe distance from collector plate was maintained at 15 cm. The electrospinning process was performed at room temperature (25 °C) and controlled humidity value (~50%). Electrospinning time was 30 min in order to achieve nanofiber matrices with suitable GS loading.

3.2. UV Quantification of GS

GS quantification was carried out by NH test. Briefly, NH test is a colorimetric assay for quantitative assessment of GS. It is based on the reaction of NH with the primary and secondary gentamicin amino groups leading to the formation of purple compound. The color intensity is directly proportional to gentamicin concentration [28,29]. GS was extracted from electrospun matrices (either the whole matrices or their portions) with the following protocol.

For GS recovery, the whole electrospun matrix was solubilized in 3 mL MC and then Phosphate Buffer Saline PBS (4 mL, pH 7.4) were added for extracting GS. The system was maintained under magnetic stirring at 1000 rpm for 1 h to promote GS extraction. The MC/PBS mixture were centrifuged (16,000 rpm, 10 min) in order to separate organic and aqueous phases and recover GS in the aqueous phase. The extraction of GS in the aqueous phase was guarantee by the high affinity of gentamicin for aqueous phase, the poor solubility of PLA-PCL in the aqueous phase, and the partial miscibility organic (MC) and aqueous phases (PBS). After centrifugation, the supernatant containing GS was recovered, and GS quantified by NH assay. A schematic representation of extraction protocol is represented in Figure 1. The extraction protocol was validated and extraction yield was confirmed to be 95 ± 3.0%.

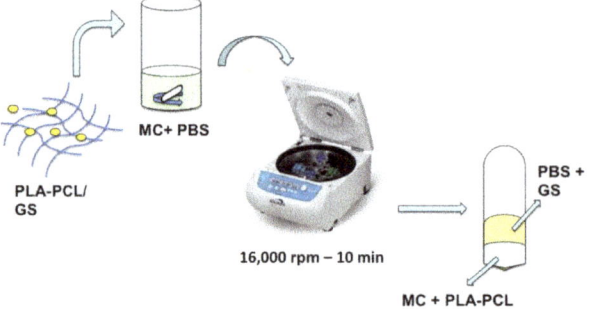

Figure 1. Schematic representation of Gentamicin (GS) extraction from polylactide-co-polycaprolactone (PLA-PCL) electrospun matrices.

A total of 500 µL of NH solution (5 mg/mL concentration), previously solubilized in PBS was added to 500 µL of supernatant. The final solution was vortexed to ensure complete mixing and subsequently heated to 95 °C for 15 min in order to induce reaction between gentamicin and NH molecules. After 15 min, the solution was stored in water/ice bath for 10 min to stop the reaction. Each sample was analyzed at UV spectrophotometer at 418 nm wavelength, using quartz cuvettes (UV-1601, UV-visible spectrophotometer, Shimadzu, ON, Canada).

PBS solution containing 1% *w/w* GS and placebo electrospun matrices were used as controls. All samples underwent the same extraction protocol as GS electrospun matrices before analysis with NH assay.

A six-points calibration curve was obtained with GS standard solutions at concentrations between 0.001 and 0.5 mg/mL. The instrument was calibrated using a blank made of 500 µL of NH solution (0.5% *w/v*) added to 500 µL of PBS at pH 7.4.

In order to evaluate drug loading uniformity, all electrospun matrices were cut in a spherical mold. The spherical mold was chosen because when electrospun fibers are collected on a plate collector, they form a circular film that widens as long as fiber deposition is prolonged over time. The reduction and/or prevention in further deposition of fibers could be due to the forming of insulator layer, which depend on electrospun membrane thickness. The mechanism of fiber formation makes that the core of circular film is made of fibers collected from the beginning of the process, while the crown of circular film is made of fiber later collected. Considering no significant differences of drug loading between the core and crown section, it is reasonable to postulate that GS feeding solution was stable during the electrospinning process.

GS extraction and quantification were performed following the protocol reported above. Each electrospun matrix, whose diameter was 7 ± 0.5 cm, was cut in two concentric parts as shown in Figure 2. Part 1 (identified as crown) having 1.75 cm external circle radius, and part 2 (identified as core) having 3.5 cm diameter. GS was extracted, and in both electrospun matrix molds was quantified.

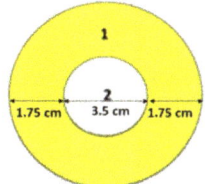

Figure 2. Representation of the two cut concentric portions of electrospun matrices: (1) crown, (2) core.

Each analysis was performed in triplicate, and average values and standard deviations (sd) were calculated. The reference for GS content percentage determination was the theoretical amount of GS loaded in the matrix calculated as follows:

$$\text{GS content (\%)} = \text{mg GS in matrix/mg GS in the electrospun polymer solution} \times 100$$

3.3. Morphology Characterization by Scanning Electron Microscopy (SEM)

SEM analysis was carried out on placebo and GS-loaded electrospun matrices in order to characterize their morphology in term of nanofiber size, shape, and orientation. Zeiss EVO MA10 apparatus (Carl Zeiss, Oberkochen, Germany) was used with 5000× magnification. Nanofiber size was determined by digital elaboration of SEM images with ImageJ software (National Institutes of Health (NIH) open source image processing program).

3.4. In Vitro GS Release Test

In vitro drug release tests were performed at 37 °C, both in static and dynamic conditions, in order to evaluate how medium flow rate and its direction affect drug release profile. The tests were carried out on both the whole electrospun matrices and on portions of the electrospun matrices that were cut as explained above.

3.4.1. In Vitro GS Release Test in Static Conditions

Each sample was placed in Erlenmeyer flasks and soaked in 10 mL of PBS (pH 7.4) at 37 °C in a thermostatic chamber. Medium was withdrawn (1 mL) at scheduled times up to GS complete release; PBS was restored with fresh buffer at each withdrawal.

3.4.2. In Vitro GS Release Test in Dynamic Conditions

In vitro release tests in dynamic conditions were performed using IVTech Livebox1 (LB1) and Livebox2 (LB2) combined with a peristaltic pump (IPC4 - ISMATEC), as shown in Figure 3. IVTech LiveBox 1 is a bioreactor made of a transparent silicon cell with a capacity of 1.5 mL and tangential flow perfusion of the incubation medium, (Figure 3A). The cell is delimited both on the upper side and on the lower side by little glass disks (Ø 20 mm), and the locking system guarantees closure and endurance during the test. IVTech LiveBox2 (LB2) has the same structural characteristics of LB1 but with vertical perfusion flow configuration (down–top), (Figure 3B).

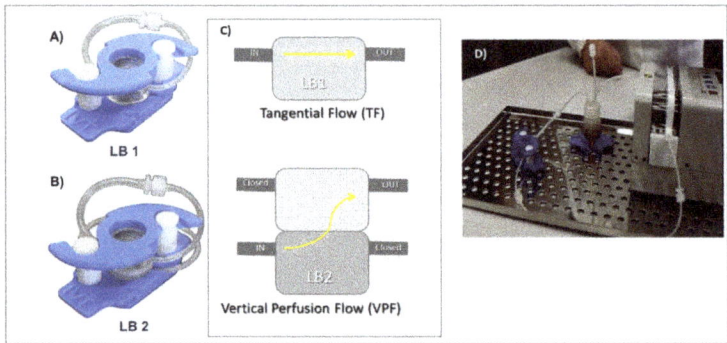

Figure 3. (**A**) Live Box1 (from IVTech website); (**B**) Live Box 2 (from IVTech website); (**C**) IVTech live Box 1 and scheme and flow configuration: Tangential Flow (TF) and Vertical Perfusion Flow (VPF); and (**D**) IVTech system equipped with pump and tubing systems.

The PBS buffer (10 mL, pH 7.4) was continuously recirculated from the reservoir vial (see Figure 3C) at two different flow rates: 0.3 mL/min and 0.6 mL/min maintaining temperature at 37 °C. IVTech LiveBox has peculiar characteristics; the sample is in contact with a small volume of incubation medium simulating the most physiologic condition of implantation into the human body. The flow through the cell creates dynamic conditions; the flow rate can be selected in the range 0.1–0.4 mL/min for LiveBox 1 (TF), and up to 0.5 mL/min in apical or basal compartments for LiveBox 2 (VPF). Flow direction can be either tangential or vertical perfusion.

In vitro release test was performed on small portions of electrospun matrix sections (1 and 2) because of the limited IVTech LiveBox chamber size. The final data were expressed as averages of the two small parts. All data were normalized against their weight in order to make them comparable with data obtained for whole matrices.

3.4.3. Kinetic Release Equations

Most common kinetic profiles considered to describe drug release are zero-order, first-order, Higuchi model, or Korsmeyer-Peppas [27–31]. The in vitro release data were elaborated using the following kinetic release equation models:

Zero-order model

$$Q_t = Q_0 + K_0 t \qquad (1)$$

where Q_t is the amount of drug determined in the incubation medium at the fixed times, t is the time spans, and K_0 is the zero-order release constant expressed in units of concentration/time. The model fits drug release from dosage forms that do not disaggregate and where drug release rate is independent of its concentration. The model is used to describe drug dissolution from several types of modified release pharmaceutical dosage forms.

First-order release model

$$\text{Log } Q_t = \text{Log} Q_0 - k_1\, t/2.303 \qquad (2)$$

where Q_t and Q_0 are the amounts of drug released at time t and at time zero respectively, K_1 is the first order release constant, and t is time. Drug release rate depends on its concentration; this model can be used to describe drug dissolution in pharmaceutical dosage forms containing water-soluble drugs in porous matrices.

Higuchi model

$$Q = K_H\, t^{1/2} \qquad (3)$$

Equation (3) represent the simplified Higuchi model where Q is the amount of drug released in time t and K_H is the Higuchi dissolution constant. The amount of drug released in the fixed time spans, represented as function of the square root of time, fits a straight line.

The Higuchi model is suitable as model for drug release from thin films, containing finely dispersed drugs into perfect sink conditions; this model suggests that drug release is by diffusion, and it takes into account matrix porosity and tortuosity. The premise of the kinetic model is that perfect sink conditions are attained in the release environment.

Korsmeyer-Peppas model

$$M_t/M = k\, t^n \qquad (4)$$

where M_t and M are the amount of drug at time t and loaded into the drug delivery system respectively, k is the kinetic constant related to the delivery system and encapsulated substance properties. n is release exponent and depends on the type of transport, geometry, and polydispersity of solute; it illustrates the solute transport mechanism as follows: (i) $n < 0.5$ corresponds to a pseudo-Fickian behavior of diffusion; (ii) $n = 0.5$ suggests Fickian behaviour; (iii) $0.5 < n < 1$ indicates an anomalous diffusion; (iv) $n = 1$ shows non-Fickian diffusion. The amount of drug released in the fixed time spans is represented on a log–log basis.

3.5. In Vitro Degradation Study: Mass Loss Analysis

Degradation study, evaluated on gravimetric basis: mass loss % (ML %) in the dissolution medium, was monitored on a parallel set of samples along all in vitro release test times, and it was determined with the following protocol. The initial mass of the matrix (M_0) was determined by weighing the lyophilized samples with an analytical balance (Mettler Toledo, AG245 mod, Milano, Italy) before being subjected to in vitro degradation tests (time zero).

The samples were incubated in PBS pH 7.4 at 37 °C, the same conditions as for the in vitro release test were followed. Each sample was taken from the buffer, at the sampling times fixed for the degradation test (3, 5, 14, 21, and 28 days), it was washed with distilled water to remove the water-soluble oligomers that can form due to copolymer degradation, and lyophilized (Lio 5P) at −48 °C at 0.4 mbar for 12 h to eliminate all water traces. The lyophilized samples were subsequently weighed (M_x). Mass loss was calculated using the following equation:

$$\text{Mass Loss (\%)} = M_0 - M_x/M_0 \times 100$$

3.6. Antibacterial Activity Measurements

The antimicrobial activity of GS-loaded electrospun matrices (EL-GS) was evaluated against the following reference bacterial strains: *Staphylococcus aureus* ATCC 6538 and *Escherichia coli* ATCC 10356. Before testing, bacteria were grown overnight in Tryptone Soya Broth (TSA, Oxoid, Basingstoke, UK) at 37 °C. The cultures were centrifuged at 224 g for 20 min, in order to separate the microorganisms from the culture broth, and then washed with purified water. Washed cells were further suspended in Dulbecco's PBS (phosphate buffered saline, Sigma-Aldrich, Milan, Italy) and optical density (OD) was adjusted to 0.3, corresponding approximately to 1×10^8 colony forming units (CFU)/mL at 650 nm wavelength.

The antimicrobial activity was evaluated in the presence of the EL-GS, or a placebo to be used as a control. Viable microbial counts were evaluated after contact for scheduled time with EL-GS and with placebo samples (electrospun matrices without GS); bacterial colonies were enumerated in TSA after incubation at 37 °C for 24 h. The microbicidal effect (ME value) was calculated for each test organisms and contact times according to the following Equation [32]:

$$ME = \log Nc - \log Nd \qquad (5)$$

where Nc is the number of CFU of the control microbial suspension and Nd is the number of CFU of the microbial suspension in presence of patches.

4. Results

4.1. Preparation of Polymeric Electrospun Fibers Loaded with GS

The GS-loaded electrospun matrices, obtained after 30 min electrospinning, were round matrices whose diameter was 7 ± 0.5 cm and with average weight value of 58 ± 2.9 mg, as determined on six replications obtained in the same experimental conditions reported in the method section.

4.2. UV Quantification of GS

The results of GS quantification in the whole electrospun matrices are reported in Figure 4.

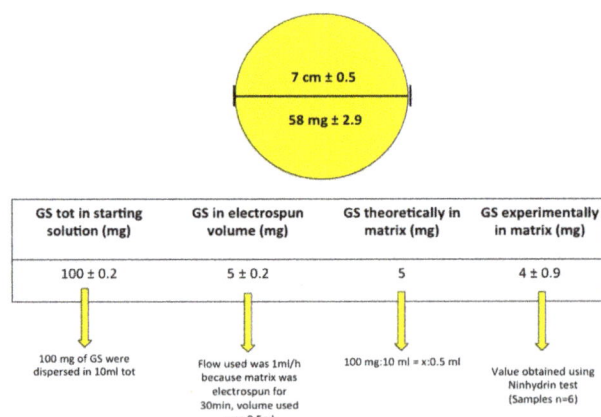

Figure 4. GS quantification in electrospun PLA-PCL matrices. The figure refers to GS amount in the whole electrospun matrix.

The amount of GS experimentally determined in the electrospun matrices, expressed as relative mass ratio of the loaded drug to the fiber, was 6.8 *w/w*%, and corresponded to the GS theoretically calculated amount. Slight loss of GS micrograms was due to the cleaning step during the electrospinning process. The results of GS determination in the matrix's portions are reported in Figure 5. GS content result was uniform compared to weight, in the two sections considered. This confirmed GS was uniformly dispersed in the polymer solution during the electrospinning process.

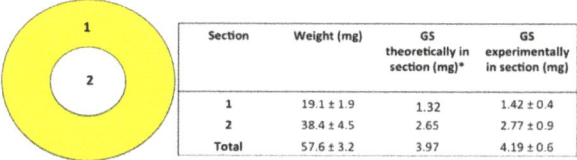

Section	Weight (mg)	GS theoretically in section (mg)*	GS experimentally in section (mg)
1	19.1 ± 1.9	1.32	1.42 ± 0.4
2	38.4 ± 4.5	2.65	2.77 ± 0.9
Total	57.6 ± 3.2	3.97	4.19 ± 0.6

* For evaluation of GS theoretical amount (mg) was used average weight of whole matrix (58 mg ± 2.9) and GS carried (4 ± 0.9)

Figure 5. GS quantification in matrices portions.

4.3. Morphologic Characterization

Data obtained by SEM analysis (Figure 5) showed that fibers morphologies were unchanged after GS addition in polymeric solution. The fibers were in a 700–800 nm range dimension with a smooth surface. No evidence of GS crystals, either on nanofibers surface (Figure 6A,B) or in the electrospun matrices (Figure 6C,D), was highlighted by SEM analysis. Electrospun matrix thickness, as measured by SEM analysis on six replications, resulted to be significantly greater for core portion, 41.81 ± 0.21 µm, with respect to external portion that was 28.61 ± 1.02 µm. The result was due to the electrospinning process on a plane collector and without any restriction, which led to the accumulation of fibers, starting from the collector central part and enlarging the radius as long as conductivity changed as a function of fiber deposition on the collector. As 30 min was fixed as the electrospinning time, this caused the fabrication of matrices with different thickness, decreasing from core to edges. Fibers entanglement, size, and shape did not change in the two different portions analyzed, while fiber density was greater in the electrospun matrices' central portions.

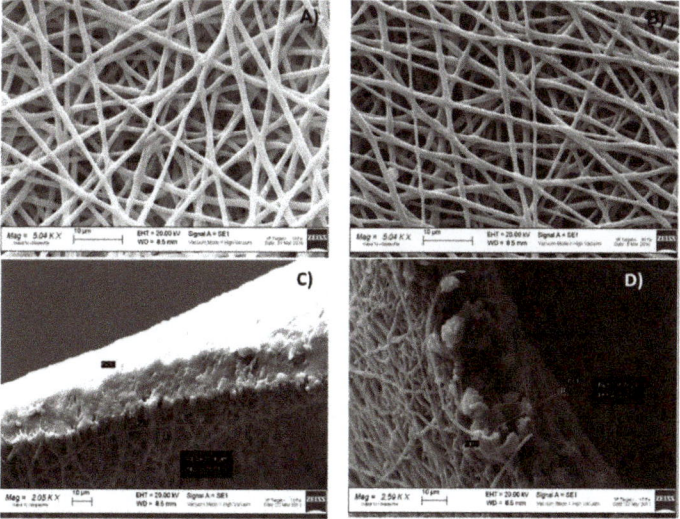

Figure 6. Scanning Electron Microscopy (SEM) images of (**A**) PLA-PCL electrospun matrices (magnification 5.04 KX); (**B**) PLA-PCL/GS electrospun matrices (magnification 5.04 KX); (**C**) orthogonal section of electrospun matrices portion 1 (external edge) (magnification 2.05 KX); and (**D**) orthogonal section of electrospun matrix portion 2 (core) (magnification 2.59 KX).

4.4. GS In Vitro Release in Static and Dynamic Conditions

GS in vitro release profiles obtained either in static or dynamic condition tests were collected in Figure 7, showing that electrospun nanofibers significantly slowed down GS release with respect to drug pristine dissolution profile (Figure 7, orange curve).

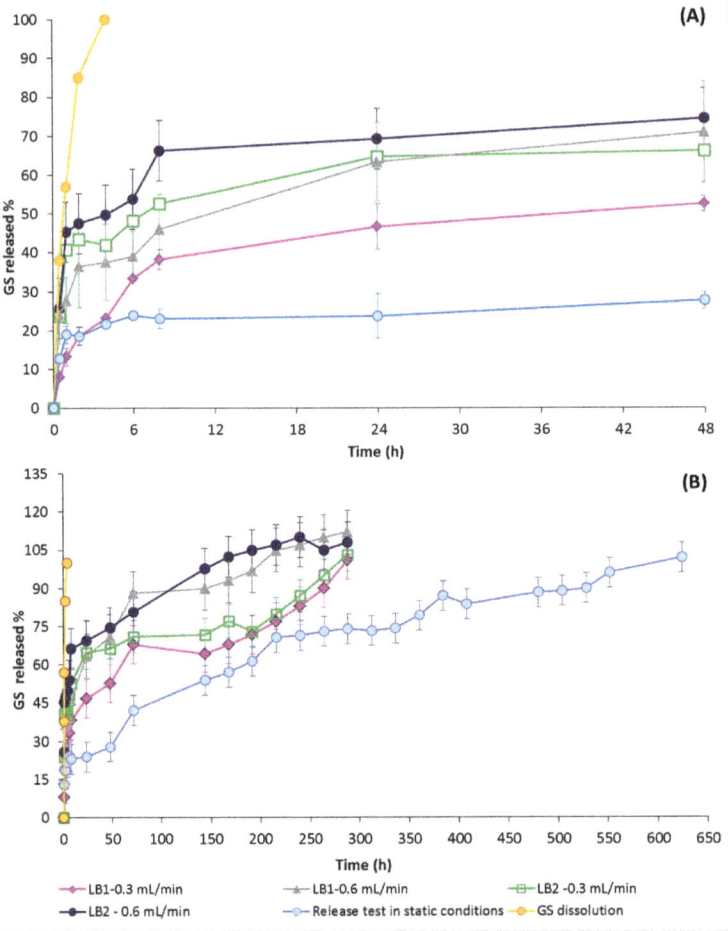

Figure 7. GS in vitro release profiles as tested in static and dynamic conditions: (**A**) GS release in the first 48 h test; and (**B**) in vitro release profiles at GS release completion.

GS release from the electrospun matrices, tested in static conditions, was completed in 624 h (26 days). No differences were highlighted between testing the whole electrospun matrices or a portion of them (data not reported), corroborating that GS was uniformly distributed in the electrospun matrix. Moreover, since GS solubility in water is 100 mg/mL, the in vitro release test on the electrospun matrices was conducted always in sink conditions. For these reasons, the different matrix thicknesses did not play a significant role in GS release. GS release profiles in dynamic conditions using IVTech bioreactors (LB1 and LB2) were reported in Figure 7.

Drug release in dynamic conditions, as expected, was significantly faster with respect to drug release rate in static conditions. In the first 24 h of testing, drug release was faster with LB2 bioreactor, which means that orthogonal flow, independently from flow rate, promoted drug release. However, drug release profiles after the first 24 h showed that the higher flow rate (0.6 mL/min) significantly sped up drug release and the higher flow rates (0.6mL/min) corresponded to significantly faster drug release with both types of flows tested (tangential for orthogonal flow). Moreover, flow direction did not seem to significantly affect the GS release profile when lower the flow rate was applied (0.3 mL/min); however, in this case, complete GS release was achieved in 288 h, both using LB1 and LB2 bioreactors.

Drug burst release (drug released in the first 8 h test) was highlighted in all the in vitro release conditions tested, and it increased by incrementing dissolution medium flow rate and changing from tangential to vertical perfusion flow direction. The results are consistent with GS high water solubility that makes drug release highly sensitive to environmental conditions.

The in vitro release data were elaborated by kinetic release equation models and results are reported in Tables 1 and 2.

Table 1. Kinetic model elaboration of GS release from EL matrices incubated in static conditions in (pH 7.4) at 37 °C.

Models	Intercept	Slope	R^2
Zero-order	0.02	1	0.94
First-order	−1.76	1.2×10^{-2}	0.93
Higuchi	0.01	2.5×10^{-3}	0.97
Korsmeyer-Peppas	−1.88	2.3×10^{-1}	0.77

Table 2. Kinetic model elaboration of GS release from electrospun matrices incubated in dynamic conditions in PBS (pH 7.4) at 37 °C.

	TF-LB1 Bioreactor						VPF – LB2 Bioreactor					
Flow Rate (mL/min)	0.3			0.6			0.3			0.6		
	Intercept	Slope	R^2	Intercept	Slope	R^2	Intercept	Slope	R^2	Intercept	Slope	R^2
Zero order	0.01	0.0001	0.77	0.01	0.0003	0.85	0.02	-7×10^{-5}	0.77	0.03	-7×10^{-5}	0.85
First order	−2.03	0.003	0.63	−1.51	0.003	0.78	−1.59	1.4×10^{-3}	0.82	−1.59	-1.3×10^{-3}	0.84
Higuchi	0.007	0.0015	0.90	0.023	0.004	0.93	0.03	-1.1×10^{-3}	0.98	0.03	-1.1×10^{-3}	0.98
Korsmeyer-Peppas	−2.15	0.25	0.87	−1.56	0.17	0.83	−1.55	-8.86×10^{-2}	0.82	−15,505	-9×10^{-2}	0.96

Electrospun matrices showed drug release was regulated from the Higuchi kinetic model, both in dynamic and static conditions. The Korsmeyer-Peppas slope exponent (n) was between 0.1 and 0.25, which confirms that the pseudo-Fickian diffusional mechanism controlled the GS release from electrospun nanofibers in all the conditions analyzed.

4.5. In Vitro Degradation Test: Mass Loss Analysis

The mass loss results in the 28 days, corresponding to in vitro release test, are reported in Figure 8. They show that matrices' mass loss reached 12% after 28 days incubation in simulated physiologic conditions. The results were consistent with data discussed by the authors in a previously published work [27] on PLA-PCL placebo electrospun matrices, showing GS-loaded PLA-PCL electrospun matrices are stable in the 28 days incubation in the simulated physiologic conditions tested.

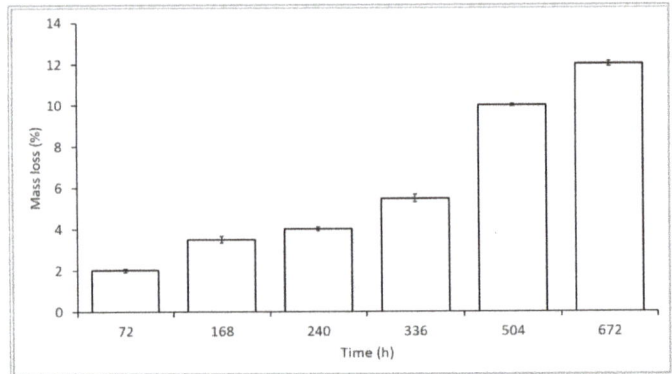

Figure 8. GS-loaded electrospun matrices' mass loss percentage in simulated physiologic conditions (PBS, pH 7.4).

4.6. Antibacterial Activity Measurements

The results of antibacterial activity measurements are reported in Table 3, they show the antimicrobial activity obtained against both *S. aureus* and *E. coli*. In particular, the values of ME were sufficiently high to reach a full antimicrobial effect at the concentrations investigated, comparable to the action of a disinfectant (ME ≥ 4) [32,33].

Table 3. Antibacterial activity of EL-GS evaluated against *S. aureus* and *E. coli*.

Sample Code	Contact Time (h)	Microbicide Effect (ME) vs. *S. aureus*	Microbicide Effet (ME) vs. *E. coli*
EL-GS *	1.0	3.79	5.86
EL-GS	6.0	7.21	8.04
EL-GS	24	10.15	10.37
EL-GS	48	10.48	10.69
EL	1.0	1.0	1.0
EL **	6.0	1.0	1.0
EL	24	0	0
EL	48	0	0

* EL-GS: Electrospun matrices loaded with GS; ** EL: placebo electrospun matrices.

CEN EN 13697 reports ME should be tested after 15 min of contact for disinfectant antibacterial activity determination. Here an antibiotic drug embedded in a polymer matrix was tested; therefore, in a different situation, slightly different time parameters were set (1 h) in order to consider GS release rate from the electrospun matrices.

The antimicrobial effect, being significant after 1 h of contact, increased with time consistently with GS release from the electrospun matrices. Placebo polymeric electrospun matrices show null antimicrobial effect against both microbial strains tested. Considering that in 48 h the EL-GS released about 27.7% GS in the same conditions (see Figure 7B, GS release in static conditions), it can be hypothesized that the antibacterial activity could prolong with time.

5. Discussion

In this work GS was solubilized in DMF, and the mixture solvent system (MC:DMF 70:30) aided the physical stabilization of GS in the polymer solution during the electrospinning process. GS concentration in the final solvent mixture, hence the amount of GS loaded into the electrospun matrices, was strictly dependent on GS solubility in the solvents used. In this experimental condition, uniform distribution of GS inside the electrospun mats was obtained, permitting an accurate dosage of GS, and no crystals were observed by SEM analysis of the electrospun matrices.

GS-loaded electrospun matrices were recently investigated by Coimbra and coll [24], demonstrating the interest in GS local delivery by polymer electrospun matrices. The authors loaded GS into electrospun matrices, starting from a suspension or an emulsion; in all cases, they highlighted similar drug release profiles with great burst release.

The results of the present experimental work highlighted that GS release rate from the electrospun matrices was slowed down with respect to in vitro dissolution of GS powder. Attention was focused on the different in vitro release tests performed, in static conditions and dynamic conditions, and results highlighted that medium flow rate significantly affects drug release rate. This could be explained by a higher differential between drug concentration at the stationary state surrounding the matrices surface and bulk drug concentration, when in vitro release test was carried out in dynamic conditions. The hypothesis was confirmed by high evidence of the phenomenon at the beginning of in vitro release test. Moreover, GS release followed a Higuchi kinetic model, typical of diffusion through porous thin films. The result is consistent with the low values of polymer mass loss obtained, demonstrating that degradation of the PLA-PCL electrospun matrix was not involved in GS release electrospun matrices.

6. Conclusions

The results indicate that there is a good and suitable chance for the future use of electrospun nanofibers as carriers for antibiotics. The electrospun matrices could be applied on severe burns, in order to prevent infections after its implantation into gingival cavities for local infection treatment, or after tooth explant. The advantage is the ability to reach high antibiotic concentrations at the site of action, in the meantime avoiding high system concentrations, thus reducing the drug side effects. Moreover, the prolonged effect of antibiotic at the site of action can reduce administration frequency and improve patient compliance. As far as GS is concerned, further studies should be conducted to ascertain how to reduce GS burst release from the electrospun matrices, meanwhile rendering drug release more independent from environmental conditions.

Author Contributions: S.P. carried out the experiment with support from E.C. Both I.G. and T.M. contributed to the implementation of the research, G.B. performed the SEM experiments, P.G. performed antibacterial activity evaluation. Both B.C. and R.D. wrote and contributed to the final version of the manuscript, B.C. supervised the project.

Funding: This research received no external funding.

Acknowledgments: The authors wish to thank PTS (Parco Tecnico Scientifico) of the University of Pavia for providing electrospinning apparatus (Polymerix S.r.l., Via Taramelli 24, Pavia, Italy).

Conflicts of Interest: The authors declare no conflict of interest.

References

1. Sankaran, S.; Deshmukh, K.; Ahamed, M.B.; Pasha, S.K.K. Electrospun Polymeric Nanofibers: Fundamental Aspects of Electrospinning Processes, Optimization of Electrospinning Parameters, Properties, and Applications. In *Polymer Nanocomposites in Biomedical Engineering*; Sadasivuni, K.K., Ponnamma, D., Rajan, M., Ahmed, B., Maadeed, M.A.S.A., Eds.; Springer International Publishing: Cham, Switzerland, 2019; pp. 375–409.
2. Hu, X.; Liu, S.; Zhou, G.; Huang, Y.; Xie, Z.; Jing, X. Electrospinning of polymeric nanofibers for drug delivery applications. *J. Control. Release* **2014**, *185*, 12–21. [CrossRef] [PubMed]
3. Chen, S.; Li, R.; Li, X.; Xie, J. Electrospinning: An enabling nanotechnology platform for drug delivery and regenerative medicine. *Adv. Drug Deliv. Rev.* **2018**, *132*, 188–213. [CrossRef]
4. Kazsoki, A.; Szabó, P.; Domján, A.; Balázs, A.; Bozó, T.; Kellermayer, M.; Farkas, A.; Balogh-Weiser, D.; Pinke, B.; Darcsi, A.; et al. Microstructural Distinction of Electrospun Nanofibrous Drug Delivery Systems Formulated with Different Excipients. *Mol. Pharm.* **2018**, *15*, 4214–4225. [CrossRef] [PubMed]

5. Radacsi, N.; Giapis, K.P.; Ovari, G.; Szabo-Revesz, P.; Ambrus, R. Electrospun nanofiber-based niflumic acid capsules with superior physicochemical properties. *J. Pharm. Biomed. Anal.* **2019**, *166*, 371–378. [CrossRef] [PubMed]
6. Modica de Mohac, L.; Keating, A.V.; De Fátima Pina, M.; Raimi-Abraham, B.T. Engineering of Nanofibrous Amorphous and Crystalline Solid Dispersions for Oral Drug Delivery. *Pharmaceutics* **2018**, *11*, 7. [CrossRef] [PubMed]
7. Padmakumar, S.; Paul-Prasanth, B.; Pavithran, K.; Vijaykumar, D.K.; Rajanbabu, A.; Sivanarayanan, T.B.; Kadakia, E.; Amiji, M.M.; Nair, S.V.; Menon, D. Long-term drug delivery using implantable electrospun woven polymeric nanotextiles. *Nanomed. Nanotechnol. Biol. Med.* **2019**, *15*, 274–284. [CrossRef]
8. Simões, M.C.R.; Cragg, S.M.; Barbu, E.; de Sousa, F.B. The potential of electrospun poly(methyl methacrylate)/polycaprolactone core–sheath fibers for drug delivery applications. *J. Mater. Sci.* **2019**, *54*, 5712–5725. [CrossRef]
9. Rychter, M.; Milanowski, B.; Grzeskowiak, B.F.; Jarek, M.; Kempinski, M.; Coy, E.L.; Borysiak, S.; Baranowska-Korczyc, A.; Lulek, J. Cilostazol-loaded electrospun three-dimensional systems for potential cardiovascular application: Effect of fibers hydrophilization on drug release, and cytocompatibility. *J. Colloid Interface Sci.* **2019**, *536*, 310–327. [CrossRef]
10. Topuz, F.; Uyar, T. Electrospinning of Cyclodextrin Functional Nanofibers for Drug Delivery Applications. *Pharmaceutics* **2019**, *11*, 6. [CrossRef]
11. Khadka, D.B.; Haynie, D.T. Protein- and peptide-based electrospun nanofibers in medical biomaterials. *Nanomed. Nanotechnol. Biol. Med.* **2012**, *8*, 1242–1262. [CrossRef] [PubMed]
12. Wang, B.; Wang, Y.; Yin, T.; Yu, Q. Applications of electrospinning technique in drug delivery. *Chem. Eng. Commun.* **2010**, *197*, 1315–1338. [CrossRef]
13. Persano, L.; Camposeo, A.; Tekmen, C.; Pisignano, D. Industrial Upscaling of Electrospinning and Applications of Polymer Nanofibers: A Review. *Macromol. Mater. Eng.* **2013**, *298*, 504–520. [CrossRef]
14. Liu, S.; Zhou, G.; Liu, D.; Xie, Z.; Huang, Y.; Wang, X.; Wu, W.; Jing, X. Inhibition of orthotopic secondary hepatic carcinoma in mice by doxorubicin-loaded electrospun polylactide nanofibers. *J. Mater. Chem. B* **2013**, *1*, 101–109. [CrossRef]
15. Angkawinitwong, U.; Awwad, S.; Khaw, P.T.; Brocchini, S.; Williams, G.R. Electrospun formulations of bevacizumab for sustained release in the eye. *Acta Biomater.* **2017**, *64*, 126–136. [CrossRef] [PubMed]
16. Goh, Y.-F.; Shakir, I.; Hussain, R. Electrospun fibers for tissue engineering, drug delivery, and wound dressing. *J. Mater. Sci.* **2013**, *48*, 3027–3054. [CrossRef]
17. Abrigo, M.; McArthur, S.L.; Kingshott, P. Electrospun Nanofibers as Dressings for Chronic Wound Care: Advances, Challenges, and Future Prospects. *Macromol. Biosci.* **2014**, *14*, 772–792. [CrossRef] [PubMed]
18. Iqbal, S.; Rashid, M.H.; Arbab, A.S.; Khan, M. Encapsulation of Anticancer Drugs (5-Fluorouracil and Paclitaxel) into Polycaprolactone (PCL) Nanofibers and In Vitro Testing for Sustained and Targeted Therapy. *J. Biomed. Nanotechnol.* **2017**, *13*, 355–366. [CrossRef]
19. Buschle-Diller, G.; Cooper, J.; Xie, Z.; Wu, Y.; Waldrup, J.; Ren, X. Release of antibiotics from electrospun bicomponent fibers. *Cellulose* **2007**, *14*, 553–562. [CrossRef]
20. Al-Enizi, A.M.; Zagho, M.M.; Elzatahry, A.A. Polymer-Based Electrospun Nanofibers for Biomedical Applications. *Nanomaterials* **2018**, *8*, 259. [CrossRef] [PubMed]
21. Wang, X.; Yuan, Y.; Huang, X.; Yue, T. Controlled release of protein from core–shell nanofibers prepared by emulsion electrospinning based on green chemical. *J. Appl. Polym. Sci.* **2015**, *132*. [CrossRef]
22. Luu, Y.K.; Kim, K.; Hsiao, B.S.; Chu, B.; Hadjiargyrou, M. Development of a nanostructured DNA delivery scaffold via electrospinning of PLGA and PLA-PEG block copolymers. *J. Control. Release* **2003**, *89*, 341–353. [CrossRef]
23. Ramalingam, R.; Dhand, C.; Leung, C.M.; Ong, S.T.; Annamalai, S.K.; Kamruddin, M.; Verma, N.K.; Ramakrishna, S.; Lakshminarayanan, R.; Arunachalam, K.D. Antimicrobial properties and biocompatibility of electrospun poly-ε-caprolactone fibrous mats containing Gymnema sylvestre leaf extract. *Mater. Sci. Eng. C* **2019**, *98*, 503–514. [CrossRef]
24. Coimbra, P.; Freitas, J.P.; Gonçalves, T.; Gil, M.H.; Figueiredo, M. Preparation of gentamicin sulfate eluting fiber mats by emulsion and by suspension electrospinning. *Mater. Sci. Eng. C* **2019**, *94*, 86–93. [CrossRef]

25. Lian, M.; Sun, B.; Qiao, Z.; Zhao, K.; Zhou, X.; Zhang, Q.; Zou, D.; He, C.; Zhang, X. Bi-layered electrospun nanofibrous membrane with osteogenic and antibacterial properties for guided bone regeneration. *Coll. Surf. B Biointerfaces* **2019**, *176*, 219–229. [CrossRef]
26. Dash, S.; Murthy, P.N.; Nath, L.; Chowdhury, P. Kinetic modeling on drug release from controlled drug delivery systems. *Acta Pol. Pharm.* **2010**, *67*, 217–223.
27. Pisani, S.; Dorati, R.; Conti, B.; Modena, T.; Bruni, G.; Genta, I. Design of copolymer PLA-PCL electrospun matrix for biomedical applications. *React. Funct. Polym.* **2018**, *124*, 77–89. [CrossRef]
28. Dorati, R.; DeTrizio, A.; Genta, I.; Grisoli, P.; Merelli, A.; Tomasi, C.; Conti, B. An experimental design approach to the preparation of pegylated polylactide-co-glicolide gentamicin loaded microparticles for local antibiotic delivery. *Mater. Sci. Eng. C* **2016**, *58*, 909–917. [CrossRef]
29. Dorati, R.; DeTrizio, A.; Spalla, M.; Migliavacca, R.; Pagani, L.; Pisani, S.; Chiesa, E.; Conti, B.; Modena, T.; Genta, I. Gentamicin Sulfate PEG-PLGA/PLGA-H Nanoparticles: Screening Design and Antimicrobial Effect Evaluation toward Clinic Bacterial Isolates. *Nanomaterials* **2018**, *8*, 37. [CrossRef] [PubMed]
30. Peppas, N.A.; Narasimhan, B. Mathematical models in drug delivery: How modeling has shaped the way we design new drug delivery systems. *J. Control. Release* **2014**, *190*, 75–81. [CrossRef] [PubMed]
31. Panotopoulos, G.P.; Haidar, Z.S. Mathematical Modeling for Pharmaco-Kinetic and -Dynamic Predictions from Controlled Drug Release NanoSystems: A Comparative Parametric Study. *Scientifica* **2019**, *2019*, 5. [CrossRef]
32. Yoo, J.H. Review of Disinfection and Sterilization—Back to the Basics. *Infect. Chemother.* **2018**, *50*, 101–109. [CrossRef] [PubMed]
33. EN 13697. *Chemical Disinfectants and Antiseptics—Quantitative Non-Porous Surface Test for the Evaluation of Bactericidal and/or Fungicidal Activity of Chemical Disinfectants Used in Food, Industrial, Domestic and Institutional Areas—Test Method and Requirements (Phase 2, Step 2)*; CEN (CEN European Committee for Standardization): Brussels, Belgium, 2015; pp. 3–34.

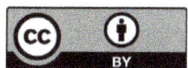

© 2019 by the authors. Licensee MDPI, Basel, Switzerland. This article is an open access article distributed under the terms and conditions of the Creative Commons Attribution (CC BY) license (http://creativecommons.org/licenses/by/4.0/).

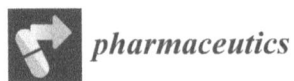

Article

Monitoring of Antimicrobial Drug Chloramphenicol Release from Electrospun Nano- and Microfiber Mats Using UV Imaging and Bacterial Bioreporters

Liis Preem [1], Frederik Bock [2], Mariliis Hinnu [3], Marta Putrinš [3], Kadi Sagor [3], Tanel Tenson [3], Andres Meos [1], Jesper Østergaard [2,4,*] and Karin Kogermann [1,*]

1. Institute of Pharmacy, Faculty of Medicine, University of Tartu, Nooruse 1, 50411 Tartu, Estonia; liis.preem@ut.ee (L.P.); andres.meos@ut.ee (A.M.)
2. Department of Pharmacy, University of Copenhagen, Universitetsparken 2, DK-2100 Copenhagen Ø, Denmark; frederik.bock@sund.ku.dk
3. Institute of Technology, Faculty of Natural Sciences, University of Tartu, Nooruse 1, 50411 Tartu, Estonia; mariliis.hinnu@ut.ee (M.H.); marta.putrins@ut.ee (M.P.); kadisagor@gmail.com (K.S.); tanel.tenson@ut.ee (T.T.)
4. LEO Foundation Center for Cutaneous Drug Delivery, Department of Pharmacy, University of Copenhagen, Universitetsparken 2, DK-2100 Copenhagen Ø, Denmark
* Correspondence: jesper.ostergaard@sund.ku.dk (J.Ø.); karin.kogermann@ut.ee (K.K.); Tel.: +372-56-509-455 (K.K.)

Received: 31 August 2019; Accepted: 16 September 2019; Published: 19 September 2019

Abstract: New strategies are continuously sought for the treatment of skin and wound infections due to increased problems with non-healing wounds. Electrospun nanofiber mats with antibacterial agents as drug delivery systems provide opportunities for the eradication of bacterial infections as well as wound healing. Antibacterial activities of such mats are directly linked with their drug release behavior. Traditional pharmacopoeial drug release testing settings are not always suitable for analyzing the release behavior of fiber mats intended for the local drug delivery. We tested and compared different drug release model systems for the previously characterized electrospun chloramphenicol (CAM)-loaded nanofiber (polycaprolactone (PCL)) and microfiber (PCL in combination with polyethylene oxide) mats with different drug release profiles. Drug release into buffer solution and hydrogel was investigated and drug concentration was determined using either high-performance liquid chromatography, ultraviolet-visible spectrophotometry, or ultraviolet (UV) imaging. The CAM release and its antibacterial effects in disc diffusion assay were assessed by bacterial bioreporters. All tested model systems enabled to study the drug release from electrospun mats. It was found that the release into buffer solution showed larger differences in the drug release rate between differently designed mats compared to the hydrogel release tests. The UV imaging method provided an insight into the interactions with an agarose hydrogel mimicking wound tissue, thus giving us information about early drug release from the mat. Bacterial bioreporters showed clear correlations between the drug release into gel and antibacterial activity of the electrospun CAM-loaded mats.

Keywords: antibacterial activity; bacterial bioreporters; drug release; electrospinning; microfibers; nanofibers; UV imaging

1. Introduction

Electrospinning is a highly versatile and robust technique that allows production of fibers with diameters from several nanometers to tens of micrometers [1]. Drug-loaded electrospun nanofiber mats have been studied intensively and show potential as drug delivery systems (DDSs) [2] and tissue engineering scaffolds [3,4] due to several advantages, such as huge specific surface area, porosity and the possibility to modify the drug release kinetics [5–7]. Compared to other delivery systems, nano- and microfiber mats enable control and tuning of the drug release kinetics [8] and, hence, design the mats with desired properties [9,10]. For example, for local antibiotic delivery, the desired drug release needs to follow two steps: initial fast release followed by the slow zero-order kinetics over a longer period of time [11]. Novel strategies for attaining sustained release have been proposed, for example via the formation of core-shell structures [12,13], beads [14], or modification of nanofiber mat thickness [15]. The drug release process is affected by several factors, such as the physicochemical properties of the drug and carrier polymer, the structural characteristics of the material system, release environment, and the possible interactions between these factors [16]. It is known that drug release from electrospun fiber mats may vary depending on the material properties and the structure of the mats [9,15,17,18].

Despite the substantial body of literature on electrospun fiber mats and their characterization, there is no standard method for the analysis of drug release from fiber mats. Traditional pharmacopoeial drug dissolution tests have been found useful for the analysis of nanofibers incorporated into capsules or pressed into a tablet [19,20]. However, when electrospun nanofiber mats are intended for the local delivery of drug, e.g., wound therapy, the amount of available liquid is low. Thus, mimicking the actual biorelevant conditions *in vitro* may be challenging using standardized dissolution testing conditions. Researchers have used methods where the amount of dissolution medium is much reduced and size of the sample is close to the actual size of the nanofiber mat used *in vivo* [18,21–23]. Samples are typically collected at predetermined time intervals and analyzed by ultraviolet-visible (UV-VIS) spectrophotometry or high performance liquid chromatography (HPLC).

The biorelevant conditions applied for the drug release studies depend on the exact problem and site of application, and may vary. Hydrogels have been widely used as DDSs for topical applications; however, hydrogels may also provide for a simplistic wound model onto which drug may be released followed by drug diffusion into the hydrogel matrix. Diffusion is one of the major transport mechanisms in the wound [16,24], although swelling and erosion may also play a role depending on the formulation. For some electrospun nanofibers, the release rate has also been explained by desorption of the embedded drug from nanopores in the fibers or from the outer surface of the fibers in contact with the water bath [25]. In addition to the actual testing, simulations have been performed and models proposed that enable prediction of the drug release behavior of the electrospun fiber mats [16,26]. These models enable the design of mats with certain structures in order to achieve a desired drug release kinetics [12].

Recently, a fully automated fiber-optics based dissolution testing systems for *in situ* monitoring of drug release from electrospun fiber mats was proposed [27]. The direct ultraviolet (UV) measurement of dissolved drug within dissolution medium provided the dissolution profile in real-time. UV imaging technology has emerged in pharmaceutical analysis [28]. It has found use for the characterization of different pharmaceutical dosage forms, including monitoring drug release from capsules [29], patches [30], and hydrogels [31,32]. Spatially resolved absorbance values are measured facilitating monitoring of concentrations and concentration gradients by UV imaging, and thereby providing the potential for new insights to the drug dissolution and release processes through real-time monitoring of swelling, precipitation, diffusion, and partitioning phenomena [31,33,34]. Drug release from electrospun fiber mats into hydrogel system has not been investigated before and was of interest within the present study.

In addition to using physical methods in drug release studies, genetically engineered whole-cell bioreporters enable to obtain valuable information during drug release studies. A few of the main advantages of using bioreporters are that they provide physiologically relevant data by measuring only biologically available fraction of the chemical. A typical bioreporter consists of a biological recognition element (i.e., sensor), a transducer, and a reporter protein. Test chemical binds to the sensor element, a transducer initiates the production of the reporter protein, and a signal is produced [35,36]. In parallel to the drug release information, such methods give direct information about the bioactivity of the developed antimicrobial DDSs.

The aim of the current study was to test and compare different drug release model systems for the characterization of electrospun nano- and microfiber antibacterial drug-loaded mats. We studied two different polymeric compositions—polycaprolactone (PCL) alone or in combination with polyethylene oxide (PEO)—with the model antibacterial drug chloramphenicol (CAM). Interestingly, we have previously shown that although these fiber mats with different carrier polymers have different drug release behavior according to the dissolution test results, their antibacterial activity was rather similar in a disc diffusion assay [22]. Therefore, in order to understand drug release from electrospun polymeric fiber mats better, novel characterization methods were acquired in order to elucidate and rationalize drug release behavior. In the current study, the drug release from electrospun fiber mats into buffer solution and agar hydrogel was investigated using HPLC, UV-VIS spectrophotometry, and bacterial bioreporters responding to the antibacterial drug CAM. UV imaging was used for the first time to monitor real-time the drug release and diffusion from electrospun fiber mats into agarose hydrogel. Antibacterial activity testing of the CAM containing fiber mats was performed using disc diffusion assay in order to shed light on the correlation between the drug release and antibacterial activity and, hence, the intended use of electrospun mats as local antibacterial DDSs for wound infections.

2. Materials and Methods

2.1. Materials, Bacteria and Release Media

Drugs, polymers, supplies. The antibacterial agent chloramphenicol (CAM) was used as a model active pharmaceutical ingredient. CAM, hydrophobic carrier polymer polycaprolactone (PCL, Mw ≈ 80,000), hydrophilic carrier polymer polyethylene oxide (PEO) (Mw ≈ 900,000), and all analytical grade reagents were purchased from Sigma-Aldrich Inc. (Darmstadt, Germany). Ampicillin sodium salt and anhydrous D-glucose used for the bacterial bioreporter preparation were obtained from Carl Roth GmbH + Co. (Karsruhe, Germany) and Fisher Scientific (Waltham, MA, USA), respectively. Type I agarose was purchased from Sigma-Aldrich (St. Louis, MO, USA). Agar hydrogel was prepared using Lennox lysogeny broth (LB) agar (Difco Laboratories, Detroit, MI, USA). FavorPrep Plasmid DNA Extraction Mini Kit and FavorPrep(TM) GEL/PCR Purification Mini Kit was purchased from Favorgen Biotech Corp. (Changzhi Township, Pingtung, Taiwan).

Bacteria. Bacteria (*Staphylococcus aureus* DSM No.: 2569) were obtained from Leibniz Institute DSMZ-German Collection of Microorganisms and Cell Cultures. *Escherichia coli* MG1655 strain [37] was used for biosensor construction. Cloning was performed in *E. coli* strain DH5α [38].

Buffers and agarose hydrogel for drug release testing by UV imaging. For the preparation of the phosphate buffer solution used as a dissolution medium, sodium dihydrogen phosphate dihydrate ($NaH_2PO_4 \cdot 2H_2O$, Merck, Darmstadt, Germany) was dissolved in distilled water. The pH of the solution (67 mM phosphate buffer) was adjusted to pH 7.40 using 5M sodium hydroxide solution. The 0.5% (w/V) agarose hydrogel was prepared by dissolving type I agarose in an appropriate volume of phosphate buffer kept at 98 °C for 45 min in a water bath. The gels were cast in the quartz cells, and allowed to settle for 30 min prior to commencing the release experiments.

Buffers and agar hydrogels for drug release and antibacterial activity testing. Drug release studies were conducted using phosphate buffered saline (1× PBS). Lennox lysogeny broth (LB) agar with a concentration of 1.5% (w/V) (*S. aureus*) and MOPS minimal medium [39] with 1.5% (w/V) agar (*E. coli*) were used for drug diffusion and antibacterial activity testing with bacteria.

2.2. Preparation and Characterization Methods

Preparation of electrospinning solutions and fiber mats. Fiber mats were prepared using an ESR200RD robotized electrospinning system (NanoNC, Seoul, Republic of Korea). Fiber mats with different compositions were prepared in order to provide different drug release kinetics. The exact compositions of the solutions used for electrospinning and electrospinning conditions are shown in Table 1.

Table 1. Composition of the electrospun formulations and electrospinning parameters.

Formulations	Materials/Polymer	Materials/Solvent	Distance (cm)	Flow Rate (ml/h)	Applied Voltage (kV)
PCL	PCL 12.5% (w/V), CONTROL	Chloroform:methanol (3:1 V/V)	14	1.0	9
PCL/CAM	PCL 12.5% (w/V) + CAM (4% w/w, solid state)	Chloroform:methanol (3:1 V/V)	14	1.0	9
PCL/PEO	PCL 10% + PEO 2% (w/V), CONTROL	Chloroform:methanol (3:1 V/V)	17	2.5	12
PCL/PEO/CAM	PCL 10% (w/V) + PEO 2% (w/V) + CAM (4% w/w, solid state)	Chloroform:methanol (3:1 V/V)	17	2.5	12

Key: CAM, chloramphenicol; CONTROL, formulation without CAM; PCL, polycaprolactone; PEO, polyethylene oxide.

A mixture of chloroform:methanol (3:1) (V/V) was used as a solvent system for the preparation of PCL and PCL/PEO systems, and a total of 10 mL was electrospun using rotation (20 rpm) and moving stage (speed 25 mm/min, distance 140 mm). For the preparation of the electrospinning solution, the polymers were dissolved in the solvent system under stirring overnight. The desired CAM concentration in the fibers was 4% (dry solid state %) and CAM was added together with the polymer into the solvent system immediately after the preparation. The electrospun fiber mats were collected onto aluminum foil and put into ziploc bags. The samples were kept in a desiccator at 0% relative humidity above silica gel to avoid humidity induced changes in the mats.

Morphology and solid state characterization of electrospun fiber mats. Morphology and diameter of electrospun fiber mats were investigated using scanning electron microscopy (SEM). Samples were mounted on aluminum stubs and magnetron-sputter coated with 3 nm gold layer in argon atmosphere prior to microscopy. Solid state characterization of the electrospun fiber mats and drug-loaded fiber mats was performed as described previously using attenuated total reflection-Fourier transform infrared (ATR-FTIR) spectroscopy (IRPrestige-21 spectrophotometer (Shimadzu Corp., Kyoto, Japan) with Specac Golden Gate Single Reflection ATR crystal (Specac Ltd., Orpington, UK) and verified with X-ray diffraction (XRD) (D8 Advance, Bruker AXS GmbH, Karlsruhe, Germany) [22]. The thickness of the fiber mats was verified using a Precision-Micrometer 533.501 (Scala Messzeuge GmbH, Dettingen, Germany) with the resolution of 0.01 mm. The thickness of the mats was 0.07 ± 0.01 mm for the PCL fiber (0.05 ± 0.01 mm with CAM) and 0.08 ± 0.01 mm for the PCL/PEO fiber (0.08 ± 0.01 mm with CAM) mats.

Drug loading and distribution in fiber mats. High performance liquid chromatography (HPLC) (Shimadzu Prominence HPLC with LC20, PDA detector SPD-M2QA, controlled by LC Solution software (1.21 SP1 Shimadzu); Shimadzu Europa GmbH, Duisburg, Germany) was used to determine the CAM concentration in the electrospun fiber mats and to evaluate its distribution uniformity throughout the fiber mats. Analyses were performed according to the official European Pharmacopoeia method for a related substance CAM sodium succinate. Briefly, CAM-loaded fiber samples were cut into 1 cm^2 pieces, weighed, and dissolved in chloroform and methanol (3:1 V/V). The HPLC measurements were performed using an octadecylsilyl column (Phenomenex, Luna C18(2), 250 × 4.6 mm, 5 µm). The flow rate was 1.0 mL/min, and injection volume was 20 µL. The mobile phase consisted of 2% phosphoric acid R, methanol R and water R in the volume ratio 5:40:55. A wavelength of 275 nm was used.

2.3. Drug Release Studies

2.3.1. Drug Release Testing into Buffer Solution and Agar Hydrogel by UV-VIS Spectrophotometry and HPLC

Drug release to buffer solution and agar hydrogel was investigated using UV-VIS spectrophotometry and HPLC, respectively.

Release to phosphate buffer solution: The *in vitro* drug release of CAM from electrospun PCL and PCL/PEO fiber mats was carried out as described previously [22]; however, a more frequent sampling protocol was used. Briefly, 4 cm^2 samples (N = 3) cut from the mats were weighed and placed into 20 mL of 1× PBS (pH 7.4) at 37 °C in 50 mL plastic tubes. The tubes were put into a dissolution apparatus vessel (Dissolution system 2100, Distek Inc., North Brunswick, NJ, USA) containing water maintained at 37 °C using rotation (paddle system, 100 rpm). Aliquots of 2 mL were removed and replaced with the same amount of 1× PBS at set time points. The aliquots were analyzed using UV-spectrophotometry (Shimadzu UV-1800, Shimadzu Europa GmbH, Duisburg, Germany) at 278 nm.

Release to agar hydrogel: The amount of drug released into agar plates was investigated by sampling different zones of the agar (illustrated with a figure in Section 3.4). Pieces of fiber mat (PCL/CAM and PCL/PEO/CAM fiber mat discs, with a diameter of 1 cm) were weighed, put onto pre-warmed LB agar plates, kept at 37 °C, and removed at set time points. Zones of the agar were cut out, the agar sample was put into ethanol (96%) and sonicated for 15 min. This extraction process was repeated twice and the obtained ethanol solutions were combined. The vials with ethanol solutions were left under a fume hood without caps, for the ethanol to evaporate. The residues left in the vials were dissolved in 1.5 mL of ethanol (96%) and the amount of CAM analyzed with HPLC. In the present study, the limit of detection for CAM was 1 µg/mL. Triplicate measurements were performed. The extraction efficacy was tested separately confirming that two times extraction resulted in 100% efficacy (Appendix A, Table A1).

2.3.2. UV Imaging for Drug Release Monitoring in Hydrogel

Complementary to the traditional HPLC method, an Actipix D200 Large Area Imager (Paraytec Ltd., York, England) controlled by Actipix D200 acquisition software ver. 3.1.7.4 was used to image the release of CAM from PCL and PCL/PEO fiber mats. These experiments were performed in a heating cabinet from Edmund Bühler TH30 (Bodelshausen, Germany) set to 37 °C. Imaging was performed at four alternating wavelengths: 525 nm, 280 nm, 255 nm, and 214 nm. Images for each wavelength were recorded at a frequency of 0.125 s^{-1} for the release experiments as well as the standard curve. The imaging area (28 × 28 mm^2; pixel size 13.8 µm^2) encompassed three quartz cells (Pion Inc., UK; 62 mm × 4 mm × 7 mm (L × H × W)), allowing three measurements to be performed simultaneously. The fibers were cut to fit the inner dimensions of the quartz cells (7.0 mm in width and 4.0 mm in height). The fibers were positioned perpendicular to the imaging direction in contact with the agarose gel. The fibers were backed by silicone plugs to ensure good contact with the gel and correct alignment. Parafilm was used to seal the quartz cells preventing evaporation of water from the gels. The release of CAM from the fibers was imaged for 3 h at 37 °C. Each imaging experiment allowed measurements of two CAM-containing fibers and one blank fiber (control). The positioning of the fibers in the imaging system (top, middle or bottom row) was randomized.

Standard Curve for quantification by UV imaging. A CAM stock solution (5 mM) in phosphate buffer was used to make the dilutions for the standard curve in 0.5% (*w/V*) agarose gel. These were made by mixing 1.5 mL 1% (*w/V*) agarose in phosphate buffer with a defined volume of CAM solution and phosphate buffer to obtain 3 mL of the mixture. The 1% (*w/V*) agarose solution and the phosphate buffer were both heated in water bath (98 °C) to facilitate mixing leading to a homogeneous mixture. The gels were cast in the quartz cells, and allowed to settle for 30 min prior to the experiments. As reference, a 0.5% (*w/V*) agarose gel in phosphate buffer without CAM was used.

2.4. Antibacterial Activity Studies—Drug Release and Effect on Bacterial Growth

2.4.1. Antibacterial Activity Testing

The antibacterial activity of released CAM on agar plates was investigated at different time points mimicking the drug diffusion tests into agarose hydrogel during UV imaging studies. Overnight culture (20 h) of *S. aureus* DSM No.: 2569 was grown from DMSO stock (100 uL to 3 mL of LB). Preparation of all bacterial DMSO stocks used in the present study is described in Appendix B. The culture was diluted to optical density (OD) 0.05 in LB and 100 µL was plated onto pre-warmed LB agar plates (1.5% (w/V)). PCL/CAM and PCL/PEO/CAM fiber discs, and a positive CAM filter paper control were applied onto each plate. At specific time points, the discs were removed and the LB plates were incubated at 37 °C for 24 h prior to measurement of the inhibition zones.

2.4.2. Bioreporter Plasmid and Strain Preparation

All cloning was performed using CPEC cloning method [40]. Plasmid vector backbone was low-copy pSC101 plasmid. *Timer* reporter gene in plasmid pSC101-Ptet-Timer [41] was replaced with two fluorescent reporter genes *GFPmut2* [42] and *mScarlet-I* [43]. In order to increase the expression of the green fluorescence protein (GFP) during antibiotic stress additional stress-inducible dnaK1 promoter (PdnaK1) originating from *E. coli* MG1655 genomic DNA was added upstream of the tet-promoter (Ptet). In addition, kanamycin resistance gene *kanR* was replaced with ampicillin resistance gene *ampR*. In order to reduce the expression of *ampR* resulting from reverse direction transcription initiation from PdnaK1, additional rrnB T2 terminator was added between *ampR* and PdnaK1.

In order to construct the ribosomal stalling reporter plasmid pSC101-CAM-bioreporter transcription attenuation-based regulatory *trpL2Ala* region together with a terminator and constitutive T5 promoter from plasmid, pRFPCER-TrpL2A [44] was inserted between *GFPmut2* and *mScarlet-I* ribosomal binding site. mRNA from the reporter gene *mScarlet-I*, and therefore, red fluorescence is only produced when ribosomal stalling occurs, e.g., due to CAM presence (Appendix C).

CPEC products were transformed into *E. coli* DH5α and plasmids were purified using FavorPrep Plasmid DNA Extraction Mini Kit. All plasmids were verified by sequencing. Purified bioreporter plasmid pSC101-CAM-bioreporter was transformed into *E. coli* MG1655 chemical competent cells via heat shock. The transformants were selected on ampicillin (100 µg/mL) containing LB-agar plates after overnight incubation. The full nucleotide sequence of the pSC101-CAM-bioreporter plasmid is provided as Supplementary Materials in GeneBank (gb) file format.

2.4.3. Bioreporter Disc Diffusion Assay

For bacterial bioreporter disc diffusion assay agar plates with defined MOPS minimal medium [39] supplemented with 0.4% (w/V) glucose as the carbon source and 1.5% (w/V) agar were prepared in sterile conditions by measuring 20 mL of warm agar medium per plate, and plates were dried for 30 min under laminar flow hood.

Bioreporter strain DMSO stock was thawed, diluted 20× into sterile 1× PBS and 75 µL was plated on each minimal plate. A sterile cotton bud dipped into 1× PBS was used to spread the cells evenly. Plates were left to incubate at 37 °C for 10 h. After incubation, the weighted fiber mats (PCL/PEO/CAM and PCL/CAM) were added to each plate. Individual plates were first scanned with the Amersham Typhoon scanner (GE Healthcare Europe GmbH, Freiburg, Germany) (pixel size 100 µm; green fluorescence: 488 nm laser, 525BP20 filter, PMT voltage 352V; red fluorescence: 532 nm laser, 570BP20 filter, PMT voltage 621V) after adding the mats and re-scanned every hour for 6 h. Scan time for each plate was approximately 6 min. The plates were incubated at 37 °C between the scans.

2.5. Data Analysis

Data are given as average ± standard deviation (SD), unless stated otherwise. Data were analyzed and figures plotted using MS Excel 2017 and/or 2016, GraphPad Prism 7 ver. 7.04 or OriginPro 8.5.

Statistical analysis was performed by two-tailed Student's *t*-test assuming unequal variances ($p < 0.05$) where applicable.

The SDI Data analysis software ver. 2.0.60624 (Paraytec Ltd., York, England) was used to analyze the recordings made on the Actipix D200 system. The CAM molar absorption coefficient determined from the standard curve was used to calculate CAM concentrations in the gels. The analysis was performed at 255 nm, because the linear range of the standard curve covered the absorbance values encountered in the release experiments in contrast to 280 nm. A 6.25 mm wide zone starting from the fiber-gel interface protruding into the gel in the CAM transport direction was defined. For each pixel column, the absorbance was averaged, converted to concentration and plotted as a function of distance from the fiber mat to attain concentration-distance profiles. From the concentration-distance profiles, the area under curve (AUC) was calculated to determine the total amount of CAM released from the fibers.

The inhibition zones free of bacterial growth (diameters, mm) were determined using ImageJ software [45] program version 1.52n. Tests were run at least in triplicate. ImageJ software was also used for obtaining numerical values of fluorescent zones from disc diffusion assay images. Green and red fluorescence images were analyzed separately. 0.8 mm wide lines were chosen as regions of interest for analysis. The 1.5 cm long line was drawn starting from the fiber mat and plot profiles of grey values for these regions were recorded.

3. Results and Discussion

3.1. Preparation and Characterization of Electrospun Fiber Mats

In order to test the suitability of the UV imaging technique and different drug release model systems for monitoring drug release from electrospun fiber mats, different mats were electrospun by varying the polymers (hydrophilic PEO vs. hydrophobic PCL) and incorporating the antibacterial drug CAM into the fibers (Table 1). The preparation and morphological and physicochemical characterization of these electrospun antibacterial CAM-loaded fibers has been performed previously [22]. As shown previously, the prepared PCL and PCL/CAM mats consisted of nanofibers within the average size range from 370 to 496 nm (SD ± 339 nm), whereas PCL/PEO and PCL/PEO/CAM mats were in the micrometer size range with an average diameter of 2.9 µm (SD ± 1.1 µm). Solid state transformation from crystalline CAM to amorphous CAM was confirmed with drug-loaded electrospun fiber mats (data not shown). In agreement with previous findings [22], CAM was homogeneously distributed within the electrospun fiber mats (data not shown) and CAM content matched with the theoretical values (Table 2).

Table 2. Average CAM concentrations within the electrospun fiber mats ($N = 3–7$). Formulation compositions and electrospinning parameters are shown in Table 1.

Electrospun Fiber Formulations	Theoretical CAM Content/%	Measured CAM Content/% ± SD
PCL/CAM	4	4.0 ± 0.2
PCL/PEO/CAM	4	3.8 ± 0.3

Key: CAM, chloramphenicol; SD, standard deviation.

3.2. Drug Release into Buffer Measured by UV-VIS Spectrophotometry

Initially, traditional dissolution testing into buffer solution was performed and CAM concentrations were determined using UV-VIS spectrophotometry. The PCL/CAM and PCL/PEO/CAM mats are different in terms of their wettability and swelling properties. PCL/PEO/CAM mats are more hydrophilic and swell when exposed to an aqueous medium [22]. The PCL/CAM mats are more hydrophobic, although the presence of CAM tends to increase the wetting of the mat and provide access for the buffer to enter the fibers. Thus, PCL/CAM fiber mats provided the expected and desired prolonged

CAM release whilst PCL/PEO/CAM mats due to the hydrophilic nature of PEO exhibited a faster drug release in buffer solution (Figure 1).

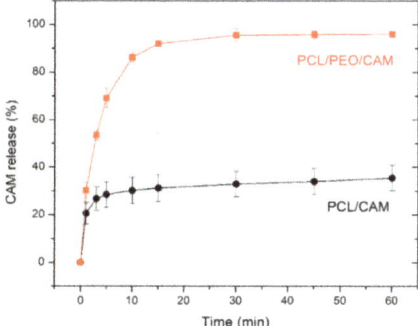

Figure 1. Relative release of CAM from PCL/PEO/CAM (■) and PCL/CAM (●) fiber mats into phosphate buffered saline at pH 7.40 and 37 °C. Data are averages ± SD of at least triplicate samples. Analyses performed using UV-VIS spectrophotometry (reference is made to Table 1 for fiber composition and preparation conditions).

Frequent sampling revealed a significant CAM burst release (up to 15 min of release testing) from both fiber mats. There were only minor differences in triplicate measurements and in the behavior of the fiber mats verifying the reproducibility of the measurements. In a recent study, the free drug (terbinafine hydrochloride) on the surface of fibers was removed after rinsing in distilled water and the amount of released drug quantified in a wound dressing-skin model utilizing filter paper as a matrix [21]. The rinsing procedure most likely removed the drug burst release. In the present study, no pretreatment of the mats was performed and the mats were analyzed directly. It is likely that if burst released amounts were removed the drug release would be even more different between the mats and most of CAM would be removed from PCL/PEO/CAM fibers mats during the pretreatment. For understanding drug release and *in vivo* activity relationships, the mats should not be pretreated; however, such pretreatment might be important if *in vitro* tests are performed to illustrate only the differences between the fiber mats in respect of their prolonged drug release.

3.3. Antibacterial Activity of Electrospun Fiber Mats

Despite the different morphologies and behavior (e.g., swelling, drug release into buffer), statistically significant differences in the inhibition zones on agar plate between the PCL/CAM and PCL/PEO/CAM fiber mats were not observed during previous antibacterial activity testing [22]. In the present study, it was of interest to investigate further how the drug is released from the electrospun mat into a gel which more closely resembles the wound matrix (e.g., agar and agarose hydrogels) and how this translates into antibacterial effect. Hydrogels have more similar hydrodynamic conditions to wound tissue as compared to aqueous solutions and thus provide more biorelevant testing option. We developed a modified disc diffusion assay, where the mats were physically removed from the surface of the solid growth medium at specified time points and the antibacterial effect of the released drug on model bacteria *S. aureus* DSM No.: 2569 was determined by measuring the size of the inhibition zones after 24 h. The faster CAM release from PCL/PEO/CAM mats compared to the PCL/CAM mats observed in buffer solution (Figure 1) correlated with larger inhibition zones (Figure 2). The differences were larger at the earlier time points. Control filter paper impregnated with CAM confirmed that the wetting of the sample is the major triggering factor for further drug release and diffusion.

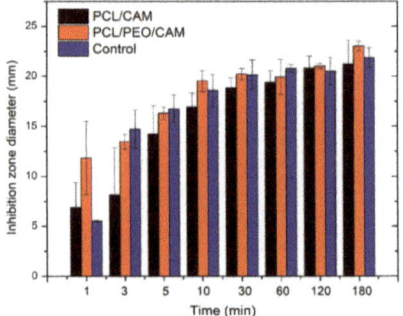

Figure 2. Inhibition zone diameters measured after 24 h on agar plates. X-axis indicates exposure time of discs (PCL/PEO/CAM or PCL/CAM fiber mats) onto the hydrogel. *S. aureus* DSM No.: 2569 was used for the study. Filter paper wetted with CAM solution and dried (same CAM concentration) served as a control. Key: CAM, chloramphenicol; PCL, polycaprolactone; PEO, polyethylene oxide. Data are averages ± SD of at least triplicate samples.

3.4. Drug Release into Agar Hydrogel Measured by HPLC

The extent of CAM release from the mats and diffusion into the agar hydrogel was quantified using HPLC upon extraction of CAM from the agar hydrogel. The agar on the plates was divided into five concentric circular zones (Figure 3A) and the CAM concentration in each zone was determined. The experimental design is detailed in the Materials and Methods and Appendix A (Tables A1 and A2). The amount of drug released from electrospun mats to the agar plates at different time points at 37 °C is summarized in Figure 3.

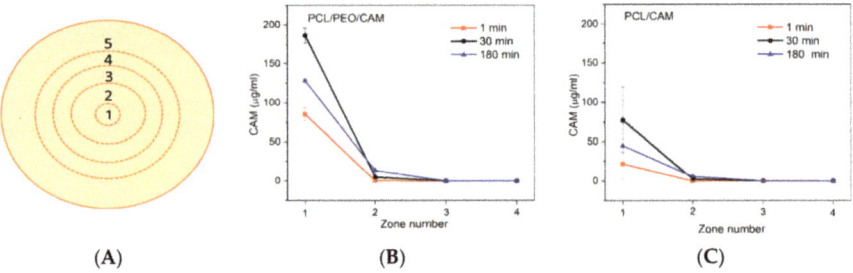

Figure 3. (**A**) Schematic illustrating the division of the agar plate into zones. Zones 1-5 are numbered starting from the inner circle. Zone diameters: 1.0 cm, 3.0 cm, 4.4 cm, 5.8 cm, and 8.6 cm. Concentrations of released CAM (detection limit of 1 µg/mL) from PCL/PEO/CAM (**B**) and PCL/CAM fiber mats (**C**) into 1.5% (*w/V*) agar hydrogel at 37 °C in different time points (1 min, 30 min, 180 min) and into different zones (1–4). Error bars represent standard deviation, $N = 3$. Key: CAM, chloramphenicol; PCL, polycaprolactone; PEO, polyethylene oxide.

The drug diffusion patterns for PCL/CAM and PCL/PEO/CAM fiber mats were qualitatively similar (Figure 3). These findings are consistent with the disc diffusion assay results (see for Figure 2). It is clear that most of the drug is present in the 1 cm diameter section (zone 1) right below the fiber mat at the early time points of the release experiment. As time passed, less drug was recovered in the inner circle (zone 1) and relatively more in zone 2 (larger circle around the mat). CAM release from PCL/PEO/CAM fiber mat was fast followed by slower diffusion further into the agar hydrogel (Figure 3B). Interestingly, after 120 min, the drug was not detectable in the 3rd zone. After 24 h (1440 min), the CAM had reached the outer circle (Appendix A, Table A2). PCL/CAM fiber mats on the other hand showed that less drug was released within the same time period compared to the

PCL/PEO/CAM fiber mat (Figure 3C). The CAM concentration distribution differences are visible in Figure 3, mainly for zone 1 but to some extent also for zone 2. This may explain why it is not always possible to detect differences in the inhibition zones between different fiber mats in a disc diffusion assay although the drug may be released differently from the delivery vehicle and, therefore, lead to different antibacterial efficacy *in vivo* [46].

3.5. Detecting CAM Release into Agar Hydrogel with Bioreporter Strain

In addition to chemical and physical methods for determining the CAM concentrations during the release, it is also possible to use bacterial bioassays. Hence, simultaneously to the antibacterial effects, the drug release can be monitored. We genetically engineered reporter bacteria (*E. coli* MG1655) to produce dose-dependent quantifiable green and red fluorescent signals in the presence of antibacterial drug CAM. The CAM-bioreporter has GFP as a control protein for expression and a red mScarlet-I as a reporter protein. Exact working mechanism of the bacterial bioreporter is provided in Appendix C. In the presence of CAM GFP signal (green) will be reduced due to protein synthesis inhibition, and mScarlet-I signal (red) will increase due to transcription continuation as a result of ribosomal stalling in the transcription attenuation system. Therefore, the CAM release and diffusion can be illustrated in different time points (selected time points 60, 180, and 360 min) using fluorescence data (Figure 4).

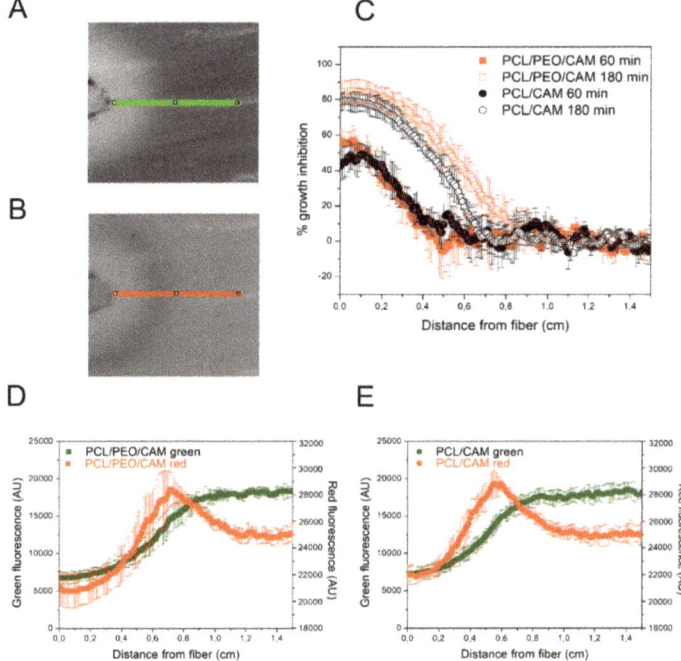

Figure 4. (**A**,**B**). Shows the analyzed region of interest (0.8 mm × 1.5 cm) of bioreporter chloramphenicol (CAM)-containing fiber disc diffusion assay from green fluorescence (**A**) and red fluorescence (**B**) scan images. Green fluorescence images in different time points (60 min and 180 min) allow estimating bacterial growth inhibition due to CAM released from PCL/PEO/CAM and PCL/CAM fiber mats (**C**). Combined green and red fluorescent figures at 6 h reveal the fluorescence levels that can be correlated with the released CAM from PCL/PEO/CAM (**D**) and PCL/CAM fiber mats (**E**). Data are presented as average of three experiments (± SD). Key: CAM, chloramphenicol; PCL, polycaprolactone; PEO, polyethylene oxide.

It is clearly seen that bacterial growth is inhibited close to the fiber mats (inhibition zones surrounding the mats) where CAM concentrations are the highest, which matches with the agar diffusion test results (Figures 2 and 3). Fluorescent bacteria surrounding the inhibition zones reveal the distance from the mat where the CAM levels above the minimum inhibitory concentration (MIC) can still be detected. Compared to the agar hydrogel diffusion tests (Figures 2 and 3), bacterial bioreporter study results on agar hydrogel did not reveal large differences between the PCL/CAM and PCL/PEO/CAM fiber mats with the respect of released drug amounts and its effect on bacteria (Figure 4C). Growth inhibition was very slightly more pronounced in PCL/PEO/CAM fiber mat (fast release) after 60 min of incubation; however, this difference was statistically insignificant and disappears in later time points (180 min). In later time points (6 h) red fluorescence detected from bacteria enabled determining the CAM concentrations even below MIC (in sub-MIC concentrations) (Figure 4D,E). After 6 h of incubation, the peak of the reporter protein signal is located further (approximately 0.75 cm) from the mat in case of PCL/PEO/CAM fiber mat (fast release) (Figure 4D) compared from PCL/CAM fiber mat (slow release; located approximately 0.60 cm) (Figure 4E). This indicates that effective CAM concentration was achieved on larger area (at a further distance from the fiber mat) with PCL/PEO/CAM fiber mat, although the difference between the two fiber mats was minor. Most likely, this is due to the fact that most of the differences between the two different electrospun fiber mats can only be seen in early time points which cannot be distinguished using fluorescent bacteria in these settings.

3.6. Drug Release into Agarose Hydrogel Using UV Imaging

The assessment of CAM release by cutting of zones from agar plates followed by extraction and analysis of the drug is both a destructive and laborious sampling procedure. The fast release of CAM cannot be monitored using bioreporter bacteria that require time for growth and detectable signal production. Therefore, UV imaging was investigated as a potentially less labor intensive and more robust (reproducible/repeatable) approach for monitoring CAM release from the electrospun fiber mats. An additional benefit of the non-intrusive imaging method is the high spatial as well as temporal resolution offered. Due to a lack of transparency of the agar plates used in antibacterial activity tests, a hydrogel matrix based on agarose was applied instead. Moreover, the Actipix D200 Large Area Imager allowed imaging of three samples in parallel enabling comparison. Images visualizing the release and diffusion of CAM at different time points are shown in Figure 5A.

Diffusion into the viscous agarose hydrogel resembles the conditions encountered both during *in vitro* disc diffusion testing (agar hydrogel) as well as *in vivo* where the drug has to be released from the electrospun fiber and diffuse into the wound. The UV imaging results reveal that PCL/CAM fibers provide slower drug release into the gel whereas PCL/PEO/CAM fibers release the drug faster (Figure 5A). The concentration-distance profiles shown in Figure 5B,C correspond to the images in Figure 5A. In addition, the average amount of CAM released was quantified based on the UV images (Figure 6). When comparing the two mats, differences were observed with respect to the total amount of released drug mainly at the early time points (Figure 6).

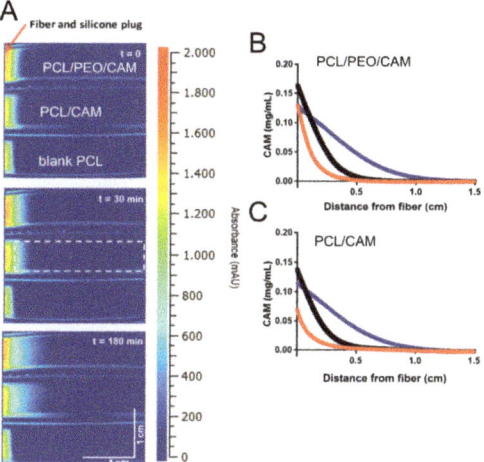

Figure 5. (**A**) Representative images of CAM release from fibers and diffusion into 0.5% (*w*/*V*) agarose hydrogel at 37 °C. Top is PCL/PEO/CAM, middle is PCL/CAM and bottom is PCL/Blank fibers (control). The zone used for the quantification of the CAM absorbance is shown in the middle row at 30 min. Representative concentration-distance profiles for PCL/PEO/CAM (**B**) and PCL/CAM (**C**) fibers diffusing into 0.5% (*w*/*V*) agarose hydrogel at 37 °C. The red, black and blue line is for 0 min (immediately after starting the experiment), 30 min and 180 min, respectively. Key: CAM, chloramphenicol; PCL, polycaprolactone; PEO, polyethylene oxide.

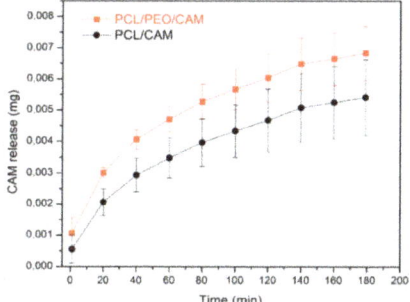

Figure 6. Amount of CAM released from PCL/PEO/CAM (■) and PCL/CAM (●) fiber mats into 0.5% (*w*/*V*) agarose hydrogel at 37 °C based on UV imaging experiment data. Error bars represent one standard deviation, $N = 5$. Key: CAM, chloramphenicol; PCL, polycaprolactone; PEO, polyethylene oxide.

Only slight differences between the PCL/CAM and PCL/PEO/CAM fiber mats with respect to their drug release behavior were detected in average drug release profiles, although these were not statistically significant and can be considered as more of a tendency.

3.7. Comparison between Different Drug Release Model Systems

Irrespective of the *in vitro* release model system (testing approach) employed, the release of CAM was found to be faster from the PCL/PEO fiber mats as compared to the PCL fiber mats (Figure 7). However, the extent to which the release differed tended to vary between the model systems.

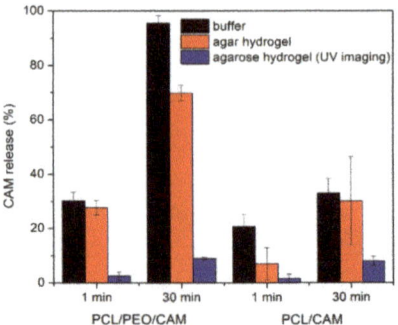

Figure 7. Amount of CAM released from PCL/PEO/CAM and PCL/CAM fiber mats into phosphate buffered saline at pH 7.40 and 37 °C and 1.5% (*w/V*) agar hydrogel at 37 °C and 0.5% (*w/V*) agarose hydrogel at 37 °C. Data are averages ± SD of at least triplicate samples. Analyzes performed using UV-VIS spectrophotometry (CAM concentration in a buffer solution), HPLC (CAM concentration extracted from hydrogel) and UV imaging (CAM concentration within hydrogel) (reference is made to Table 1 for fiber composition and preparation conditions). Key: CAM, chloramphenicol; PCL, polycaprolactone; PEO, polyethylene oxide.

Drug release into buffer revealed that after 30 min the PCL/PEO/CAM fibers had released nearly all CAM into the buffer, whereas only a minor amount (approximately 30%) of drug was released from PCL/CAM fiber mats (Figure 7). When the CAM release into hydrogel was monitored by agar disc diffusion and extraction method, the amount of CAM released from PCL/PEO/CAM fiber mat after 30 min was approximately 70% and the released CAM amount from PCL/CAM mat was similarly approximately 30% (with huge variability between 17–48% for individual PCL/CAM fiber mats). UV imaging, however, showed that the differences with respect to the amount of drug released into the agarose hydrogel between PCL/CAM and PCL/PEO/CAM fiber mats after 30 min were less pronounced as compared to the differences in CAM release into buffer (Figure 7). It was also seen that much less CAM was released and diffused to the region of analysis from both fiber mats (approximately 9% and 8% for PCL/PEO/CAM and PCL/CAM fiber mats, respectively) within the same time period. Most likely, less CAM is released from the fiber mats into the hydrogel according to the UV imaging due to the different geometries of the setup. In the UV imaging setup, diffusion is limited to one direction perpendicular to the mat, whereas diffusion in the agar setup may occur in three dimensions. The latter will favor a relatively larger release of CAM. We believe that the concentration may be more likely to build up at the interface in the UV imaging setup. As might be expected due to the similarity of the release matrices (hydrogel), the UV imaging drug release and diffusion profiles matched more with the drug release into agar hydrogel extraction (Figures 3–5) than release and dissolution into buffer test (Figure 1). The contact and/or of the mats with the hydrogels may be different between the agar and agarose hydrogels. It is not known whether the agar hydrogel may contain components interacting, and thereby facilitating the release of CAM. Similarly to UV imaging, less pronounced differences between the two different electrospun CAM-loaded fiber mats were also observed with bacterial bioreporters (Figure 4C). It is due to the fact that the drug has to diffuse away from the mat before it will be detected (UV imaging and bacterial bioreporters), whereas in the agar hydrogel extraction method, the area under the fiber mat will be included into the total released and detected drug amount.

The differences with respect to CAM release from the mats observed using the *in vitro* release testing model systems are related to the different properties of the release media (volume, agitation, and viscosity), its capability to penetrate into the fiber mat, the sample size of fiber mats, effect of shaking, and geometry of the setup. It is believed that drug diffusion and wetting of the samples were the rate-limiting steps for the drug release from fiber mat into agar and agarose hydrogels. The release into buffer solution, however, was more affected by the hydrodynamics of the buffer measurements. For the different fiber mats agitation led to increased erosion and/or disintegration of the PCL/PEO/CAM fiber mats as compared to the PCL/CAM fiber mats.

In terms of repeatability the model systems and analytical methods were all comparable. It can be seen that larger variations in drug release between replicates were detected for PCL/CAM fiber mats compared to PCL/PEO/CAM fiber mats. This was seen with both drug release model systems (buffer vs. hydrogel) as well as different techniques (UV-VIS spectrophotometry, HPLC, UV imaging, and bacterial bioreporters). This might be explained by the different wettability of the PCL/CAM fiber mats compared to PCL/PEO/CAM fiber mats as discussed previously for PCL and PCL-drug loaded fiber mats [15]. The hydrophilicity of the PCL/PEO/CAM fiber mats makes them wet more homogeneously, whereas for PCL/CAM fiber mats the sample-to-sample variations in wettability may also cause variability in the drug release behavior.

Compared to agar diffusion assay (extraction of CAM from hydrogel), the UV imaging was easier to conduct. Although for both these methods the size of sample, the release environment (hydrogel) and static conditions resembled the *in vitro* antibacterial activity testing conditions. Bacterial bioreporter study enabled to monitor the CAM release into agar hydrogel during diffusion in later time points where even sub-MIC concentration of CAM was determined based on the green and red fluorescence intensity. The method has the advantage of revealing the released antibacterial drug effect directly on bacteria.

For polymer fiber mats as wound matrices it is favorable to have the burst effect. The extent of the burst release is often associated with device geometry, surface characteristics of host material, heterogeneous distribution of drug within the polymer matrix, intrinsic dissolution rate of drug, and heterogeneity of matrices [16]. From the drug release experiments we see that the burst release is smaller with the hydrogels for hydrophilic PCL/PEO/CAM and hydrophobic PCL/CAM fiber mats compared to the buffer solution (Figure 7). Larger differences in the burst release between the samples were observed with hydrophobic PCL/CAM fiber mats (Figure 7). For the drug release to occur from the PCL fiber mat, the medium needs to penetrate into the electrospun fiber mat to cause the diffusion of the drug to the exterior. Initially, the diffusion is affected by the electrospun mat composition and the fiber characteristics, as for PCL/PEO/CAM fiber mats the release was also affected by swelling and dissolution of PEO. As a second step, the diffusion further into the wound and reaction with the surrounding tissue and environment is important [47]. It is clear that the buffer release method shows higher burst release as compared to the *in vitro* antibacterial activity testing. Sadri et al. have measured tetracycline release in a dialysis bag mimicking the human skin-like conditions and shown that the burst release effect is reduced most likely due to the diffusion through the bag, which modified the release [48]. The gels *in vitro* and the wound tissue *in vivo* can be envisioned to provide a diffusion barrier or matrix minimizing burst release effects. Local transport mechanisms determine the volume in which the drug is distributed; thus, understanding these mechanisms is essential for optimizing the effectiveness of local delivery [47]. The *in vitro* methods that enable to most closely mimic the *in vivo* conditions are likely to enable accurate predictions of the drug release and transport in the wound environment. Moreover, it is important to understand the effect on bacteria. Therefore, the response of the bacteria to the active antibiotic concentration has to be measured directly. Here, we have shown that genetically engineered bioreporter systems can be used for this purpose.

4. Summary and Conclusions

All tested drug release model systems enabled to study the drug release from electrospun fiber mats. UV imaging provided faster, non-intrusive real-time information on chloramphenicol (CAM) release and diffusion with higher spatial and temporal resolution as compared to the release methods relying on release from fiber mats directly into buffer solution as well as to the agar plates followed by destructive sampling. The data were similar in terms of sensitivity in detecting differences between the electrospun fiber mat compositions in comparison to the more laborious drug release testing setups. Furthermore, the UV imaging and release into hydrogel method appeared to mimic the *in vitro* antibacterial activity testing conditions to a large degree, while release into buffer solution overestimated the burst release effects.

Advanced antibacterial disc diffusion assays enabled to distinguish small differences in the antibacterial activity of the differently designed electrospun fiber mats, these slight differences were also visualized using UV imaging as well as modified drug release and diffusion into hydrogel model systems. These results suggest that diffusional resistance to drug release observed in the hydrogel based systems may emulate the *in vivo* conditions of the wound matrix.

Supplementary Materials: The following are available online at http://www.mdpi.com/1999-4923/11/9/487/s1. The full nucleotide sequence of the pSC101-CAM-bioreporter plasmid is provided in GeneBank (gb) file format.

Author Contributions: Conceptualization, M.P., T.T., J.Ø., and K.K.; methodology, L.P., F.B., M.H., K.S., M.P., T.T., A.M., J.Ø., and K.K.; validation, L.P., F.B., M.H., M.P., A.M., J.Ø., and K.K.; formal analysis, L.P., F.B., M.H., and K.S.; investigation, L.P., F.B., M.H., K.S., M.P., T.T., A.M., J.Ø., and K.K.; resources, T.T., J.Ø., and K.K.; data curation, M.P., J.Ø., and K.K.; writing—original draft preparation, J.Ø. and K.K.; writing—review and editing, L.P., F.B., M.H., M.P., T.T., A.M., J.Ø., and K.K.; visualization, L.P., F.B., M.H., M.P., J.Ø., and K.K.; supervision, M.P., T.T., J.Ø., and K.K.; project administration, K.K.; funding acquisition, T.T., J.Ø., and K.K.

Funding: This research was funded by the Estonian Research Council and Estonian Ministry of Education and Research for funding of ETF7980 and PUT1088 projects (K.K.), by the European Regional Development Fund through the Centre of Excellence for Molecular Cell Technology (M.P. and T.T.), and by the Estonian Research Council grant PRG335 (M.P. and T.T.).

Acknowledgments: K.K. would like to thank the Estonian National Commission for UNESCO and the Estonian Academy of Sciences and the L'ORÉAL–UNESCO international L'ORÉAL Baltic program "For Women In Science" for the fellowship in 2018. MSc Georg-Marten Lanno and MSc Aleksandr Simaško (University of Tartu) and M.I. Andersen (University of Copenhagen) are thanked for the laboratory work. MSc J. Aruväli and Prof K. Kirsimäe are acknowledged for their help in conducting the SEM measurements.

Conflicts of Interest: The authors declare no conflict of interest.

Appendix A. Drug Release Into Agar Hydrogel

Table A1. Confirmation of extraction efficacy.

mg/Samples	% Extracted		
0.119	66.6%	E1	1x extraction
0.122	68.2%	E2	
0.119	66.6%	E3	
	67.1%		
0.186	103.9%	E1	2x extraction
0.191	106.8%	E2	
0.177	98.9%	E3	
	103.2%		

Two times extraction used in the present study provides approximately 100% efficacy.

Table A2. Percentage of total amount of drug CAM recovered from all sections on the agar plate. The release of CAM into agar hydrogel was monitored from PCL/PEO/CAM fiber mats.

Zone	5 min	10 min	15 min	30 min	60 min	120 min	1440 min
1	86.8	80.6	78.1	88.5	66.6	62.6	11.8
2	13.2	19.4	21.9	11.5	33.4	37.4	54.6
3	0.0	0.0	0.0	0.0	0.0	0.0	26.9
4	0.0	0.0	0.0	0.0	0.0	0.0	6.3
5	0.0	0.0	0.0	0.0	0.0	0.0	0.4

Appendix B

DMSO stocks preparation. Overnight culture was diluted 100 times into fresh LB medium (100 µL on bacteria in 10 mL medium) and grown aerobically at 37 °C to an OD of 0.8–1 (OD600), cultures were chilled on ice and dimethylsulfoxide (DMSO) was added to a final concentration of 8%. 120 µL of suspension was added to PCR tubes and frozen in liquid nitrogen. The tubes were stored at −80 °C and used within 6 months.

Appendix C

Bacterial bioreporters. Bacterial bioreporters are genetically engineered cells, which will produce a measurable signal in response to some chemical or physical environmental change [36]. In the present study, bacteria were developed to report the presence of antibacterial drug CAM by producing fluorescent proteins. Schematics explaining the working principle of bacterial bioreporters are provided in Figure A1.

Our developed CAM-bioreporter has GFP as a control protein for expression and a red mScarlet-I as a reporter protein. When there is no CAM present, only GFP (green) signal is produced by bacteria (Figure A2).

Bacteria exhibit fast translation and green protein production. In the presence of CAM GFP signal (green) will be reduced due to protein synthesis inhibition, and reporter protein mScarlet-I signal (red) will increase due to transcription continuation as a result of ribosomal stalling in the transcription attenuation system.

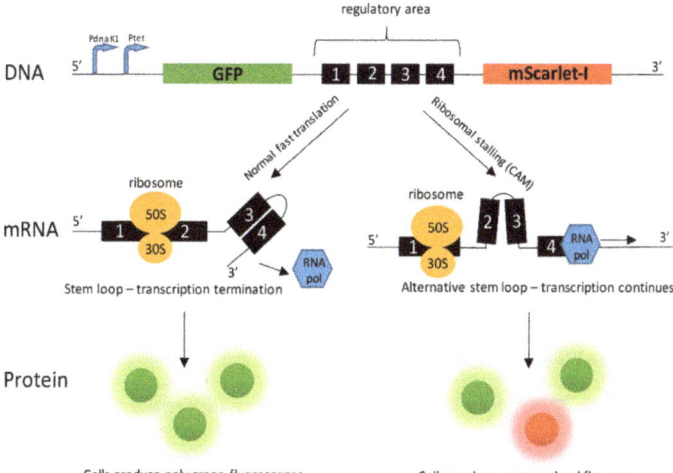

Figure A1. Schematics about bacterial bioreporter system working principle. Key: CAM—chloramphenicol; GFP—green fluorescent protein; mRNA—messenger RNA; 30S/50S—ribosomal subunits; RNA pol—RNA polymerase; PdnaK1 and Ptet—transcription promoters.

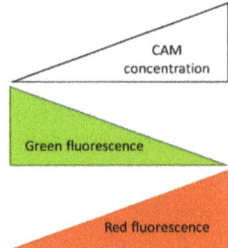

Figure A2. Simplified schematics about bacterial bioreporter system working principle. Key: CAM—chloramphenicol.

References

1. Weng, L.; Xie, J. Smart electrospun nanofibers for controlled drug release: Recent advances and new perspectives. *Curr. Pharm. Des.* **2015**, *21*, 1944–1959. [CrossRef] [PubMed]
2. Torres-Martinez, E.J.; Cornejo Bravo, J.M.; Serrano Medina, A.; Pérez González, G.L.; Villarreal Gómez, L.J. A summary of electrospun nanofibers as drug delivery system: Drugs loaded and biopolymers used as matrices. *Curr. Drug Deliv.* **2018**, *15*, 1360–1374. [CrossRef] [PubMed]
3. Sill, T.J.; von Recum, H.A. Electrospinning: Applications in drug delivery and tissue engineering. *Biomaterials* **2008**, *29*, 1989–2006. [CrossRef] [PubMed]
4. Ye, K.; Kuang, H.; You, Z.; Morsi, Y.; Mo, X. Electrospun nanofibers for tissue engineering with drug loading and release. *Pharmaceutics* **2019**, *11*, 182. [CrossRef] [PubMed]
5. Liu, Y.; He, J.-H. Bubble electrospinning for mass production of nanofibers. *Int. J. Nonlinear Sci. Numer. Simul.* **2007**, *8*, 393–396. [CrossRef]
6. Sultanova, Z.; Kaleli, G.; Kabay, G.; Mutlu, M. Controlled release of a hydrophilic drug from coaxially electrospun polycaprolactone nanofibers. *Int. J. Pharm.* **2016**, *505*, 133–138. [CrossRef] [PubMed]
7. Thakkar, S.; Misra, M. Electrospun polymeric nanofibers: New horizons in drug delivery. *Eur. J. Pharm. Sci.* **2017**, *107*, 148–167. [CrossRef]
8. Gao, S.; Tang, G.; Hua, D.; Xiong, R.; Han, J.; Jiang, S.; Zhang, Q.; Huang, C. Stimuli-responsive bio-based polymeric systems and their applications. *J. Mater. Chem. B* **2019**, *7*, 709–729. [CrossRef]
9. Chou, S.F.; Carson, D.; Woodrow, K.A. Current strategies for sustaining drug release from electrospun nanofibers. *J. Control. Release* **2015**, *220*, 584–591. [CrossRef]
10. Singh, A.; Rath, G.; Singh, R.; Goyal, A.K. Nanofibers: An effective tool for controlled and sustained drug delivery. *Curr. Drug Deliv.* **2018**, *15*, 155–166. [CrossRef]
11. Blanchemain, N.; Laurent, T.; Chai, F.; Neut, C.; Haulon, S.; Krump-konvalinkova, V.; Morcellet, M.; Martel, B.; Kirkpatrick, C.J.; Hildebrand, H.F. Polyester vascular prostheses coated with a cyclodextrin polymer and activated with antibiotics: Cytotoxicity and microbiological evaluation. *Acta Biomater.* **2008**, *4*, 1725–1733. [CrossRef]
12. Liu, X.; Shao, W.; Luo, M.; Bian, J.; Yu, D.-G. Electrospun blank nanocoating for improved sustained release profiles from medicated gliadin nanofibers. *Nanomaterials* **2018**, *8*, 184.
13. Chew, S.Y.; Wen, J.; Yim, E.K.; Leong, K.W. Sustained release of proteins from electrospun biodegradable fibers. *Biomacromolecules* **2005**, *6*, 2017–2024. [CrossRef] [PubMed]
14. Gaharwar, A.K.; Mihaila, S.M.; Kulkarni, A.A.; Patel, A.; Di Luca, A.; Reis, R.L.; Gomes, M.E.; Van Blitterswijk, C.; Moroni, L.; Khademhosseini, A. Amphiphilic beads as depots for sustained drug release integrated into fibrillar scaffolds. *J. Control. Release* **2014**, *187*, 66–73. [CrossRef] [PubMed]
15. Zupančič, Š.; Preem, L.; Kristl, J.; Putriņš, M.; Tenson, T.; Kocbek, P.; Kogermann, K. Impact of PCL nanofiber mat structural properties on hydrophilic drug release and antibacterial activity on periodontal pathogens. *Eur. J. Pharm. Sci.* **2018**, *122*, 347–358. [CrossRef]
16. Fu, Y.; Kao, W.J. Drug release kinetics and transport mechanisms of non-degradable and degradable polymeric delivery systems. *Expert Opin. Drug Deliv.* **2010**, *7*, 429–444. [CrossRef] [PubMed]
17. Natu, M.V.; de Sousa, H.C.; Gil, M.H. Effects of drug solubility, state and loading on controlled release in bicomponent electrospun fibers. *Int. J. Pharm.* **2010**, *397*, 50–58. [CrossRef] [PubMed]

18. Chou, S.-F.; Woodrow, K.A. Relationships between mechanical properties and drug release from electrospun fibers of PCL and PLGA blends. *J. Mech. Behav. Biomed. Mater.* **2017**, *65*, 724–733. [CrossRef] [PubMed]
19. Brettmann, B.K.; Cheng, K.; Myerson, A.S.; Trout, B.L. Electrospun formulations containing crystalline active pharmaceutical ingredients. *Pharm. Res.* **2013**, *30*, 238–246. [CrossRef]
20. Radacsi, N.; Giapis, K.P.; Ovari, G.; Szabó-Révész, P.; Ambrus, R. Electrospun nanofiber-based niflumic acid capsules with superior physicochemical properties. *J. Pharm. Biomed. Anal.* **2019**, *166*, 371–378. [CrossRef]
21. Paskiabi, F.A.; Bonakdar, S.; Shokrgozar, M.A.; Imani, M.; Jahanshiri, Z.; Shams-Ghahfarokhi, M.; Razzaghi-Abyaneh, M. Terbinafine-loaded wound dressing for chronic superficial fungal infections. *Mater. Sci. Eng. C* **2017**, *73*, 130–136. [CrossRef] [PubMed]
22. Preem, L.; Mahmoudzadeh, M.; Putriņš, M.; Meos, A.; Laidmäe, I.; Romann, T.; Aruväli, J.; Härmas, R.; Koivuniemi, A.; Bunker, A.; et al. Interactions between chloramphenicol, carrier polymers, and bacteria–implications for designing electrospun drug delivery systems countering wound infection. *Mol. Pharm.* **2017**, *14*, 4417–4430. [CrossRef] [PubMed]
23. Hu, J.; Prabhakaran, M.P.; Tian, L.; Ding, X.; Ramakrishna, S. Drug-loaded emulsion electrospun nanofibers: Characterization, drug release and *in vitro* biocompatibility. *RSC Adv.* **2015**, *5*, 100256–100267. [CrossRef]
24. Fu, Y.; Kao, W.J. Drug release kinetics and transport mechanisms from semi-interpenetrating networks of gelatin and poly (ethylene glycol) diacrylate. *Pharm. Res.* **2009**, *26*, 2115–2124. [CrossRef] [PubMed]
25. Srikar, R.; Yarin, A.L.; Megaridis, C.M.; Bazilevsky, A.V.; Kelley, E. Desorption-limited mechanism of release from polymer nanofibers. *Langmuir* **2008**, *24*, 965–974. [CrossRef] [PubMed]
26. Nakielski, P.; Kowalczyk, T.; Zembrzycki, K.; Kowalewski, T.A. Experimental and numerical evaluation of drug release from nanofiber mats to brain tissue. *J. Biomed. Mater. Res. Part B Appl. Biomater.* **2015**, *103*, 282–291. [CrossRef] [PubMed]
27. Seif, S.; Graef, F.; Gordon, S.F.; Windbergs, M. Monitoring drug release from electrospun fibers using an in situ fiber-optic system Diss. *Technol.* **2016**, *23*, 6–12.
28. Østergaard, J. UV imaging in pharmaceutical analysis. *J. Pharm. Biomed. Anal.* **2018**, *147*, 140–148. [CrossRef]
29. Asare-Addo, K.; Walton, K.; Ward, A.; Totea, A.-M.; Taheri, S.; Alshafiee, M.; Mawla, N.; Bondi, A.; Evans, W.; Adebisi, A.; et al. Direct imaging of the dissolution of salt forms of a carboxylic acid drug. *Int. J. Pharm.* **2018**, *551*, 290–299. [CrossRef]
30. Østergaard, J.; Meng-Lund, E.; Larsen, S.W.; Larsen, C.; Petersson, K.; Lenke, J.; Jensen, H. Real-time UV imaging of nicotine release from transdermal patch. *Pharm. Res.* **2010**, *27*, 2614–2623. [CrossRef]
31. Ye, F.; Yaghmur, A.; Jensen, H.; Larsen, S.W.; Larsen, C.; Østergaard, J. Real-time UV imaging of drug diffusion and release from Pluronic F127 hydrogels. *Eur. J. Pharm. Sci.* **2011**, *43*, 236–243. [CrossRef] [PubMed]
32. Ye, F.; Larsen, S.W.; Yaghmur, A.; Jensen, H.; Larsen, C.; Østergaard, J. Real-time UV imaging of piroxicam diffusion and distribution from oil solutions into gels mimicking the subcutaneous matrix. *Eur. J. Pharm. Sci.* **2012**, *46*, 72–78. [CrossRef] [PubMed]
33. Østergaard, J.; Lenke, J.; Jensen, S.S.; Sun, Y.; Ye, F. UV imaging for *in vitro* dissolution and release studies: Initial experiences. *Diss. Technol.* **2014**, *21*, 27–38. [CrossRef]
34. Ye, F.; Larsen, S.W.; Yaghmur, A.; Jensen, H.; Larsen, C.; Ostergaard, J. Drug release into hydrogel-based subcutaneous surrogates studied by UV imaging. *J. Pharm. Biomed. Anal.* **2012**, *71*, 27–34. [CrossRef] [PubMed]
35. Daunert, S.; Barrett, G.; Feliciano, J.S.; Shetty, R.S.; Shrestha, S.; Smith-Spencer, W. Genetically engineered whole-cell sensing systems: Coupling biological recognition with reporter genes. *Chem. Rev.* **2000**, *100*, 2705–2738. [CrossRef] [PubMed]
36. Van der Meer, J.R.; Belkin, S. Where microbiology meets microengineering: Design and applications of reporter bacteria. *Nat. Rev. Microbiol.* **2010**, *8*, 511–522. [CrossRef]
37. Blattner, F.R.; Plunkett, G.; Bloch, C.A.; Perna, N.T.; Burland, V.; Riley, M.; Collado-Vides, J.; Glasner, J.D.; Rode, C.K.; Mayhew, G.F.; et al. The complete genome sequence of *Escherichia coli* K-12. *Science* **1997**, *277*, 1453–1462. [CrossRef]
38. Sambrook, J.; Russell, D. *Molecular Cloning: A Laboratory Manual*, 3rd ed.; Cold Spring Harbor Laboratory Press: New York, NY, USA, 2012.
39. Neidhardt, F.C.; Bloch, P.L.; Smith, D.F. Culture medium for enterobacteria. *J. Bacteriol.* **1974**, *119*, 736–747.
40. Quan, J.; Tian, J. Circular polymerase extension cloning for high-throughput cloning of complex and combinatorial DNA libraries. *Nat. Protoc.* **2011**, *6*, 242–251. [CrossRef]

41. Murina, V.; Kasari, M.; Takada, H.; Hinnu, M.; Saha, C.K.; Grimshaw, J.W.; Seki, T.; Reith, M.; Putriņš, M.; Tenson, T.; et al. ABCF ATPases involved in protein synthesis, ribosome assembly and antibiotic resistance: Structural and functional diversification across the tree of life. *J. Mol. Biol.* **2019**, *431*, 3568–3590. [CrossRef]
42. Cormack, B.P.; Valdivia, R.H.; Falkow, S. FACS-optimized mutants of the green fluorescent protein (GFP). *Gene* **1996**, *173*, 33–38. [CrossRef]
43. Bindels, D.S.; Haarbosch, L.; van Weeren, L.; Postma, M.; Wiese, K.E.; Mastop, M.; Aumonier, S.; Gotthard, G.; Royant, A.; Hink, M.A.; et al. mScarlet: A bright monomeric red fluorescent protein for cellular imaging. *Nat. Methods* **2016**, *14*, 53–56. [CrossRef] [PubMed]
44. Osterman, I.A.; Prokhorova, I.V.; Sysoev, V.O.; Boykova, Y.V.; Efremenkova, O.V.; Svetlov, M.S.; Kolb, V.A.; Bogdanov, A.A.; Sergiev, P.V.; Dontsova, O.A. Attenuation-based dual-fluorescent-protein reporter for screening translation inhibitors. *Antimicrob. Agents Chemother.* **2012**, *56*, 1774–1783. [CrossRef] [PubMed]
45. Schneider, C.A.; Rasband, W.S.; Eliceiri, K.W. NIH image to ImageJ: 25 years of image analysis. *Nat. Methods* **2012**, *9*, 671–675. [CrossRef] [PubMed]
46. Mekkawy, A.I.; El-Mokhtar, M.A.; Nafady, N.A.; Yousef, N.; Hamad, M.A.; El-Shanawany, S.M.; Ibrahim, E.H.; Elsabahy, M. *In vitro* and *in vivo* evaluation of biologically synthesized silver nanoparticles for topical applications: Effect of surface coating and loading into hydrogels. *Int. J. Nanomed.* **2017**, *12*, 759–777. [CrossRef] [PubMed]
47. Weiser, J.R.; Saltzman, W.M. Controlled release for local delivery of drugs: Barriers and models. *J. Control. Release* **2014**, *190*, 664–673. [CrossRef] [PubMed]
48. Sadri, M.; Mohammadi, A.; Hosseini, H. Drug release rate and kinetic investigation of composite polymeric nanofibers. *Nanomed. Res. J.* **2016**, *1*, 112–121.

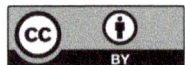

© 2019 by the authors. Licensee MDPI, Basel, Switzerland. This article is an open access article distributed under the terms and conditions of the Creative Commons Attribution (CC BY) license (http://creativecommons.org/licenses/by/4.0/).

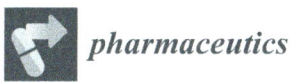

Article

Quasi-Dynamic Dissolution of Electrospun Polymeric Nanofibers Loaded with Piroxicam

Urve Paaver [1,*], Jyrki Heinämäki [1], Ivan Kassamakov [2], Tuomo Ylitalo [2], Edward Hæggström [2], Ivo Laidmäe [1] and Karin Kogermann [1]

1. Institute of Pharmacy, Faculty of Medicine, University of Tartu, Nooruse 1, 50411 Tartu, Estonia; jyrki.heinamaki@ut.ee (J.H.); ivo.laidmae@ut.ee (I.L.); karin.kogermann@ut.ee (K.K.)
2. Electronics Laboratory, Department of Physics, P.O. Box 64 (Gustaf Hällströmin katu 2a), University of Helsinki, FI-00014 Helsinki, Finland; ivan.kassamakov@helsinki.fi (I.K.); tuomo.ylitalo@helsinki.fi (T.Y.); edward.haeggstrom@helsinki.fi (E.H.)
* Correspondence: urve.paaver@ut.ee; Tel.: +372-5649-0280

Received: 31 August 2019; Accepted: 19 September 2019; Published: 24 September 2019

Abstract: We investigated and monitored in situ the wetting and dissolution properties of polymeric nanofibers and determined the solid-state of a drug during dissolution. Piroxicam (PRX) was used as a low-dose and poorly-soluble model drug, and hydroxypropyl methylcellulose (HPMC) and polydextrose (PD) were used as carrier polymers for electrospinning (ES). The initial-stage dissolution of the nanofibers was monitored in situ with three-dimensional white light microscopic interferometry (SWLI) and high-resolution optical microscopy. The physical solid-state characterization of nanofibers was performed with Raman spectroscopy, X-ray powder diffraction (XRPD), and scanning electron microscopy (SEM). We showed that PRX recrystallizes in a microcrystalline form immediately after wetting of nanofibers, which could lead to enhanced dissolution of drug. Initiation of crystal formation was detected by SWLI, indicating: (1) that PRX was partially released from the nanofibers, and (2) that the solid-state form of PRX changed from amorphous to crystalline. The amount, shape, and size of the PRX crystals depended on the carrier polymer used in the nanofibers and dissolution media (pH). In conclusion, the present nanofibers loaded with PRX exhibit a quasi-dynamic dissolution via recrystallization. SWLI enables a rapid, non-contacting, and non-destructive method for in situ monitoring the early-stage dissolution of nanofibers and regional mapping of crystalline changes (re-crystallization) during wetting. Such analysis is crucial because the wetting and dissolution of nanofibers can greatly influence the performance of nanofibrous drug delivery systems in pharmaceutical and biomedical applications.

Keywords: wetting; in situ drug release; nanofibers; electrospinning; poorly water-soluble drug; piroxicam; hydroxypropyl methyl cellulose; polydextrose; scanning white light interferometry

1. Introduction

In recent years, advanced polymeric nanofibrous drug delivery systems (DDSs) have been of increasing use in pharmaceutical and biomedical applications. Such systems include oral dispersible thin films, ophthalmic preparations, multifunctional wound dressings, and implanted DDSs [1–3]. These hybrid polymer nanofibers hold great promise with respect to drug therapy and tissue engineering in both human and veterinary medicine. Nanofibers have a unique capability to modify material properties, which could have a paramount effect on drug delivery performance. They possess fiber structure dimensions at the nanoscale and a large outer surface-to-volume ratio, enabling multiple alternatives in drug delivery. The conversion of polymer solutions to nanofibers by solution electrospinning (ES) is affected by material, process, and ambient parameters [3–5]. The geometric and physicochemical properties of nanofibers depend, for example, on the nature of the solution, polymer type, polymer chain conformation, viscosity, elasticity, and electrical conductivity, as well as on solvent polarity and surface tension [4,5]. These structural fiber properties in turn can have a great impact on the dissolution and drug release of fibers [6–11]. To date, however, our understanding on the dissolution (drug release) behavior of polymeric nanofibers and related physicochemical mechanisms is still limited. This is partially due to the fact that the nanofibers are challenging samples for analysis due to their nanoscale size and brittleness.

In the state-of-the art literature there are many examples of how the geometric nanofiber properties (size, size distribution, surface morphology, orientation) and porosity can greatly affect the dissolution (drug release) and therapeutic efficiency of nanofibrous DDSs [6,12–14]. With poorly water-soluble drugs, the limitations in drug release of the nanofibrous DDSs can delay the onset of drug action, cause poor oral bioavailability, and ultimately decrease therapeutic effect. The geometric nanofiber properties can be governed by the adjustment and control of the critical material, process, and environmental parameters in an ES process [5,15,16]. Lately, increasing interest has been focused on developing ES processes which could produce drug-loaded nanofibers of a specific quality and with reproducible drug release. Due to the nanoscale size, controlling the quality and performance of such nanofibers is still challenging. Consequently, the mechanisms of drug release associated with such novel polymeric nanofibrous DDSs remain poorly understood.

Scanning white light microscopic interferometry (SWLI) is a high-depth resolution imaging technique suitable for determining the geometric properties (i.e., fiber shape, diameter, and length), porosity, and surface topography of nanofibrous DDSs [17]. Three-dimensional (3D) SWLI permits rapid, non-contacting and non-destructive imaging of nanofibrous samples, since it requires neither sample preparation nor modification. Recently, we applied SWLI and high-resolution scanning electron microscopy (SEM) equipped with a customized measurement program for 3D surface topography analysis of non-woven nanofibrous mats [17]. In pharmaceutical research, the use of SWLI for investigating and non-contact imaging of the manufacturing processes and final products is still limited. Sandler et al. and Genina et al. used SWLI to image 3D printed multi-layered DDSs [18,19]. Hanhijärvi et al. applied SWLI to investigate the film surface properties of hydroxypropyl methylcellulose (HPMC)-coated tablets [20], while O'Bryan et al. used it to image 3D printed microgels intended for bioprinting applications [21]. Recently, Wickström et al. applied SWLI to characterize the surface texture and surface roughness of antibiotic-loaded fiber-reinforced composite implants [22].

The aim of the present study was to provide insight into the wetting and early-stage dissolution of drug loaded polymeric nanofibers. To gain an understanding of such phenomena, we monitored in situ the wetting and drug release of fibers loaded with a poorly water-soluble drug (piroxicam, PRX), and determined the solid-state of the drug during dissolution. Two hydrophilic polymers were investigated in nanofibers: hydroxypropyl methylcellulose (HPMC) intended for the sustained drug release and polydextrose (PD) intended for the immediate drug release of a poorly water-soluble drug [23,24]. We combined SWLI and high-resolution optical microscopy to image PRX-loaded nanofibers in contact with an aqueous medium, and the physical appearance and solid-state changes of nanofibers were verified with scanning electron microscopy (SEM), Raman spectroscopy, and X-ray diffraction (XRD), respectively. To our knowledge, this is the first time when such imaging and solid-state analyses are applied in a complimentary fashion to investigate the dissolution of polymeric nanofibers.

2. Materials and Methods

2.1. Materials

Commercially available cellulose ether, hydroxypropyl methylcellulose, HPMC (Methocel K100M premium CR, Colorcon Ltd., Dartford, Kent, UK), and polydextrose, PD (STA-LITE L90, 70% aqueous solution of PD, Tate & Lyle Netherlands B.V., Koog Aan De Zaan, KA, Netherlands) (Figure 1) were used as carrier polymers for the ES of nanofibers. The organic solvents were 1,1,1,3,3,3-hexa-fluoro-2-propanol (HFIP) (≥99.0%) (Sigma-Aldrich C.C., St. Louis, MO, USA) and methanol (Lach-Ner, s.r.o., Neratovice,

Czech Republic). Anhydrous piroxicam, (PRX, pure form I, PRXAH I, Letco Medical, Inc., N Livonia, MI, USA) was selected as a model drug for a low-dose poorly water-soluble active substance in nanofibers. In the wetting and dissolution experiments, purified water, hydrochloric acid buffer solution, USP 28 (pH 1.2), and phosphate buffer solution (pH 7.2) were used as dissolution media. The materials for the preparation of buffer solutions were of analytical grade and purchased from Lach-Ner, s.r.o., Neratovice, Czech Republic.

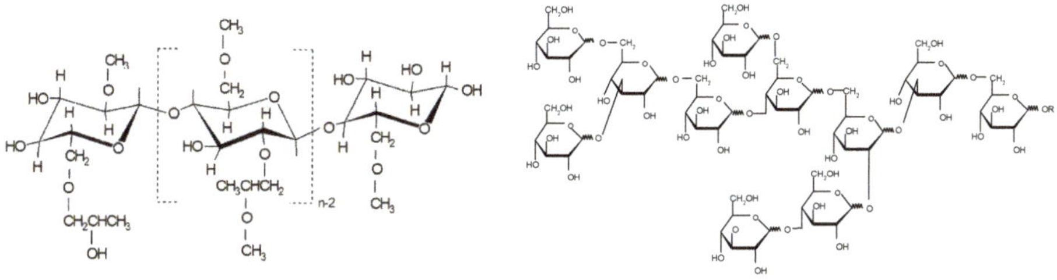

Figure 1. Structural formula of (**A**) hydroxypropyl methylcellulose (HPMC) and (**B**) polydextrose (PD).

2.2. Preparation of Fiber Mats

The carrier polymer (HPMC) and model drug (PRX) were first manually dry mixed with a mortar and pestle at three different ratios (1:1, 1:2, and 1:4). Next, the pre-mixtures were dissolved in organic solvent to obtain the 0.8% (*w/V*) solution of HPMC in HFIP as described in our previous study [16]. With PD, the aqueous solution of PD (70%) alone or the mixture of the aqueous solution of PD (70%) and methanol (5:1) were used for ES. The amount of PRX in the 70% aqueous solution of PD (0.75 mL) used for ES was 20 mg, and 0.75 mL contained 530 mg PD. The drug-loaded nanofibers were fabricated with an in-house ES set-up equipped with a syringe system, automatic syringe pump, spinneret, high-voltage power supply, and a grounded collector plate. The high-voltage power supply system was a Gamma (Gamma High Voltage Research, Model ES3OP-10W/DAM, Ormond Beach, FL, USA). For HPMC solutions, the ES distance and voltage between the spinneret and the collector plate were 8.0 cm and 7 kV, respectively. The pump rate of the automatic syringe pump (KdScientific, Model No: KDS-250-CE, Geneq Inc, Montreal, Quebec, Canada) was 1.0 mL/h. For PD solutions, the ES distance, voltage, and pump rate were 17 cm, 14 kV, and 2.0 mL/h, respectively. The prepared fibers were stored in desiccators (above silica gel, with relative humidity (RH) of 0%) at ambient room temperature (21 ± 2 °C) and in a refrigerator (6 ± 2 °C/RH 0%) prior to use.

2.3. Physical Appearance and Solid-State Characterization

The size and surface morphology of fibers were investigated with scanning electron microscopy, SEM (Helios NanoLab 600, FEI Company, Hillsboro, OR, USA). The samples were coated with a 3-nm gold layer in an argon atmosphere using a magnetron sputter prior to SEM imaging. Solid-state characterization of the starting materials and the electrospun fibers were carried out with X-ray diffraction, XRD (D8 Advance, Bruker AXS GmbH, Karlsruhe, Germany), and Raman spectroscopy (B&W Tek Inc., Newark, DE, USA). In XRD, Cu Kα1 radiation (λ= 1.5418 Å, 40 kV, and 40 mA) was used, and data were collected in the range of 5° and 35° 2θ with a step size of 0.2° 2θ. The brittleness of the fibrous mats was detected by visual inspection and manual palpation with tweezers.

2.4. In Situ Wetting and Dissolution Tests of Fibers

For in-situ wetting tests, we applied the fiber mats as such and the tablets compressed from these fibers. The initial-stage dissolution of the fiber mats were monitored by a high-resolution optical microscopy (Microscope Leica DMLB equipped with the Leica Germany 5.0× and L50×/0.50 objectives and Canon Power Shot 550 digital camera). A standardized drop (50 µL) of aqueous dissolution media was gently placed in contact with a fiber mat at room temperature (21 ± 2 °C), and the dissolution was monitored by taking micrographs at regular intervals.

Pieces of a fiber mat were manually compressed into small flat-faced tablets (discs) with a miniaturized press (Specac Ltd., Orpington BR5 3FQ, UK) intended for preparing sample discs for infrared (IR) spectroscopy analysis. The compression pressure was 196 MPa (2t/cm^2) and the compression time was 5 s. The tablets (discs) were 12.7 mm in diameter and 0.8–1.0 mm in thickness. For in situ initial-stage dissolution experiments, one micro-pipette drop of purified water (2 µL) was gently placed onto the surface of fibrous tablets at room temperature (21 ± 2 °C). The contact point of the drop onto the tablet surface was kept as constant as possible.

The wetting and early-stage dissolution of fibrous tablets were monitored in situ with an in-house 3D scanning white light microscopic interferometry (SWLI). In SWLI, a light beam passes through an interferometric objective (Nikon, Michelson type, magnification 120×) containing a beam splitter that reflects half the incident beam onto a reference surface and passes the other half onto the test surface (Figure 2). Light reflected from the test and reference surfaces recombines and interferes to form an interferogram. The working principle and structure of SWLI is described elsewhere. For details see Kassamakov et al. [25,26], Hanhijärvi et al. [20], and Paaver et al. [17]. In the present study, we obtained three-dimensional (3D) images featuring 29 nm × 29 nm active pixel size from a 55 × 40 µm^2 area. The time period of 10 min prior to a subsequent drop was required for the complete SWLI analysis of the tablets. Purified water (pH 5.6) and the USP 28 buffer solutions (hydrochloric acid buffer pH 1.2 and phosphate buffer solution pH 7.2) were used as dissolution media. The total number of optical microscopy and SWLI images taken on the course of the in situ dissolution experiments was over 500 (including short video-clips). The number of samples was 3–6 in each analysis.

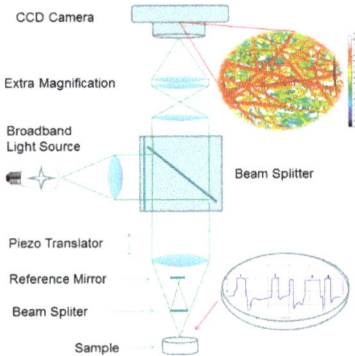

Figure 2. Schematic diagram of scanning white light interferometer (SWLI) and the experimental setup for the in situ wetting and early-stage dissolution of nanofibers.

A high-resolution scanning electron microscope (SEM) (Helios NanoLab 600, FEI Company, Hillsboro, OR, USA) was used as a reference method to the SWLI. A software-based measurement function xT Microscope Control (FEI) was used to measure the horizontal dimensions of the nanofibers. Samples were mounted on aluminum stubs with silver paint and were magnetron-sputter coated with a 3-nm gold layer in an argon atmosphere prior to microscopy. ImageJ (vers. 1.50i) was used for fiber size distribution analysis.

2.5. Dissolution Test

The in vitro dissolution tests of the electrospun nanofiber mats and the pure PRX powder samples were performed using an USP dissolution apparatus I (basket method) in a semi-automated dissolution system (Termostat-Sotax AT7, Sotax AG, Aesch, Switzerland). The concentration of PRX in the dissolution medium was measured at 354 nm by using a UV-VIS spectrophotometer (Ultrospec III, Biochrom Ltd, Cambourne, Cambridge, UK). The dissolution medium was 900 mL of purified water (pH 5.6) and buffer solution (pH 1.2 or pH 7.2) maintained at 37 ± 0.5 °C as described in the USP 28. The basket rotation speed was 50 rpm. The amount of PRX in the powder and nanofiber samples used in the dissolution test was 20 mg. Six parallel tests were performed for each sample.

3. Results and Discussion

3.1. Physical Appearance of Nanofibers

The ES of PRX-loaded fibers with both HPMC and PD polymers resulted in yellowish and white thin fiber mats with a porous internal structure, respectively (Figure 3). HPMC generated fibrous mats with a nanoscale fiber diameter ranging from 100 nm to 400 nm and uniform fiber thickness (Figure 3A,B,E). With PD, we found that due to the hygroscopic nature of PD, the ES of PRX-loaded fibers was possible only in precisely controlled and optimized temperature and humidity conditions (below 30 °C and 40% RH). The PD fiber mat consisted of individual short fibers reaching micron size and a large spread in diameters (Figure 3C,D,F). The diameter of these fibers ranged from 400 nm to 5 μm, and the corresponding fiber mats were brittle (based on palpation with tweezers). A number of spherical beads were observed (SEM) in the electrospun PD fiber mats (Figure 3C). This was due to the high surface tension and low viscosity of the solution. The fiber mats prepared from the mixtures of an aqueous PD solution and methanol, were smaller in diameter, more uniform in radial size, and less brittle (based on visual inspection and palpation with tweezers). The thickness of an entire PD fiber mat ranged from few microns to several tens microns (SWLI).

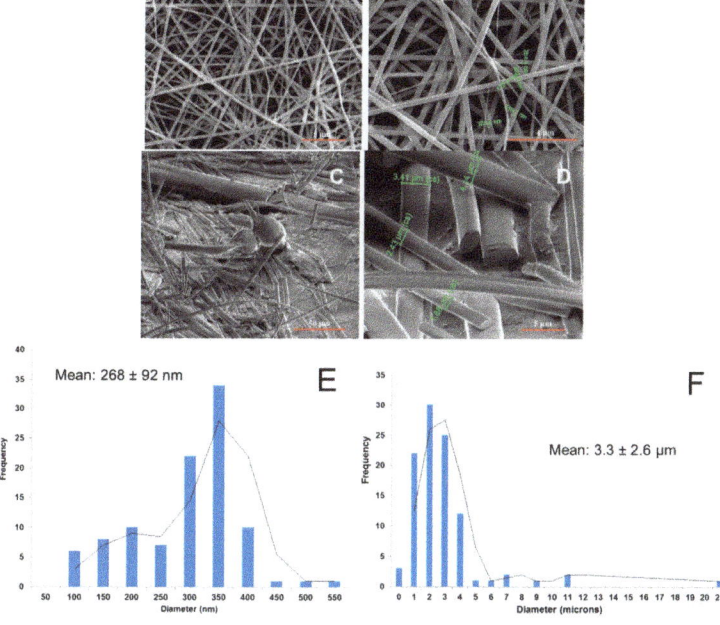

Figure 3. SEM images of piroxicam (PRX)-loaded hydroxypropyl methylcellulose (HPMC) (**A,B**) nanofibers and polydextrose (PD) (**C,D**) fibers. Magnification of SEM: 5000× (**A**), 10000× (**B**), 600× (**C**), and 5000× (**D**). (**E**) Fiber size distribution of the PRX-loaded HPMC nanofibers; (**F**) Fiber size distribution of the PRX-loaded PD fibers.

3.2. Physical Solid-State Properties of Nanofibers

Recently, we reported that the electrospun HPMC nanofibers loaded with PRX are amorphous, and they remain as an amorphous form during a short storage period [16]. In the present study, we found that the ES of PD fibers loaded with PRX did not generate the corresponding amorphous structure, or the produced PRX amorphous structure was very unstable and immediately recrystallized as also discussed previously [27]. The solid-state properties of the electrospun PD fibers loaded with PRX were investigated immediately after the preparation and after a 1-month short-term storage at 0% RH and low temperature (6 °C). As seen in Figure 4 (I), the XRD patterns of electrospun fiber mats showed an amorphous halo together with the characteristic crystalline reflections of PRX anhydrate form I (PRXAH I) immediately after preparation. The XRD and Raman spectroscopy results (Figure 4 (II)) confirmed that PRX (PRXAH I) had lost some of its crystallinity during ES, but did not stay amorphous. No other crystalline reflections (XRD) or spectral features (Raman) characteristic to the known anhydrous PRX solid-state forms were observed in XRD diffractograms or Raman spectra.

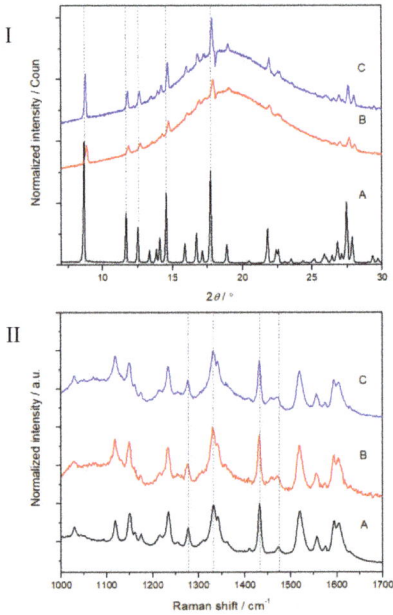

Figure 4. XRD patterns (**I**) and Raman spectra (**II**) of piroxicam (PRX)-loaded polydextrose (PD) fibers. Key: (**A**) PRX anhydrate form I (PRXAH I); (**B**) Fibers immediately after preparation; (**C**) Fibers stored for 30 days at 0% room humidity (RH) and low temperature (6 °C).

3.3. In Situ Wetting and Initial Dissolution of Fibers

Figures 5 and 6 show the high-resolution optical microscopy and SWLI results on the initial stages of the release and dissolution of PRX from the HPMC and PD fiber mats. Since PRX was completely dissolved in the HPMC solution, it is evident that the drug is homogeneously dispersed within nanofibers after ES, and hence the release would be uniform from fiber mats. Figure 5A shows a time-lapse-like snapshot from a high-resolution optical microscope of what happens to the PRX-loaded HPMC nanofiber mats during wetting and initial-stage dissolution. As shown in Figure 5A, the polymeric HPMC-PRX nanofibers dissolved within 1–5 s in the aqueous dissolution media used. According to the literature, PRX exists in an amorphous form in electrospun HPMC nanofibers [16,17,28,29], and the amorphous state of PRX hastened the onset of wetting and premature drug release. In our study, in situ wetting and dissolution monitoring indicated that PRX recrystallizes in a microcrystalline form immediately after wetting and release from the HPMC nanofibers. The PRX microcrystals ranging from 0.2 µm to 12 µm in size were formed after the addition of a standardized drop (50 µL) of purified water, hydrochloric acid (pH 1.2) or phosphate buffer (pH 7.2) solutions onto the HPMC nanofiber mats (Figure 5A,C). The recrystallization of PRX was associated with the formation of larger clusters of microcrystals.

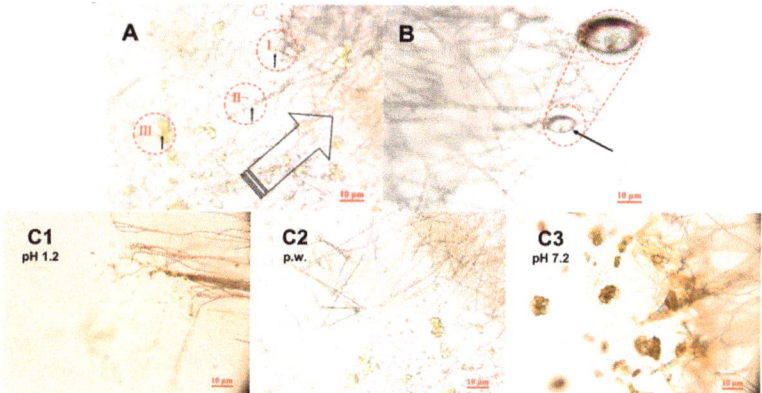

Figure 5. (A) Three phases identified in the release and crystallization of piroxicam (PRX) from hydroxylpropyl methylcellulose (HPMC) nanofibers. High-resolution light microscopy image (magnification 50×) validates the results obtained with SWLI (shown in Figure 6): I. PRX embedded in the nanofibers. II. Crystallization inside or on the nanofibers. III. Recrystallization of PRX. The large arrow indicates the propagation direction of the water front. Magnification 50×. (B) Representative micrograph on the initial dissolution of PRX–loaded polydextrose (PD) fibers. Visible crystals of PRX evident (highlighted with a black arrow) inside a red circle. Magnification 50×. (C) The PRX crystals visible at 30 s after wetting of nanofibers (HPMC:PRX 1:4) by placing a small drop of different dissolution media onto the surface of the fibrous sample: (C1) hydrochloric acid buffer solution pH 1.2; (C2) purified water, p.w. (pH 5.6); (C3) phosphate buffer solution pH 7.2 (22 ± 2 °C). Magnification 50×.

The overall initial-stage dissolution behavior of freely water-soluble PD fibers loaded with PRX was similar, but faster than that observed with the corresponding HPMC nanofibers. As seen in Figure 5B, individual PRX crystals entrapped inside the PD fibers, and the release and dissolution of PRX from the PD fibers progressed via crystal formation. The rapid dissolution of a carrier polymer (PD) fostered the dissolution of PRX. The number and size of the PRX crystals differed from those observed with HPMC nanofibers. With PD, the number of crystals detected was smaller and the size of the crystals slightly larger (ranging from 0.3 µm to 15 µm) than with the HPMC nanofibers. The PRX crystals were located (clustered) inside the PD fibers (Figure 5B), which evidently could advance the dissolution of PRX since PD is a freely water-soluble carrier material. Consequently, this is an interesting approach to use freely water-soluble carrier polymer in electrospun fibers for the improvement of drug dissolution rate. The dissolution behavior of both types of drug-loaded fibers was verified with an established in vitro dissolution test (USP), and the results are shown in the next section (Figures 7–9).

Figure 5C illustrates the status of the HPMC:PRX (1:4) nanofibers at 30 s after wetting the surface of a thin nanofibers sample layer by a small drop (2 µL) of different dissolution media (hydrochloric acid buffer solution at pH 1.2, purified water, or phosphate buffer solution at pH 7.2). The number, shape, and size of the PRX crystals depended on the pH of the dissolution media used. With all dissolution media, the dissolution of nanofibers occurred via immediate crystal formation of PRX (i.e., recrystallization to microcrystals). Rapid changes in the solubility of PRX were also observed with a high-resolution optical microscope. The largest PRX microcrystals and clusters (ranging from few micrometers up to 10 µm) were present with phosphate buffer solution at pH 7.2 (Figure 5C3) and the smallest (0.2–1 µm in size) with hydrochloric acid buffer solution at pH 1.2 (Figure 5C1). It is evident that the recrystallization of PRX associated with the dissolution of HPMC nanofibers is dependent on both the pH and viscosity of dissolution media (in the microenvironment of dissolving nanofibers). Based on our findings, the lower pH of the dissolution media (pH 1.2) induces PRX to recrystallize into small 0.2–1 µm microcrystals in the vicinity of dissolving HPMC nanofibers. In addition, the subsequent formation of microcrystalline clusters occurred slower than that observed with the corresponding nanofibers in the higher pH of dissolution media (pH 7.2). The release of drug from nanofiber mat is shown to be also dependent on the mat thickness [30]. In the present study, the thickness of the HPMC fiber mat was in the range of 2–3 µm (measured by SEM and SWLI).

The SWLI images on the surface of the tablets compressed from the drug-loaded HPMC nanofibers are presented in Figure 6. Figure 6A shows a SWLI image of a tablet surface, where individual fibers are visible: A(I) initial state of tablet (magnification 30×) and A(II) after wetting with 2 µL of water and evaporating for 1 min. In the initial stage, the tablet surface is flat and there is no crystal formation visible. This indicates that PRX is located in nanofibers and most likely is still amorphous. Point A(II) is the first wetting point after adding 2 µL of water and evaporating for 1 min. Figure 6B illustrates the surface of the same tablet after wetting with another 2 µL of water and evaporating for 10 min. Initiation of crystal formation is visible indicating that PRX is partially released from the nanofibers (as seen in Figure 6B). This indicates also that the solid-state form of PRX has changed from amorphous to crystalline form. In contact with water, PRX anhydrate form I transfers to PRX monohydrate before dissolving [27]. It is obvious that PRX monohydrate crystals are visible in SWLI images (Figure 6B,C). Figure 6C shows that the surface of the same tablet after the identical wetting procedure applied to the same spot for a third time. The release of PRX and crystallization occur rapidly, and most likely the crystals of PRX monohydrate are instantly formed in the vicinity of nanofibers. This in turn leads to the retarded quasi-dynamic dissolution of PRX. The present finding is in good agreement with our previous study describing the dissolution behavior of PRX anhydrate and monohydrate forms [31].

In summary, the three phases of the initial-stage dissolution of PRX-loaded HPMC nanofibers were observed with the present compressed tablets and with the corresponding free nanofiber mats studied by SWLI and high-resolution optical microscopy, respectively. These phases are as follows (as shown in Figures 5 and 6): (A) PRX is embedded in the nanofibers (in an amorphous state confirmed by our earlier study [16]), and all nanofibers are intact prior to the water front moving into them; (B) Crystallization of PRX starts inside the nanofibers; (C) Recrystallization of PRX is finalized after drug release from nanofibers.

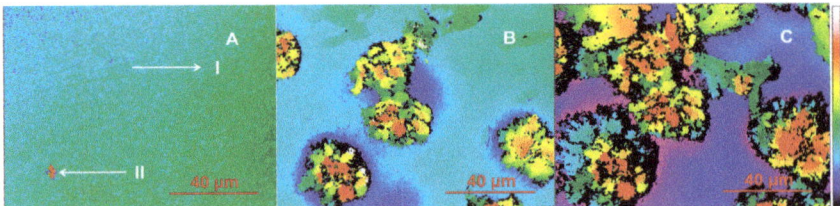

Figure 6. Time-lapse of wetting induced piroxicam (PRX) crystallization on the fixed surface of the tablet consisting of PRX-loaded hydroxypropyl methylcellulose (HPMC) nanofibers. The PRX release is visualized by scanning white light interferometry (SWLI). Key: (**A-I**) Initial state of the tablet; (**A-II**) After wetting with 2 µL of water and evaporating for 1 min; (**B**) After wetting a second time with 2 µL of water and evaporating for 10 min; (**C**) After wetting a third time with 2 µL water and evaporating for 10 min. The scale for height differences is changed according to changes in surface altitude (A—0 to 8 µm; C—0 to 90 µm). The diameter and thickness of tablet (disc) are 12.7 mm and 0.8–1.0 mm, respectively. Magnification 30×.

3.4. Dissolution of Fibers

Figures 7–9 show the early-phase dissolution curves for the PRX anhydrate form I (PRXAH I) in a powder form, the PRX-loaded HPMC nanofibers, and PRX-loaded PD fibers. PRXAH I in a powder form exhibited clearly a longer lag-time in the early-phase dissolution than that observed with the drug-loaded HPMC or PD fiber mats. The early-phase dissolution of PRX anhydrous form I powder was also dependent on the dissolution media used (the amount of PRX dissolved in purified water within the first 15 min was only less than 3%). The present results are also supported by the results on the dissolution behavior of PRX obtained in our previous study [31].

As shown in Figures 7 and 8, the HPMC nanofibers accelerated the immediate dissolution of PRX compared to that obtained with pure PRX anhydrous form I in a powder form. With the drug-loaded HPMC nanofibers, the early-phase dissolution of PRX was fast within the first 3 min followed by a sustained-release phase (Figures 7 and 8). This accelerated dissolution is obviously due to an immediate release of amorphous PRX from the surface of nanofibers and formation of PRX microcrystals in the vicinity of nanofibers (as shown in Figure 5A). The initial drug release from the HPMC nanofibers depended on the dissolution medium, and this finding was in line with the optical microscopy images on the dissolution of HPMC nanofiber mats shown in Figure 5C. The subsequent sustained dissolution phase of PRX observed with the HPMC nanofibers (Figures 7 and 8) is most likely partially due to the gel formation of HPMC as the nanofibers are dissolved, thus forming a hydrophilic gel barrier for the release of drug.

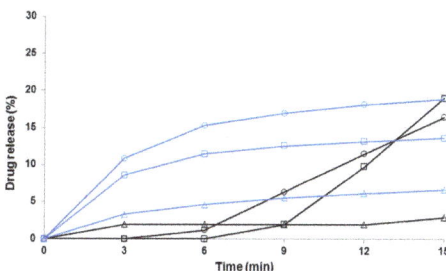

Figure 7. Early-phase dissolution of piroxicam (PRX)-loaded hydroxypropyl methylcellulose (HPMC) nanofibers freely set into the dissolution baskets ($n = 6$). The ratio of a carrier polymer (HPMC) and PRX is 1:1 in the nanofibers. Key: black curve—PRX anhydrate form I (PRXAH I) in a powder form; blue curve—HPMC:PRX nanofibers 1:1; △—purified water; ○—pH 7.2; □—pH 1.2. Standard deviation (SD) in each time point is less than 0.5%.

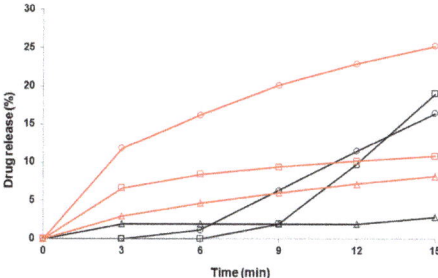

Figure 8. Early-phase dissolution of piroxicam (PRX)-loaded hydroxypropyl methylcellulose (HPMC) nanofibers freely set into the dissolution baskets ($n = 6$). The ratio of a carrier polymer (HPMC) and PRX is 1:4 in the nanofibers. Key: black curve—PRX anhydrate form I (PRXAH I) in a powder form; red curve—HPMC: PRX nanofibers 1:4; △—purified water; ○—pH 7.2; □—pH 1.2. Standard deviation (SD) in each time point is less than 0.5%.

With the drug-loaded PD fibers, the initial-stage dissolution of PRX within the first 3 min was somewhat slower than that obtained with the PRX-loaded HPMC nanofibers (Figure 9). This is obviously due to the crystalline state PRX in the PD fibers, thus resulting in a short delay in the onset of dissolution. In spite of a 3-min lag-time, over 70% of PRX was dissolved within 15 min in acidic dissolution medium (pH 1.2) when formulated as PD fibers. The use of methanol as a co-solvent for ES slightly improved the dissolution of PRX from the PD fibers compared to the corresponding fibers electrospun with pure aqueous solution of PD (i.e., without any organic solvent component) (Figure 9).

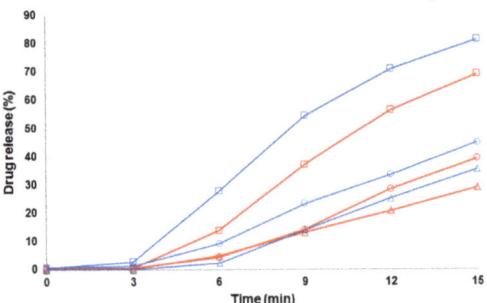

Figure 9. Early-phase dissolution of piroxicam (PRX)-loaded polydextrose (PD) fibers freely set into the dissolution baskets ($n = 6$). Key: red curve—the fibers containing PRX anhydrate form I (PRX AH I) and PD (electrospun from water solution); blue curve—the fibers containing PRXAH I and PD (electrospun from a water-in-methanol 5:1 solution); ∆—purified water; ○—pH 7.2; □—pH 1.2. Standard deviation (SD) in each time point is less than 1.4%.

4. Conclusions

A solution electrospinning (ES) can be used to prepare composite hydroxypropyl methyl cellulose (HPMC) and polydextrose (PD) nanofibers loaded with piroxicam (PRX). The wetting and early-phase dissolution of PRX from these fiber mats are accelerated compared to PRX anhydrate form I in a powder form. With PRX-loaded HPMC nanofiber mats, the dissolution of drug progressed via immediate wetting of the polymeric matrix followed by a lucid recrystallization and dissolution of the drug. A poorly water-soluble PRX recrystallizes in a microcrystalline form after wetting of nanofiber mats, and the further dissolution of PRX is dependent on the pH of the dissolution media. The accelerated dissolution of PRX from freely water-soluble PD nanofibers occurs also via immediate microcrystals formation after wetting. We propose that the present electrospun nanofibers mats loaded with PRX exhibit a quasi-dynamic dissolution behavior. SWLI provides rapid non-contacting and non-destructive in situ monitoring of early-stage dissolution of nanofibers and regional mapping of crystalline changes (re-crystallization) during wetting.

Author Contributions: Conceptualization, U.P., J.H., I.K., T.Y., K.K., and E.H.; methodology, U.P., I.K., T.Y., K.K., and I.L.; investigation, U.P., I.K., and T.Y.; resources, J.H., K.K., and E.H.; writing—original draft preparation, U.P. and J.H.; writing—review and editing, U.P., J.H., I.K., I.L., E.H., and K.K.; visualization, U.P., I.K., and T.Y.; supervision, J.H., I.K., and E.H.; project administration, J.H., E.H., and K.K.; funding acquisition, J.H., E.H., and K.K.

Funding: The research work was funded by the national research projects in Estonia IUT34-18 and PUT1088. Estonian Research Council and the Ministry of Education and Research are acknowledged for funding.

Acknowledgments: J. Aruväli is kindly acknowledged for performing XRPD analyses, J. Kozlova for taking SEM images, and Helder A. Santos for consulting in optical microscopy experiments.

Conflicts of Interest: The authors declare no conflict of interest.

References

1. Rošic, R.; Kocbek, P.; Pelipenko, J.; Kristl, J.; Baumgartner, S. Nanofibers and their biomedical use. *Acta Pharm.* **2013**, *63*, 295–304. [CrossRef] [PubMed]
2. Schiffman, J.D.; Schauer, C.L. A Review: Electrospinning of biopolymer nanofibers and their applications. *Polym. Rev.* **2008**, *48*, 317–352. [CrossRef]
3. Bhardwaj, N.; Kundu, S.C. Electrospinning: A fascinating fiber fabrication technique. *Biotechnol. Adv.* **2010**, *28*, 325–347. [CrossRef] [PubMed]
4. Rošic, R.; Pelipenko, J.; Kocbek, P.; Baumgartner, S.; Bešter-Rogač, M.; Kristl, J. The role of rheology of polymer solutions in predicting nanofiber formation by electrospinning. *Eur. Polym. J.* **2012**, *48*, 1374–1384. [CrossRef]
5. Pelipenko, J.; Kocbek, P.; Kristl, J. Critical attributes of nanofibers: Preparation, drug loading, and tissue regeneration. *Int. J. Pharm.* **2015**, *484*, 57–74. [CrossRef] [PubMed]
6. Sebe, I.; Szabo, P.; Kallai-Szabo, B.; Zelko, R. Incorporating small molecules or biologics into nanofibers for optimized drug release: A review. *Int. J. Pharm.* **2015**, *494*, 516–530. [CrossRef]
7. Torres-Martinez, E.J.; Cornejo Bravo, J.M.; Serrano Medina, A.; Pérez González, G.L.; Villarreal Gómez, L.J. A Summary of Electrospun Nanofibers as Drug Delivery System: Drugs Loaded and Biopolymers Used as Matrices. *Curr. Drug Deliv.* **2018**, *15*, 1360–1374. [CrossRef]
8. Patra, J.K.; Das, G.; Fraceto, L.F.; Campos, E.V.R.; Rodriguez-Torres, M.D.P.; Acosta-Torres, L.S.; Diaz-Torres, L.A.; Grillo, R.; Swamy, M.K.; Sharma, S.; et al. Nano based drug delivery systems: Recent developments and future prospects. *J. Nanobiotechnol.* **2018**, *16*, 71. [CrossRef]
9. Thakkar, S.; Misra, M. Electrospun polymeric nanofibers: New horizons in drug delivery. *Eur. J. Pharm. Sci.* **2017**, *107*, 148–167. [CrossRef]
10. Haider, A.; Haider, S.; Kang, I.K. A comprehensive review summarizing the effect of electrospinning parameters and potential applications of nanofibers in biomedical and biotechnology. *Arab. J. Chem.* **2018**, *11*, 1165–1188. [CrossRef]
11. Lim, C.T. Nanofiber technology: Current status and emerging developments. *Prog. Polym. Sci.* **2017**, *70*, 1–17.
12. Wang, J.; Windbergs, M. Functional electrospun fibers for the treatment of human skin wounds. *Eur. J. Pharm. Biopharm.* **2017**, *119*, 283–299. [CrossRef]
13. Xue, J.; Wu, T.; Dai, Y.; Xia, Y. Electrospinning and Electrospun Nanofibers: Methods, Materials, and Applications. *Chem. Rev.* **2019**, *119*, 5298–5415. [CrossRef]
14. Hu, X.; Liu, S.; Zhou, G.; Huang, Y.; Xie, Z.; Jing, X. Electrospinning of polymeric nanofibers for drug delivery applications. *J. Control. Release* **2014**, *185*, 12–21. [CrossRef]
15. Wang, J.; Hu, X.; Xiang, D. Nanoparticle drug delivery systems: An excellent carrier for tumor peptide vaccines. *Drug Deliv.* **2018**, *25*, 1319–1327. [CrossRef]
16. Paaver, U.; Heinämäki, J.; Laidmäe, I.; Lust, A.; Kozlova, J.; Sillaste, E.; Kirsimäe, K.; Veski, P.; Kogermann, K. Electrospun nanofibers as a potential controlled-release solid dispersion system for poorly water-soluble drugs. *Int. J. Pharm.* **2015**, *479*, 252–260. [CrossRef]
17. Paaver, U.; Heinämäki, J.; Kassamakov, I.; Haeggstrom, E.; Ylitalo, T.; Nolvi, A.; Kozlova, J.; Laidmäe, I.; Kogermann, K.; Veski, P. Nanometer depth resolution in 3D topographic analysis of drug-loaded nanofibrous mats without sample preparation. *Int. J. Pharm.* **2014**, *462*, 29–37. [CrossRef]
18. Sandler, N.; Kassamakov, I.; Ehlers, H.; Genina, N.; Ylitalo, T.; Haeggstrom, E. Rapid interferometric imaging of printed drug laden multilayer structures. *Sci. Rep.* **2014**, *4*, 4020. [CrossRef]
19. Genina, N.; Fors, D.; Vakili, H.; Ihalainen, P.; Pohjala, L.; Ehlers, H.; Kassamakov, I.; Haeggstrom, E.; Vuorela, P.; Peltonen, J.; et al. Tailoring controlled-release oral dosage forms by combining inkjet and flexographic printing techniques. *Eur. J. Pharm. Sci.* **2012**, *47*, 615–623. [CrossRef]
20. Hanhijärvi, K.; Majava, T.; Kassamakov, I.; Heinämäki, J.; Aaltonen, J.; Haapalainen, J.; Haeggström, E.; Yliruusi, J. Scratch resistance of plasticized hydroxypropyl methylcellulose (HPMC) films intended for tablet coatings. *Eur. J. Pharm. Biopharm.* **2010**, *74*, 371–376. [CrossRef]
21. O'Bryan, C.S.; Bhattacharjee, T.; Hart, S.; Kabb, C.P.; Schulze, K.D.; Chilakala, I.; Sumerlin, B.S.; Sawyer, W.G.; Angelini, T.E. Self-assembled micro-organogels for 3D printing silicone structures. *Sci. Adv.* **2017**, *3*, e1602800. [CrossRef]

22. Wickström, H.; Hilgert, E.; Nyman, O.J.; Desai, D.; Şen Karaman, D.; De Beer, T.; Sandler, N.; Rosenholm, M.J. Inkjet Printing of Drug-Loaded Mesoporous Silica Nanoparticles—A Platform for Drug Development. *Molecules* **2017**, *22*, 2020. [CrossRef]
23. Florek, C.A.; Kohn, J.B.; Michniak-Kohn, B.B.; Thakur, R.A. Electrospun Matrices for Delivery of Hydrophilic and Lidophilic Compounds. Available online: https://patentsgooglecom/patent/EP2079416A2/en (accessed on 9 August 2019).
24. Baier, S.; Given, P.; Kanjanapongkul, K.; Weiss, J. Formation of Conjugated Protein by Electrospinning. Available online: https://patentsgooglecom/patent/WO2013151694A1/de (accessed on 9 August 2019).
25. Kassamakov, I.V.; Seppänen, H.O.; Oinonen, M.J.; Hæggström, E.O.; Österberg, J.M.; Aaltonen, J.P.; Saarikko, H.; Radivojevic, Z.P. Scanning white light interferometry in quality control of single-point tape automated bonding. *Microelectron. Eng.* **2007**, *84*, 114–123. [CrossRef]
26. Kassamakov, I.; Hanhijärvi, K.; Abbadi, I.; Aaltonen, J.; Ludvigsen, H.; Haeggström, E. Scanning white-light interferometry with a supercontinuum source. *Opt. Lett.* **2009**, *34*, 1582–1584. [CrossRef]
27. Kogermann, K.; Veski, P.; Rantanen, J.; Naelapää, K. X-ray powder diffractometry in combination with principal component analysis—A tool for monitoring solid state changes. *Eur. J. Pharm. Sci.* **2011**, *43*, 278–289. [CrossRef]
28. Brewster, M.E.; Verreck, G.; Chun, I.; Rosenblatt, J.; Mensch, J.; Van Dijck, A.; Noppe, M.; Ariën, A.; Bruining, M.; Peeters, J. The use of polymer-based electrospun nanofibers containing amorphous drug dispersions for the delivery of poorly water-soluble pharmaceuticals. *Pharmazie* **2004**, *59*, 387–391.
29. Verreck, G.; Chun, I.; Rosenblatt, J.; Peeters, J.; Dijck, A.V.; Mensch, J.; Noppe, M.; Brewster, M.E. Incorporation of drugs in an amorphous state into electrospun nanofibers composed of a water-insoluble, nonbiodegradable polymer. *J. Control. Release* **2003**, *92*, 349–360. [CrossRef]
30. Zupančič, Š.; Preem, L.; Kristl, J.; Putrinš, M.; Tenson, T.; Kocbek, P.; Kogermann, K. Impact of PCL nanofiber mat structural properties on hydrophilic drug release and antibacterial activity on periodontal pathogens. *Eur. J. Pharm. Sci.* **2018**, *122*, 347–358. [CrossRef]
31. Paaver, U.; Lust, A.; Mirza, S.; Rantanen, J.; Veski, P.; Heinamaki, J.; Kogermann, K. Insight into the solubility and dissolution behavior of piroxicam anhydrate and monohydrate forms. *Int. J. Pharm.* **2012**, *431*, 111–119. [CrossRef]

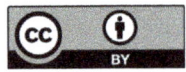

© 2019 by the authors. Licensee MDPI, Basel, Switzerland. This article is an open access article distributed under the terms and conditions of the Creative Commons Attribution (CC BY) license (http://creativecommons.org/licenses/by/4.0/).

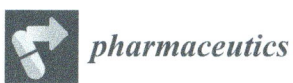

Article

Formulation and Characterization of Aceclofenac-Loaded Nanofiber Based Orally Dissolving Webs

Emese Sipos [1], Nóra Kósa [1], Adrienn Kazsoki [2], Zoltán-István Szabó [1,*] and Romána Zelkó [2]

[1] Department of Drugs Industry and Pharmaceutical Management, University of Medicine, Pharmacy, Sciences and Technology of Targu Mures, Gheorghe Marinescu 38, 540139 Targu Mures, Romania
[2] University Pharmacy Department of Pharmacy Administration, Semmelweis University, H-1092 Hőgyes Endre utca 7-9, 1092 Budapest, Hungary
* Correspondence: zoltan.szabo@umfst.ro; Tel.: +40-744-231-522

Received: 5 July 2019; Accepted: 12 August 2019; Published: 17 August 2019

Abstract: Aceclofenac-loaded poly(vinyl-pyrrolidone)-based nanofiber formulations were prepared by electrospinning to obtain drug-loaded orally disintegrating webs to enhance the solubility and dissolution rate of the poorly soluble anti-inflammatory active that belongs to the BCS Class-II. Triethanolamine-containing ternary composite of aceclofenac-poly(vinyl-pyrrolidone) nanofibers were formulated to exert the synergistic effect on the drug-dissolution improvement. The composition and the electrospinning parameters were changed to select the fibrous sample of optimum fiber characteristics. To determine the morphology of the nanofibers, scanning electron microscopy was used. Fourier transform infrared spectroscopy (FT-IR), and differential scanning calorimetry (DSC) were applied for the solid-state characterization of the samples, while the drug release profile was followed by the in vitro dissolution test. The nanofibrous formulations had diameters in the range of few hundred nanometers. FT-IR spectra and DSC thermograms indicated the amorphization of aceclofenac, which resulted in a rapid release of the active substance. The characteristics of the selected ternary fiber composition (10 mg/g aceclofenac, 1% w/w triethanolamine, 15% w/w PVPK90) were found to be suitable for obtaining orally dissolving webs of fast dissolution and potential oral absorption.

Keywords: aceclofenac; nanofiber; electrospinning; scanning electron microscopy; fourier transform infrared spectroscopy; differential scanning calorimetry

---

1. Introduction

Nonsteroidal anti-inflammatory drugs (NSAIDs) are often used in the therapy of osteoarthritis and rheumatoid arthritis for pain relief and to reduce inflammation. NSAIDs inhibit both isoforms of cyclooxygenase enzyme (COX), but their analgesic and anti-inflammatory effects are due to inhibition of COX-2 [1]. The adverse effects such as gastrointestinal bleeding and ulcer, stroke, heart attacks are primarily caused by the inhibition of COX-1 [2,3]. The risk of side effects increases with high doses and long duration of systemic exposure to NSAIDs [4].

Aceclofenac is a potent NSAID with significant anti-inflammatory and analgesic properties. Its effect is achieved by inhibiting the production of inflammatory mediators including prostaglandin E2 (PGE2), tumor necrosis factors (TNF) and different interleukins (IL1-β, IL-2) [5,6]. Aceclofenac also has chondroprotective effects by the synthesis of glycosaminoglycan [6–8]. It is reported to be more potent or at least to have similar anti-inflammatory effects than conventional NSAIDs in double-bind studies [9,10]. Aceclofenac has a better gastric tolerance, explained by its higher selectivity towards COX-2 than COX-1, which explains its safety compared to traditional NSAIDs and COX-2 selective inhibitors [1,6,8].

The drug is practically insoluble in water, belongs to the Biopharmaceutical Classification System (BCS) Class II. [6] After oral administration aceclofenac is well absorbed, however, its bioavailability is reduced due to high first pass metabolism and poor aqueous solubility of the drug [6,8].

There are numerous technological methods to increase the bioavailability of a drug. For BCS class II drugs, this can be achieved by enhancing the dissolution of the poorly water-soluble active substance by reducing particle size, preparation of water-soluble complexes, using surfactant systems, liposomes, and formulation of solid dispersions [11]. Among the different kinds of solid dispersion strategies new type of solid dispersions, typically ternary or quaternary systems, with one or two additives (such as surfactants and other polymeric excipients) that, together with the drug and host polymer, are combined to exert a synergistic effect on drug-dissolution improvement. The polymer-based solid dispersions are amorphous composites [12].

The oral bioavailability of aceclofenac could be enhanced using chitosan cocrystals trapped into the alginate matrix as a supersaturated drug delivery system (SDDS) or using polymeric microspheres, which can act as delivery systems for sustained drug release [13–16]. The production of nanocrystals using the surface solid dispersion technique is also an appropriate method to improve the dissolution rate of aceclofenac [17,18]. Triethanolamine was also used to prepare aceclofenac salt to improve the solubility [19]. In order to minimize the gastrointestinal side effects and to attain controlled release delivery of the drug, the development of starch-blended Ca^{2+}-Zn^{2+}-alginate microparticles and aceclofenac-loaded interpenetrating network (IPN) nanocomposites were also described [20,21].

Nowadays nanotechnology is an evolving area for the development of drug delivery systems with dimensions between 1–100 nm [22]. Nano-carriers have high surface area to volume ratio, can reduce the side effects of conventional pharmaceuticals and they are successful carriers for insoluble active ingredients [23]. Core/shell nanoscale particles were prepared with a modified coaxial electrospraying process in which a very thin shell layer was employed to give very rapid dissolution of a poorly water soluble helicid [24]. Nanofiber-based drug delivery systems own their high drug uptake due to their large surface area and porosity, but they are also able to simultaneously deliver more than one drug or can be used as transdermal drug delivery systems, as well [25].

These nanofibers can be successfully used to prepare orally dissolving webs, an innovative group of drug delivery systems with several advantages over existing oral formulations such as:

- rapid disintegration and high dissolution rate in the oral cavity due to the large surface area,
- no need of water for administration; this could be an advantage in geriatrics, pediatrics, but also for dysphagic patients or patients who are unable to swallow tablets and capsules or a large amount of water,
- precise dosage administration in each film,
- rapid absorption from the highly vascularized buccal mucosa—drugs are absorbed directly to the superior vena cava, entering into the systemic circulation without pre-systemic metabolism,
- increase in bioavailability and rapid onset of action by avoiding the first-pass hepatic metabolism, while the dose can be reduced, which can lead to a reduction of side effects [26,27].

The nanofibrous formulations enable sustained drug release, as well. Aceclofenac/pantoprazole loaded zein/eudragit S 100 nanofibers were developed using a single nozzle electrospinning process to obtain the sustained release of both the drugs up to 8 h to reduce the gastrointestinal side-effect of aceclofenac [28]. In contrast to the combined formulation, our concept was to enhance the bioavailability and reduce the gastrointestinal side effect of aceclofenac with orally dissolving nanofibrous webs, which can provide fast buccal absorption of active. The present study aimed to formulate and characterize aceclofenac-loaded nanofiber-based orally dissolving webs from triethanolamine-containing polyvinylpyrrolidone (PVP) by electrospinning. The morphology, thermal properties, drug content and drug release profile of the ternary systems were analyzed in order to select the right polymer and active substance concentrations concerning the properties of potential orally dissolving webs.

2. Materials and Methods

2.1. Materials

The active pharmaceutical, aceclofenac (Figure 1a) was provided by Richter Gedeon Plc. (Budapest, Hungary). For the preparation of the viscous polymeric solutions, poly(vinyl-pyrrolidone) (PVP K90, Kollidon K90, Figure 1b) was used, which was obtained from Sigma Aldrich (Merck, Darmstadt, Germany). Triethanolamine (trolamine) and ethanol were from Molar Chemicals (Budapest, Hungary). Ultrapure, distilled water was prepared in-house by a MilliQ water purification system. Potassium dihydrogen phosphate and disodium hydrogen phosphate (Merck KGaA, Darmstadt, Germany) were employed for the preparation of the phosphate buffer solution (1 M, pH 6.8) used for the in vitro dissolution study.

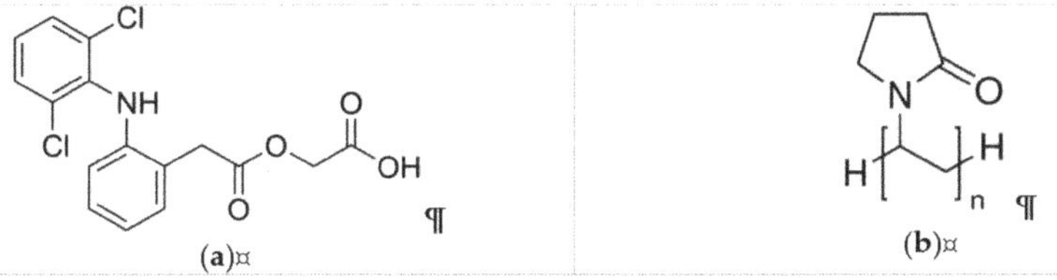

Figure 1. Chemical structures of (**a**) aceclofenac and (**b**) polyvinylpyrrolidone (PVP).

2.2. Methods

2.2.1. Preparation of PVP Solutions Containing Aceclofenac

The active substance was dissolved in a solvent mixture consisting of ethanol and distilled water in a ratio of 75:25 (*w/w*), obtaining a final concentration of 10 mg/g. Trolamine and PVP was dissolved in the obtained solution (amounts described in Table 1) under magnetic stirring until a clear gel was obtained (700 rpm, 1 h with an Ikamag RET magnetic stirrer).

Table 1. Composition of viscous polymeric solutions used for the preparation of nanofibers, diameters of the obtained fibers and estimation of the glass transition temperatures.

Sample No.	Aceclofenac Concentration (mg/g)	PVP Concentration (*w/w*%)	Trolamine Concentration (*w/w*%)	Diameters (nm)	Predicted T_{gmix} (°C)
N1	10	13	1	435 ± 159	139.7
N2	10	15	1	596 ± 215	143.6
N3	10	17	1	1046 ± 113	147.1
N4	10	13	3	757 ± 157	89.9
N5	10	15	3	786 ± 322 *	97.9
N6	10	17	3	812 ± 244 *	104.5

* The average diameters were determined from the fibrous elements of the sample, bias.

2.2.2. Electrospinning Process

The resulting gel was transferred into a 1 mL plastic syringe equipped with a metallic needle (22G–0.7 mm inner diameter). The needle to the collector distance was 10, 12.5 and 15 cm, while the applied voltage was examined at 14, 15 and 16 kV. For the final formulation, the distance between the spinneret and the collector was set to 12.5 cm and the applied voltage to 15 kV, the flow rate was set at 0.1 µL/s. The nanofibers were obtained using the eSpin Cube device (SpinSplit Ltd., Budapest, Hungary), equipped with an NT-35 high voltage DC supply (Unitronik Ltd., Nagykanizsa, Hungary) and collected on a vertically-positioned, grounded aluminum plate covered with parchment paper.

2.2.3. Scanning Electron Microscopic Analysis (SEM)

The morphology of the nanofibers was investigated with a scanning electron microscope (SEM). The samples were fixed by a double-sided carbon adhesive tape and then coated by a sputtered gold conductive layer (JEOL JFC-1200 Fine Coater, JEOL Ltd., Tokyo, Japan). SEM images were taken with a JEOL JSM-6380LA scanning electron microscope (JEOL Ltd., Tokyo, Japan) at 500×, 1500× and 5000× magnifications.

The diameters of the fibers were measured with the aid of the ImageJ software (US National Institutes of Health, Bethesda, MD, USA) and the average fiber diameter was calculated based on 50 different randomly selected individual filaments at 5000× magnification.

2.2.4. Fourier-Transform Infrared (FT-IR) Spectroscopy

Physicochemical properties of the nanofibers were studied using the Jasco FT/IR-4200 spectrophotometer equipped with the Jasco ATR PRO470-H single reflection accessory (Jasco Corporation, Tokyo, Japan). The measurements were accomplished in the absorbance mode, and spectra were collected over a wavenumber range of 4000 and 400 cm^{-1}. 100 scans were performed at a resolution of 4 cm^{-1}.

2.2.5. Differential Scanning Calorimetry (DSC)

Thermograms of aceclofenac, PVP, physical mixture and nanofibers with and without the drug were recorded on a Shimadzu DSC-60 type of thermal analyzer (Shimadzu Corporation, Kyoto, Japan). Samples were accurately weighted in aluminium pans, sealed and scanned from 27 to 250 °C under air atmosphere with a rate of 10 °C/min. Al_2O_3 was used as reference.

2.2.6. Determination of Drug Content of Aceclofenac-Loaded Nanofibers

The absorbance of samples was measured on 277 nm absorption band of aceclofenac using the Shimadzu UV-1601PC UV spectrophotometer (Shimadzu Corporation, Kyoto, Japan). The stock solution was prepared by dissolving 10 mg aceclofenac in 10 mL ethanol, then diluting 1 mL to 50 mL with distilled water, resulting in a final concentration of 20 μg/mL. The drug content was measured by following the absorbance of the solution prepared by dissolving the nanofibers in the same way. Samples were assayed from three consecutive electrospinning runs ($n = 3$).

2.2.7. In Vitro Drug Dissolution Test

Small volume dissolution tests were performed in an in-house assembled dissolution setup, as described in our earlier publication [29]. In order to demonstrate the small-volume dissolution in the oral cavity, dissolution tests of aceclofenac-loaded nanofibers were investigated in 20 mL of dissolution medium, at 37.0 ± 1 °C. As dissolution medium phosphate buffer (pH 6.8, 1 M, Ph. Eur. 8) was prepared. Aceclofenac samples (around 3 mg) and N2 fiber samples (corresponding to 3 mg aceclofenac, around 50 mg nanofiber, each) were put into six test tubes equipped with a magnetic stirring bar. The stir rate was set to 200 rpm. The dissolution was followed for 30 min. At predetermined time points (1 min, 3 min, 5 min, 10 min, 15 min, 30 min), 1 mL samples were withdrawn and filtered through a 10 μm Whatman filter. 300 μL sample was diluted to 3.0 mL with dissolution media. Aceclofenac concentration was determined spectrophotometrically at 277 nm.

3. Results and Discussion

3.1. Morphology of the Aceclofenac-Loaded Nanofibers

Morphology of the obtained nanofibers were examined by SEM. Figure 2 represents the SEM images of samples with 13%, 15% and 17% PVP content with different trolamine proportions, with 12.5 cm emitter to collector distance.

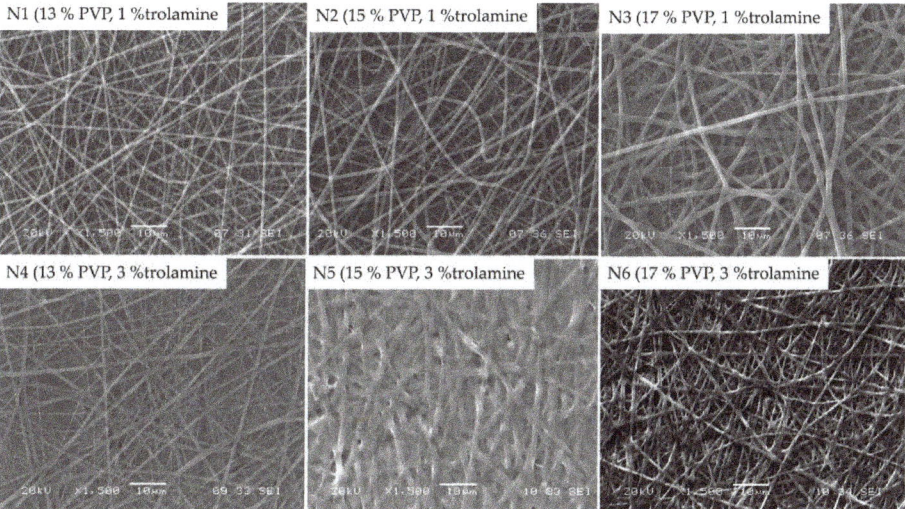

Figure 2. SEM morphology of different samples at 1500× magnification.

When compared to the 1% trolamine content, on the images of samples with 3% trolamine, the deterioration of nanofibers can be observed, which could be the consequence of the plasticization effect of higher trolamine content. The latter is in good agreement with the results of the authors' previous works [29,30], where the film formation occurred as a result of the glassy-to-rubbery transition of the polymeric carriers. The moisture absorbed from the environment acts also as a plasticizer leading to a significant decrease of the T_g of the fiber-forming polymers. Among the samples with 1% trolamine content, the fibers with 15% PVP content proved to be the most suitable for their intended use. The obtained fibers presented diameters from approximately 200 to 800 nanometers with an average of 596 ± 215 nm, with smooth, uniform surfaces. Thus, the composition N2 was used for further studies. Along with the increase of the trolamine concentration the nanofiber structure was shifted to film formation, depending on the polymer-trolamine ratio of the composite fibers. This phenomenon was visualized on the SEM photos (Figure 2, 3% trolamine-containing samples) and can be explained by the enhanced molecular mobility of the plasticized fibers and thus the decreased inner cohesion within the polymeric chains.

3.2. FT-IR Analysis

FT-IR spectra of the components and aceclofenac-loaded nanofibers are represented in Figure 3. In accordance with earlier reports, the IR spectrum of pure aceclofenac shows characteristic peaks at around 3318 cm^{-1} (Figure 3A), which can be attributed to the secondary amine N-H stretching or carboxylic acid band (O-H stretching), two ketone bands at around 1714 and 1770 cm^{-1} and multiple phenyl ring bands in the fingerprint region (Figure 3B) [31]. In the case of the fiber-forming polymer, PVP presents a strong absorption peak at 1650 cm^{-1}, characteristic for the carbonyl group (C=O stretching). The band at 1419 cm^{-1} is the –CH$_2$ bending vibration, while the band at 1285 cm^{-1} is usually assigned to the C-N stretching vibrations [32]. The IR spectrum of trolamine displays a broad absorption peak at around 3330 cm^{-1}, which corresponds to O-H stretching, while those at 2817, 2874 and 2947 cm^{-1}, respectively are assigned to fundamental vibrations of the CH bond. IR spectrum of the nanofibrous sample displays the abovementioned characteristic bonds of both PVP and trolamine, however, none of the absorption peaks of aceclofenac is clearly distinguishable. The latter could refer to that the dissolved initially crystalline aceclofenac remained amorphous in the nanofibrous formulation. On the other hand, in the region of 1500–500 cm^{-1} (fingerprint region) the characteristic peaks of trolamine can be identified (882, 909, 1032 and 1071 cm^{-1}, respectively).

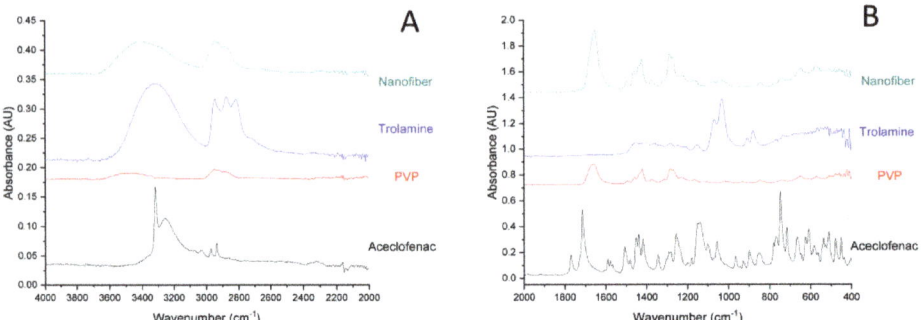

Figure 3. Expanded FT-IR spectra (**A**) 4000–2000 cm^{-1}; (**B**) 2000–400 cm^{-1}) of individual components and the nanofibrous formulation (composition N2: 10 mg/g aceclofenac, 15 *w/w*% PVP, 1 *w/w*% trolamine in ethanol:water 75:25 *w/w*%).

3.3. DSC Measurements

Figure 4 shows the DSC curves of aceclofenac, PVP, physical mixture, neat fiber and aceclofenac-loaded nanofiber.

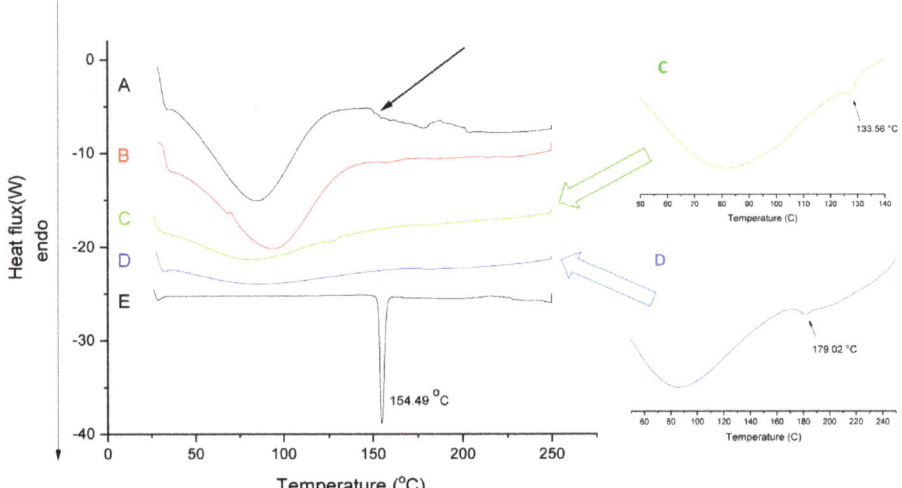

Figure 4. Differential scanning calorimetry (DSC)thermograms of the (A) nanofibrous formulation (composition N2 of polymeric solution: 10 mg/g aceclofenac, 15 *w/w*% PVP, 1 *w/w*% trolamine in ethanol:water 75:25 *w/w*%); (B) neat fiber; (C) physical mixture (same amount of PVP and aceclofenac as in composition N2); (D) PVP and (E) aceclofenac.

The thermogram of aceclofenac presents a sharp endotherm peak at 154.49 °C, indicating its melting point. The melting-point depression of aceclofenac (approximately 133.6 °C) can be observed in the physical mixture (see green insert) showing the effect of the adsorption of PVP and trolamine on the surface of aceclofenac and consequently modifying its thermal properties. The small peak intensity of the aceclofenac melting endotherm refers to its proportion in the physical mixture. On the curves of aceclofenac-loaded nanofibers, there is a lack of melting endotherm, probably due to the amorphization of aceclofenac. Broad endothermic peaks below 100 °C on the thermograms of neat, placebo fibers and aceclofenac-loaded fibers can be associated with the moisture content of the prepared samples. The increased moisture content of the fibrous samples is associated with their larger surface area compared to the powder substances; thus, they are prone to absorb more water. Based on the extent of the peaks, it can be concluded, that the increased hygroscopicity of the fibers, on the one hand, can have a significant impact on the dissolution improvement of the active, but on the other hand it could initiate a glassy-to-rubbery transition of the PVP, thus destroying the fibrous structure. Similar pseudopolymorphism of the fiber-base polymer composite can be seen in the authors' previous stability studies of papaverine hydrochloride-loaded electrospun nanofibrous buccal sheets [30]. The glass transition temperature of PVP K90 denoted by an endothermic change in the baseline thermal profiles (see blue insert) of reversible heat flow was 179 °C [33], which can be more sensitively detected at 5 °C/min heating rate. The presence of solvent residues (e.g., water) and other excipients, like the solubilizing agent trolamine, decreased the glass transition temperature (indicated with black arrow) and thus modifying the glassy-to-rubbery transition of the fibrous polymeric carriers. The estimated glass transition temperature of ternary fibers (T_{gmix}) calculated based on the Fox equation (Equation (1), [34]) are as follows

$$1/T_{gmix} = (w_1/T_{g1}) + (w_2/T_{g2}) \tag{1}$$

where w = weight fraction of components, T_g = glass transition temperature of the components.

The predicted glass transition temperature of various fibers, calculated by Equation (1), together with the average diameters, are summarized in Table 1. The presence of low molecular weight additive, trolamine lowers the T_g of the ternary composite fibers and consequently increases their free volumes. The average diameters of the different composite nanofibers (see Table 1) indicated that along with the increase of the polymer concentration, the obtained fiber diameter also increased at a given plasticizer content of the initial polymer solution. The increased free volume of the fibers results in enhanced water absorption, which enables further lowering of the T_{gmix} and showing rubbery properties at lower temperatures by creating ribbon-like fibers.

3.4. Determination of Drug Content of Aceclofenac-Loaded Nanofibers

In order to confirm the presence of the active in the prepared nanofibers, comparative UV spectra were recorded for ethanolic solutions of neat aceclofenac and the nanofibrous web obtained from composition N2 (Figure 5). The obtained spectra are similar, except the low UV region, where the solution obtained from the nanofibrous formulation displays a higher absorption due to the matrix components. For both spectra, λ_{max} values were recorded at 277 nm (i.e., the expected UV maximum for aceclofenac). Based on the UV spectrometric measurements, the nanofibrous webs contain 5.77 ± 0.12 w/w% aceclofenac, which corresponds to 98.19 ± 2.04% of the theoretical aceclofenac content (5.88 w/w%).

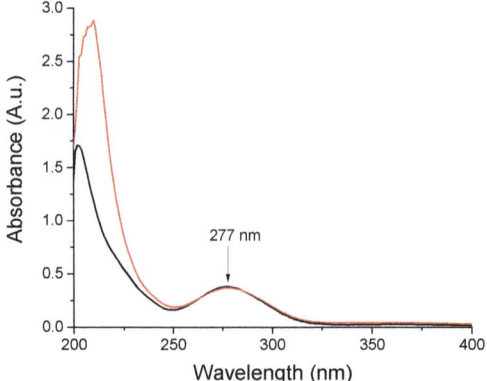

Figure 5. Comparative UV spectra recorded of ethanolic solutions of-red trace-the nanofibrous formulation (composition N2 of polymeric solution: 10 mg/g aceclofenac, 15 *w/w*% PVP, 1 *w/w*% trolamine in ethanol:water 75:25 *w/w*%); black trace–neat aceclofenac.

3.5. Dissolution Measurements of the Nanofibers

Figure 6 illustrates the obtained comparative dissolution profiles of the drug-loaded nanofibers (composition N2 of polymeric solution) and neat aceclofenac. As it can be observed, drug release is spontaneous from the nanofibrous webs and complete even at the first minute of the low volume dissolution test. Although, around 90% of the selected dose of the pure active substance dissolves throughout the dissolution test, the dissolution rate is slower in comparison to the nanofibrous formulation (51% and 85% at 1 min and 3 min, respectively). The faster dissolution rate of the fibrous formulation can be explained by the increased specific surface area of the nanofibers, the amorphous state of the active and the highly hydrophilic nature of the fiber-forming polymer.

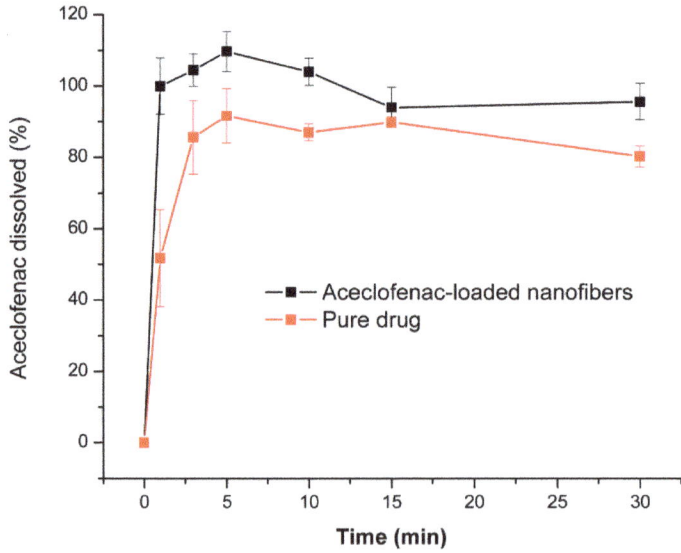

Figure 6. Dissolution profile of aceclofenac-loaded nanofibers (composition N2 of polymeric solution: 10 mg/g aceclofenac, 15 *w/w*% PVP, 1 *w/w*% trolamine in ethanol:water 75:25 *w/w*%) and pure active substance (average of three measurements ± SD).

4. Conclusions

This study demonstrated that the nanofiber forming process is influenced by multiple parameters such as the composition of the aceclofenac-containing viscous solution and the electrospinning parameters. The SEM studies confirmed the nanofibrous structure, while the FT-IR and DSC tests can indicate that the originally crystalline aceclofenac was in the amorphous form in the nanofibrous formulations. Upon exposure to aqueous media, dissolution is believed to generate a supersaturated state due to the amorphous state of the drug. The dissolution of the polymer matrix was fast and complete. The selected composition of the triethanolamine-aceclofenac-poly(vinyl-pyrrolidone) ternary composite resulted in an amorphous drug-loaded electrospun nanofibrous structure of fast and complete dissolution in aqueous media. Based on the results the formulated aceclofenac-loaded orally dissolving webs provide a promising alternative in the therapy of osteoarthritis and rheumatoid arthritis with an enhanced rate and extent of absorption due to the improved wettability and dissolution rate thus providing smaller effective doses and causing fewer potential side effects.

Author Contributions: Conceptualization, E.S. and R.Z.; Data curation, Z.-I.S.; Formal analysis, Z.-I.S. and R.Z.; Investigation, N.K. and A.K.; Methodology, E.S., A.K. and Z.-I.S.; Project administration, E.S., Z.-I.S. and R.Z.; Resources, R.Z.; Writing—original draft, E.S., N.K. and A.K.; Writing—review and editing, Z.-I.S. and R.Z.

Funding: This research was funded by Richter Gedeon Plc. (Budapest, Hungary), Erdélyi Múzeum Egyesület-EME—SE Tender.

Acknowledgments: The authors are grateful to Balogh Diána for the Scanning Electron Microscopic images.

Conflicts of Interest: The authors declare no conflict of interest.

References

1. Aceclofenac. Available online: https://www.drugbank.ca/drugs/DB06736 (accessed on 23 April 2019).
2. Lanas, A.; Chan, F.K. Peptic ulcer disease. *Lancet* **2017**, *390*, 613–624. [CrossRef]
3. Day, R.; Graham, G. The vascular effects of COX-2 selective inhibitors. *Aust. Prescr.* **2004**, *27*, 142–145. [CrossRef]
4. Kienzler, J.L.; Gold, M.; Nollevaux, F. Systemic bioavailability of topical diclofenac sodium gel 1% versus oral diclofenac sodium in Healthy Volunteers. *J. Clin. Pharmacol.* **2010**, *50*, 50–61. [CrossRef] [PubMed]
5. Dooley, M.; Spencer, C.M.; Dunn, C.J. Aceclofenac. A reappraisal of its use in the management of pain and rheumatic disease. *Drugs* **2001**, *61*, 1351–1378. [CrossRef] [PubMed]
6. Legrand, E. Aceclofenac in the management of inflammatory pain. *Expert Opin. Pharmacother.* **2004**, *5*, 1347–1357. [CrossRef] [PubMed]
7. Diaz-Gonzalez, F.; Sanchez-Madrid, F. NSAIDs: Learning new tricks from old drugs. *Eur. J. Immunol.* **2015**, *45*, 679–686. [CrossRef]
8. Raza, K.; Kumar, M.; Kumar, P.; Ruchi, M.; Gajanand, S.; Manmeet, K.; Katare, O.P. Topical delivery of aceclofenac: Challenges and promises of novel drug delivery systems. *BioMed Res. Int.* **2014**, *2014*, 406731. [CrossRef]
9. Pareek, A.; Chandurkar, N. Comparison of gastrointestinal safety and tolerability of aceclofenac with diclofenac: A multicenter, randomized, double-blind study in patients with knee osteoarthritis. *Curr. Med. Res. Opin.* **2013**, *29*, 849–859. [CrossRef]
10. Pareek, A.; Chandurkar, N.; Gupta, A.; Sirsikar, A.; Dalal, B.; Jesalpura, B.; Mehrotra, A.; Mukherjee, A. Efficacy and safety of aceclofenac-CR and aceclofenac in the treatment of knee osteoarthritis: A 6-week, comparative, randomized, multicentric, double-blind study. *J. Pain* **2011**, *12*, 546–553. [CrossRef]
11. Khadka, P.; Ro, J.; Kim, H.; Kim, I.; Kim, J.T.; Kim, H.; Cho, J.M.; Yun, G.; Lee, J. Pharmaceutical particle technologies: An approach to improve drug solubility, dissolution and bioavailability. *Asian J. Pharm. Sci.* **2014**, *9*, 304–316. [CrossRef]
12. Huang, W.; Yang, Y.; Zhao, B.; Liang, G.; Liu, S.; Liu, X.L.; Yu, D.G. Fast dissolving of ferulic acid via electrospun ternary amorphous composites produced by a coaxial process. *Pharmaceutics* **2018**, *10*, 115. [CrossRef]

13. Mutalik, S.; Anju, P.; Manoj, K.; Nayak Usha, A. Enhancement of dissolution rate and bioavailability of aceclofenac: A chitosan-based solvent change approach. *Int. J. Pharm.* **2008**, *350*, 279–290. [CrossRef]
14. Ganesha, M.; Jeona, U.J.; Ubaidullab, U.; Hemalatha, P.; Saravanakumar, A.; Peng, M.M.; Jang, H.T. Chitosan cocrystals embedded alginate beads for enhancing the solubility and bioavailability of aceclofenac. *Int. J. Biol. Macromol.* **2015**, *74*, 310–317. [CrossRef]
15. Deshmukh, R.; Naik, J. Aceclofenac microspheres: Quality by design approach. *Mater. Sci. Eng. C Mater. Biol. Appl.* **2014**, *36*, 320–328. [CrossRef]
16. Deshmukh, R.; Naik, J. Optimization of sustained release aceclofenac microspheres using response surface methodology. *Mater. Sci. Eng. C Mater. Biol. Appl.* **2015**, *48*, 197–204. [CrossRef]
17. Pattnaik, S.; Swain, K.; Manaswini, P.; Divyavani, E. Venkateswar Rao, J.; Talla, V.; Subudhi, S.K. Fabrication of aceclofenac nanocrystals for improved dissolution: Process optimization and physicochemical characterization. *J. Drug. Deliv. Sci. Tec.* **2015**, *29*, 199–209. [CrossRef]
18. Maulvi, F.; Dalwadi, S.; Thakkar, V.; Soni, T.G.; Gohel, M.C.; Gandhi, T.R. Improvement of dissolution rate of aceclofenac by solid dispersion technique. *Powder. Technol.* **2011**, *207*, 47–54. [CrossRef]
19. Sevukarajan, M.; Parveen, S.S.; Nair, R.; Badivaddin, T.M. Preparation and characterization of aceclofenac salt by using triethanolamine. *J. Pharm. Sci. Res.* **2011**, *3*, 1280–1283.
20. Nayak, A.K.; Malakar, J.; Pal, D.; Hasnain Saquib, B.; Beg, S. Soluble starch-blended Ca2+-Zn2+-alginate composites-based microparticles of aceclofenac: Formulation development and in vitro characterization. *Future J. Pharm. Sci.* **2018**, *4*, 63–70. [CrossRef]
21. Jana, S.; Sen, K.K. Chitosan—Locust bean gum interpenetrating polymeric network nanocomposites for delivery of aceclofenac. *Int. J. Biol. Macromol.* **2017**, *102*, 878–884. [CrossRef]
22. Chakraborty, C.; Pal, S.; Doss, G.P.; Wen, Z.H.; Lin, C.S. Nanoparticles as 'smart' pharmaceutical delivery. *Front. Biosci. (Landmark Ed.)* **2013**, *18*, 1030–1050. [CrossRef]
23. McNeil, S.E. Unique Benefits of Nanotechnology to Drug Delivery and Diagnostics. In *Characterization of Nanoparticles Intended for Drug Delivery*; McNeil, S.E., Ed.; Humana Press (Springer Science+Business Media): New York, NY, USA, 2010; pp. 3–8. [CrossRef]
24. Yu, D.-G.; Zheng, X.-L.; Yang, Y.; Li, X.-Y.; Williams, G.R.; Zhao, M. Immediate release of helicid from nanoparticles produced by modified coaxial electrospraying. *Appl. Surf. Sci.* **2019**, *473*, 148–155. [CrossRef]
25. Pillay, V.; Dott, C.; Choonara, Y.E.; Tyagi, C.; Tomar, L.; Kumar, P.; du Toit, L.C.; Ndesendo, V.M.K. A review of the effect of processing variables on the fabrication of electrospun nanofibers for drug delivery applications. *J. Nanomater* **2013**, *2013*, 789289. [CrossRef]
26. Irfan, M.; Rabel, S.; Bukhtar, Q.; Qadir, M.I.; Jabeen, F.; Khan, A. Orally disintegrating films: A modern expansion in drug delivery system. *Saudi Pharm. J.* **2016**, *24*, 537–546. [CrossRef]
27. Dixit, R.P.; Puthli, S.P. Oral strip technology: Overview and future potential. *J. Control. Release.* **2009**, *139*, 94–107. [CrossRef]
28. Karthikeyan, K.; Guhathakarta, S.; Rajaram, R.; Korrapati, P.S. Electrospun zein/eudragit nanofibers based dual drug delivery system for the simultaneous delivery of aceclofenac and pantoprazole. *Int. J. Pharm.* **2012**, *438*, 117–122. [CrossRef]
29. Sipos, E.; Szabó, Z.I.; Rédai, E.; Szabó, P.; Sebe, I.; Zelkó, R. Preparation and characterization of nanofibrous sheets for enhanced oral dissolution of nebivolol hydrochloride. *J. Pharm. Biomed. Anal.* **2016**, *129*, 224–228. [CrossRef]
30. Kazsoki, A.; Szabó, P.; Süvegh, K.; Vörös, T.; Zelkó, R. Macro- and microstructural tracking of ageing-related changes of papaverine hydrochloride-loaded electrospun nanofibrous buccal sheets. *J. Pharm. Biomed. Anal.* **2017**, *143*, 62–67. [CrossRef]
31. Aigner, Z.; Heinrich, R.; Sipos, E.; Farkas, G.; Ciurba, A.; Berkesi, O.; Szabó-Révész, P. Compatibility studies of aceclofenac with retard tablet excipients by means of thermal and FT-IR spectroscopic methods. *J. Therm. Anal. Calorim.* **2010**, *104*, 265–271. [CrossRef]
32. Bagazini, D.R.; Nyairo, E.; Duncan, S.A.; Singh, S.R.; Dennis, V.A. Interleukin-10 conjugation to carboxylated PVP-coated silver nanoparticles for improved stability and therapeutic efficacy. *Nanomaterials* **2017**, *7*, 165. [CrossRef]

33. Gupta, S.S.; Meena, A.; Parikh, T.; Serajuddin, A.T.M. Investigation of thermal and viscoelastic properties of polymers relevant to hot melt extrusion, I: Polyvinylpyrrolidone and related polymers. *J. Excipients Food Chem.* **2014**, *5*, 32–45.
34. Sperling, L.H. *Introduction to Physical Polymer Science*, 4th ed.; John Wiley & Sons: Hoboken, NJ, USA, 2015.

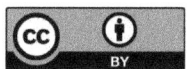

© 2019 by the authors. Licensee MDPI, Basel, Switzerland. This article is an open access article distributed under the terms and conditions of the Creative Commons Attribution (CC BY) license (http://creativecommons.org/licenses/by/4.0/).

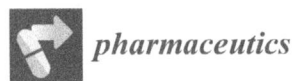

Article

Preformulation Study of Electrospun Haemanthamine-Loaded Amphiphilic Nanofibers Intended for a Solid Template for Self-Assembled Liposomes

Khan Viet Nguyen [1,2], Ivo Laidmäe [2], Karin Kogermann [2], Andres Lust [2], Andres Meos [2], Duc Viet Ho [1], Ain Raal [2], Jyrki Heinämäki [2,*] and Hoai Thi Nguyen [1]

[1] Faculty of Pharmacy, Hue University of Medicine and Pharmacy, Hue University, 06 Ngo Quyen, Hue City 530000, Viet Nam; nvietkhan@gmail.com (K.V.N.); hovietduc661985@gmail.com (D.V.H.); hoai77@gmail.com (H.T.N.)
[2] Institute of Pharmacy, Faculty of Medicine, University of Tartu, Nooruse str. 1, 54011 Tartu, Estonia; ivo.laidmae@ut.ee (I.L.); kkogermann@gmail.com (K.K.); andres.lust@ut.ee (A.L.); andres.meos@ut.ee (A.M.); ain.raal@ut.ee (A.R.)
* Correspondence: jyrki.heinamaki@ut.ee; Tel.: +37-2737-5281

Received: 31 August 2019; Accepted: 27 September 2019; Published: 29 September 2019

Abstract: Haemanthamine (HAE) has been proven as a potential anticancer agent. However, the therapeutic use of this plant-origin alkaloid to date is limited due to the chemical instability and poorly water-soluble characteristics of the agent. To overcome these challenges, we developed novel amphiphilic electrospun nanofibers (NFs) loaded with HAE, phosphatidylcholine (PC) and polyvinylpyrrolidone (PVP), and intended for a stabilizing platform (template) of self-assembled liposomes of the active agent. The NFs were fabricated with a solvent-based electrospinning method. The chemical structure of HAE and the geometric properties, molecular interactions and physical solid-state properties of the NFs were investigated using nuclear magnetic resonance (NMR) spectroscopy, scanning electron microscopy (SEM), photon correlation spectroscopy (PCS), Fourier transform infrared (FTIR) spectroscopy, X-ray powder diffraction (XRPD) and differential scanning calorimetry (DSC), respectively. An in-house dialysis-based dissolution method was used to investigate the drug release in vitro. The HAE-loaded fibers showed a nanoscale size ranging from 197 nm to 534 nm. The liposomes with a diameter between 63 nm and 401 nm were spontaneously formed as the NFs were exposed to water. HAE dispersed inside liposomes showed a tri-modal dissolution behavior. In conclusion, the present amphiphilic NFs loaded with HAE are an alternative approach for the formulation of a liposomal drug delivery system and stabilization of the liposomes of the present alkaloid.

Keywords: haemanthamine; plant-origin alkaloid; electrospinning; amphiphilic nanofibers; self-assembled liposomes; physical solid-state properties; drug release

1. Introduction

Today, nanoscale drug delivery systems (DDSs) provide a novel alternative for conventional therapeutic approaches for potential new drugs of plant origin, or for established synthetized drugs which have been forgotten due to their challenging properties. Compared to the conventional dosage forms, nanotechnology-based DDSs enable the enhancement of biological activity, reduce therapeutic dose, reduce side-effects, deliver active ingredients to the desired target and improve physicochemical stability. The common problems associated with the potential active agents of plant origin, e.g., poor water-solubility, physicochemical stability, permeability, safety and efficiency of challenging drug molecules, can be solved when these are formulated into nanoscale DDSs, such as liposomes, nanoparticles, dendrimers, nanocapsules, ethosomes and polymersomes [1].

Haemanthamine (HAE; Figure 1) is a crinine-type alkaloid isolated from the plant of the family Amaryllidaceae [2]. HAE is reported to have many prominent bioactivities (potential therapeutic effects), including neuromuscular transmission, antimalarial, antioxidant, anticonvulsant, butyrylcholinesterase-inhibitory activity, antiviral and anticancer activity [2,3]. Numerous studies have shown that HAE has a strong cytotoxic activity being effective against human melanoma (SK-MEL-28), human lung carcinoma (A549), human T lymphoblast leukemia (MOLT-4), human esophageal squamous carcinoma (OE21), mouse melanoma (B16-F10), human hepatocellular carcinoma (HepG2), human brain glioma (Hs683), human breast adenocarcinoma (MCF-7) and human acute T cell leukemia (Jurkat) [2–5]. Havelek et al. [2] reported that the treatment of accumulating cells at G1 and G2 stages suppressed cell viability and mitochondrial membrane potential, increased apoptosis through cell cycle progressions and slowed down proliferation. According to Pellegrino et al. [6], HAE suppressed the growth of cancer cells by binding at the A-site of the large ribosomal subunit and, consequently, activating a p53-dependent antitumoral nucleolar stress response [6].

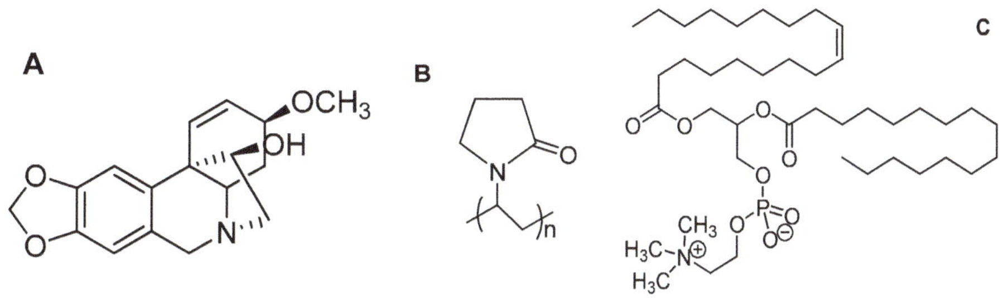

Figure 1. The chemical structure of (**A**) haemanthamine (HAE), (**B**) polyvinylpyrrolidone (PVP) and (**C**) phosphatidylcholine (PC).

From the pharmaceutical formulation point of view, HAE is a very challenging plant-origin active agent since it is a large molecule agent, chemically instable (acid-labile) and poorly soluble in water. We believe that this a major reason for the absence of the relevant formulation and clinical studies in the current literature associated with the present potentially anti-cancer drug. Our scientific hypothesis is that the development of an advanced nanoscale DDS for HAE would enhance the physicochemical stability and drug delivery of the present anticancer drug candidate, and ultimately enable effective therapy.

The drug-loaded liposomes made of lipid bilayer vesicles have been widely used as nanoscale DDSs for, e.g., combating multi-drug resistance, targeting anticancer drug, vaccine and protein delivery, developing long-term circulating DDSs and enhancing gene therapy [7]. However, the well-known limitation associated with the formulation and use of pharmaceutical liposomes is their limited physical stability under storage. Yu and coworkers [8] introduced amphiphilic electrospun nanofibers (NFs) intended for a stabilizing platform of the self-assembled liposomes. The NFs were composed of hydrophilic polyvinylpyrrolidone (PVP) and phosphatidylcholine (PC) (Figure 1), and the corresponding self-assembled PC liposomes were spontaneously formed as the NFs were exposed to water. The present approach has major advantages over the conventional fabrication methods of liposomes since no heating, cooling, agitating, sonicating or sterilizing phases are needed in a fabrication process, and the liposomes can be stored as an "inactive" solid form in the nanofibrous platform prior to use [8]. The study published by Yu et al. [8] inspired us to make attempts to develop such stabilized nanoscale DDSs also for HAE. Our study was conducted to further develop the pioneer work of Yu and co-workers, and to extend the use of such amphiphilic nanofibers in the field of Pharmacy. To date, such amphiphilic nanofibers have not been used as DDSs and as a formulation strategy for active pharmaceutical ingredients. The loading of a high-molecule active agent in such nanofibers to maintain the formation of self-assembled liposomes is a paramount challenge.

In the recent years, the interest in the development of nanofibrous DDSs for therapeutic small molecules and large molecules (biologicals) has been greatly increased [9]. Electrospinning (ES) is the technique of choice for preparing composite nanomaterials and nanofibrous DDSs. ES is a rapid, continuous and low-cost fabrication method that can be readily scaled-up to large-scale production. The active agents (including the challenging plant-origin molecular solids) can be loaded in the electrospun NFs resulting in the desirable properties of the NFs, including a thin diameter, uniform structure, high surface area and porosity [9–11]. In spite of well-known advantages, however, the use of ES and its modifications (coaxial and melt ES) in the pharmaceutical formulation development is still rather limited.

The main objectives of the present study were (1) to formulate novel amphiphilic electrospun NFs for HAE, and to use such nanofibrous platforms as a solid template for self-assembled liposomes of HAE, and (2) to investigate the formation, drug-polymer interactions and physical solid-state properties of the abovementioned nanofibrous templates and self-assembled liposomes. The present novel nanoformulation could be applicable for anticancer drug therapy and for administering via a parenteral route. The nanoscale solid template and self-assembled liposomes could provide an alternative formulation strategy for HAE, thus enabling to enhance the chemical stability and antitumor efficacy of this plant-origin alkaloid.

2. Materials and Methods

2.1. Materials

HAE (a white, crystalline powder, purity NLT 95%) was isolated from *Zephyranthes ajax* Hort. belonging to the family Amaryllidaceae in the Hue University of Medicine and Pharmacy, Hue City, Vietnam. PVP (Kollidon 90F K90) was obtained from BASF SE, Germany. Soybean PC (Lipoid S-100) was obtained from Lipoid GmbH, Ludwigshafen, Germany. Ethanol, methanol and acetonitrile were purchased from Merck GmbH, Germany. Purified water (HPLC grade) was used as an aqueous media. Sodium dodecylsulphate, sodium phosphate and ammonium acetate were purchased from Sigma-Aldrich C.C., St. Louis, MO, USA.

2.2. NMR Structure Analysis

Nuclear magnetic resonance (NMR) spectra of HAE were obtained with a Bruker Avance 500 NMR spectrometer (^{1}H NMR for 500 MHz, ^{13}C NMR for 125 MHz) (Bruker BioSpin Corporation, Billerica, MA, USA), with tetramethylsilane (TMS) as an internal reference.

2.3. Fabrication of Amphiphilic Nanofibers

For preparing the solutions for ES, soybean PC (0.15 g) was first dissolved in ethanol and stirred in a magnetic stirrer for one hour. Subsequently, PVP (0.30 g) was added in the solution and stirred for at least 17 h in a magnetic stirrer at an ambient room temperature (22 ± 2 °C). Finally, HAE (21.0 mg) was added and stirred for 6 h to form the solution for fabricating the amphiphilic NFs. The present solution consisted of soybean PC and PVP at a weight ratio of 1:2. In addition, we tested the ES of amphiphilic NFs with the solution consisting of soybean PC and PVP at a weight ratio of 1:4.

The amphiphilic NFs intended for a solid template for self-assembled liposomes were fabricated with an ESR200RD robotized ES and electrospraying system (NanoNC Co. Ltd., Seoul, Korea). The robotized ES system was composed of a programmable syringe pump, a special 2.5 mL syringe (spinneret) equipped with a metal 25G needle, a high-voltage power supply (Model HV30) and a collector plate covered with aluminum foil (Figure 2). The flow rate of the solution was set at 1.0 mL/h, and the operating voltage between the spinneret and the grounded collector plate was set at 10 kV. The distance between the needle tip and the collector plate was approximately 12 cm. The ES experiments were carried out at an ambient room temperature (22 ± 2 °C) and a relative humidity (RH) of 18–20%. The fiber samples were stored in a zip-lock plastic bag in a refrigerator (3–8 °C) prior to analysis.

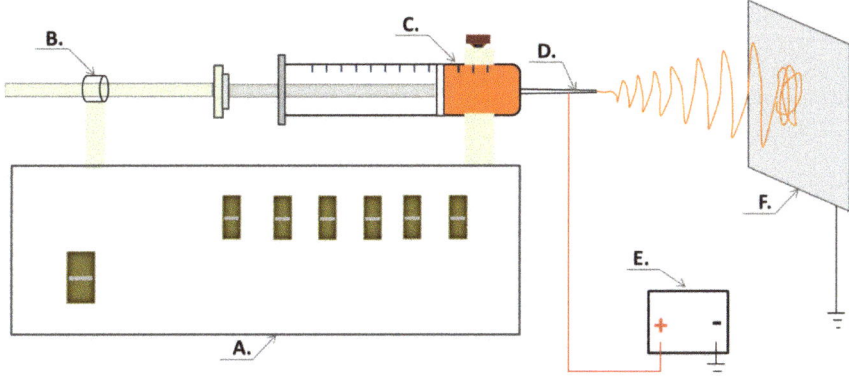

Figure 2. The electrospinning (ES) setup for generating nanofibrous templates for self-assembled liposomes of HAE. Key: (**A**) A robotized ES system; (**B**) programmable syringe pump; (**C**) polymer solution; (**D**) spinneret (a needle system); (**E**) high-voltage power supply; (**F**) collector plate.

2.4. The Geometric Properties and Surface Morphology of NFs

A digital microscope (CETI, Medline Scientific Limited, Chalgrove Oxon, UK) and a high-resolution SEM (NanoSEM 450, FEI Corp., Hillsboro, OR, USA) were used for investigating the physical appearance, geometric properties (diameter and shape) and surface morphology of the nanofibrous templates, respectively. The SEM experiments were conducted as described in our previous study, with slight modifications [12,13]. For SEM, the NF samples were attached onto aluminum stubs and coated with a 3 nm gold layer with a magnetron sputter. The SEM diameter of NFs was measured with ImageJ 1.50b software (National Institutes of Health, Rockville Pike, Bethesda, MD, USA). The measurements were performed for at least 100 individual NFs ($n = 100$).

2.5. Optical Microscopy of Self-Assembled Liposomes

For assessing the spontaneous formation of self-assembled liposomes, 1.0 mL of distilled water was added onto the pre-weighted sample (100 mg) of HAE-loaded NFs. The mixture was then gently manually shaken for about 1–2 min at an ambient room temperature (22 ± 2 °C) to obtain a homogenous dispersion. The dispersion was equilibrated for at least 10 min for forming the liposomes by self-deposition. The sample dilution was required for acquiring proper images. Then, the formation of the self-assembled liposomes was verified and imaged with an optical microscope CETI MAGTEX (Medline Scientific Limited, Chalgrove Oxon, UK).

2.6. Photon Correlation Spectroscopy (PCS)

Photon correlation spectroscopy (PCS instrument Nicomp submicron particle analyzer model 380, Nicomp Inst Corp, Santa Barbara, CA, USA) was used for measuring the size and size distribution of liposomes. The nanofibrous template was first wetted by adding 5.0 mL of distilled water onto the pre-weighted sample (100 mg) of NFs (as optimized earlier in our laboratory). After hydration of NFs, the dispersion with self-assembled liposomes was ultra-centrifuged in a Beckman Optima LE-80K ultracentrifuge (Beckman Coulter Inc., Fullerton, CA, USA) using a SW55 rotor at 50,000 rpm (at 4 °C for 1 h). The supernatant containing polymer (PVP) was discarded. The PCS analysis was performed as described by Ingebrigtsen and Brandl, with slight modifications [14]. The specific dilution of the initial dispersion was prepared for the PCS analysis (50× dilution in distilled water).

2.7. Fourier Transform Infrared Spectroscopy

For verifying drug-polymer interactions of NFs, a Fourier transform infrared (FTIR) spectroscope (IRPrestige-21, Shimadzu Corp., Kyoto, Japan) and Single Reflection ATR crystal (Specac Ltd., Orpington, UK) were used for the HAE, PC and PVP powders, as well as for the electrospun NFs. The analytical range was from 550 cm^{-1} to 4000 cm^{-1} and spectra (n = 3) were normalized and scaled.

2.8. X-ray Powder Diffraction (XRPD)

The pure materials were studied by XRPD using the Bruker D8 Advance diffractometer (Karlsruhe, Germany) with a Vario1 focusing primary monochromator (the wavelength of Cu K-alpha 1 radiation = 1.5406 Å), two 2.5 Soller slits and a LynxEye line-detector. For HAE powder, a scanning step of 0.0173°2θ from 5 to 40°2θ and a total counting time of 324 s per step was used. The electrospun NFs were measured with a Goebel mirror (the wavelength of Cu K-alpha radiation = 1.39222Å), two 2.5° Soller slits and a LynxEye line-detector. For NFs, a scanning step of 0.0194°2θ from 5 to 35°2θ and a total counting time of 328 s per step was used.

2.9. Differential Scanning Calorimetry (DSC)

The thermal properties of PVP, PC, HAE and NFs were studied with a PerkinElmer DSC 4000 differential scanning calorimeter (PerkinElmer Ltd., Shelton, CT, USA). The calorimeter was calibrated using indium as a standard. Samples were analyzed under dry nitrogen purge in crimped aluminum pans with 2 pinholes in a lid. The weight of the samples was approximately 3.0 mg. The heating rate was 20 °C/min, and the range for the temperature heating was between 30 °C and 215 °C. Each DSC run was carried out in triplicate.

2.10. In Vitro Drug Release

Drug release studies were conducted in a dialysis bag (molecular weight cut off 10 kDa, Membrane-Cel, Viskase, Inc., Chicago, IL, USA) with 20.0 mg of HAE-loaded NFs re-dispersed in 2.0 mL of phosphate buffered saline (PBS), pH 6.8, as release media. The control sample consisted of 1.0 mL HAE aqueous solution (1 mg/mL) and 1.0 mL of PBS which was placed inside dialysis bags. The dialysis bag was placed in a 50 mL tube containing 20 mL of PBS, pH 6.8. The tube was capped and placed in a dissolution apparatus vessel (Dissolution system 2100, Distek Inc., North Brunswick Township, NJ, USA) with paddles rotating at 100 rpm and maintained at 37 °C. At predetermined time points, 1.0 mL of sample was collected and replaced with a fresh media after sampling. The drug (HAE) content of samples was determined with high-performance liquid chromatography, HPLC (Shimadzu Corporation, Kyoto, Japan) equipped with a Luna C18 25 cm × 4.6 cm, 5 mm C18 analytic column (Phenomenex Inc., Torrance, CA, USA). The HPLC method is described in more detail in the literature [15]. The mobile phase consisted of a solvent A: solvent B mixture (60:40, volume ratio). Solvent A was a 7 mM sodium dodecylsulphate, 25 mM sodium phosphate and 1 mM ammonium acetate solution in a water:acetonitrile mixture (33:67, volume ratio), and solvent B was methanol. The flow rate was 1.0 mL/min and the detector was set at a wavelength of 293 nm.

3. Results and Discussion

The grand idea of the present molecular self-assembly strategy is that the active-loaded amphiphilic nanofibrous matrix could serve as a solid template for "inactivate" liposomes under storage, and for the on-demand liposome preparation ("activation") the present template could be exposed to a small amount of water for spontaneous formation of the liposomes. To date, the formulation of liposomes has encountered a challenge related to the limited physical stability of the final products under storage. The present self-assembled nanofibrous templates introduced by Yu et al. [8] inspired us to utilize such strategy in our study, and it could be a promising approach to resolve this bottleneck in pharmaceutical nanoformulation. To our best knowledge, this area is under researched to date, and would need true attempts to incorporate a therapeutic agent into the amphiphilic NFs to form self-assembled liposomes.

3.1. NMR Spectroscopy Analysis of HAE

Since the plant-origin active agent used in our study (HAE) was isolated from *Zephyranthes ajax* Hort. belonging to the family Amaryllidaceae in Vietnam, the chemical structure of the present alkaloid was verified by means of NMR spectroscopy. The results are summarized in Figure 3 and in the text below.

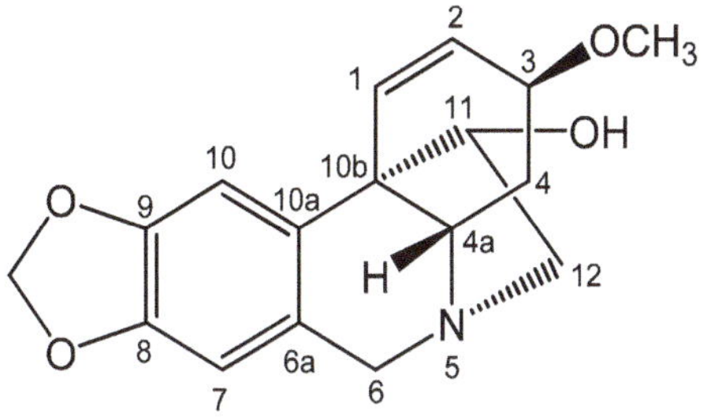

Figure 3. Chemical structure (NMR) of HAE.

Haemanthamine (HAE): Colorless crystal; ^{1}H NMR (500 MHz, CDCl$_3$): 6.41 (1H, d, J = 10.5 Hz, H-1), 6.35 (1H, dd, J = 10.5, 5.0 Hz, H-2), 3.86 (1H, m, H-3), 2.11 (1H, ddd, J = 13.5, 13.5, 4.0 Hz, H-4), 2.01 (1H, dd, J = 13.5, 4.5 Hz, H-4), 4.32 (1H, d, J = 16.5 Hz, H-6); 3.68 (1H, d, J = 16.5 Hz, H-6), 6.47 (1H, s, H-7), 6.82 (1H, s, H-10), 3.97 (1H, brd, J = 4.0 Hz, H-11), 3.35 (1H, dd, J = 13.5, 6.5 Hz, H-12), 3.22 (1H, dd, J = 13.5, 3.5 Hz, H-12), 5.88 (1H, d, J = 4.5 Hz, –OCH$_2$O–), 3.35 (1H, s, –OCH$_3$); ^{13}C NMR (125 MHz, CDCl$_3$): 127.4 (C-1), 126.9 (C-2), 72.8 (C-3), 28.3 (C-4), 62.7 (C-5), 63.6 (C-6), 132.0 (C-6a), 106.9 (C-7), 146.2 (C-8), 146.5 (C-9), 103.3 (C-10), 135.4 (C-10a), 50.1 (C-10b), 80.2 (C-11), 61.4 (C-12), 100.8 (–OCH$_2$O–), 56.7 (–OCH$_3$). The present NMR spectroscopy results obtained with HAE agreed well with the previous studies on the corresponding plant-origin alkaloid [16,17].

3.2. SEM Analysis of Amphiphilic NFs and Templates

Figure 4 shows the representative SEM images of the HAE powder and the individual amphiphilic NFs of HAE as a solid nanofibrous template for self-assembled liposomes. The isolated and milled HAE powder consisted of large irregular particles with a particle size ranging from some tenths of micrometers to several hundred micrometers (Figure 4A). We found that combining HAE and soybean PC with the ES carrier polymer PVP did not impair the performance of an ES process and the formation of NFs. The ES solutions containing HAE, soybean PC and PVP generated continuous elongated NFs with a smooth surface and uniform diameter (Figure 4B,C). The topography of the nanofibrous solid templates exhibited a non-woven and loosely packed platform with randomly oriented individual NFs. The external pore size of the present amphiphilic nanofibrous templates ranged from few micrometers to ten micrometers. Our results are in agreement with those reported by Yu et al. [8] suggesting that the amphiphilic NFs intended for the solid templates for self-assembled liposomes can be fabricated by means of ES.

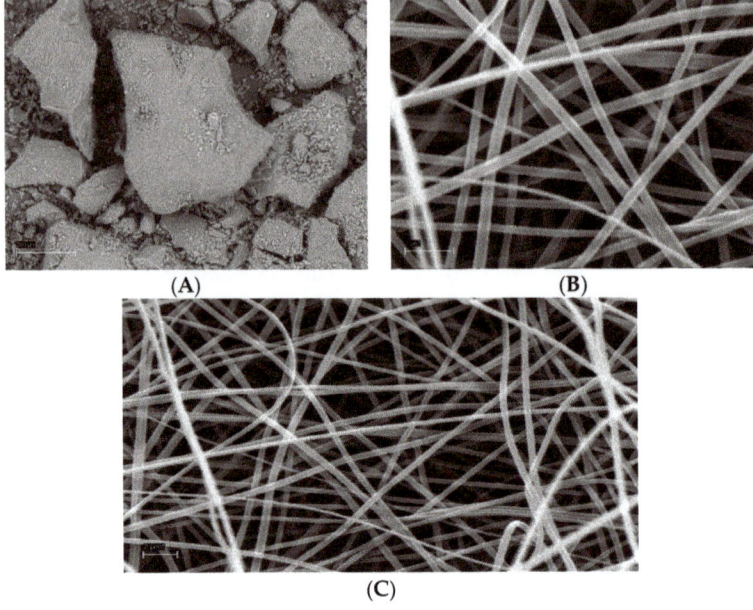

Figure 4. The SEMs of an isolated and milled HAE powder (**A**) and the amphiphilic electrospun NFs (**B**,**C**) used as a solid template for the self-assembled liposomes. Scale bar 200 μm (**A**) and 2.0 μm (**B**,**C**).

In our study, the fiber diameter of amphiphilic NFs measured on the SEM micrographs was 392 ± 66 nm ($n = 100$) (Figure 4). The diameter of individual NFs ranged from 197 nm to 534 nm. Yu and coworkers [8] reported that the average fiber diameter of the corresponding amphiphilic NFs (without HAE) ranged from 580 nm to 1250 nm, and the size of the NFs can be tailored by varying the content of PC in the NFs. According to Yu et al. [8], the average diameter of NFs fabricated from pure PVP was 910 ± 110 nm, and there was a significant decrease in the average fiber diameters as the PC content in the NFs was increased (580 ± 90 nm at 33.3% w/w of PC). However, as the PC content was increased to 50% (w/w), the average diameter of NFs was significantly increased to 1010 ± 110 nm. The presence of PC, as a zwitterionic surfactant, changes the surface tension and viscosity of the PVP solution, thus affecting the morphology and diameter of the NFs [8].

It is well known that PVP is a good carrier polymer for ES to generate NFs. When adding to PVP solutions, it is evident that PC causes electrostatic hydrophobic interactions with PVP [8]. These molecular-level interactions change the conformation of a PVP chain and PVP–PVP molecular interactions resulting in decreasing entanglements and viscosity [8,18,19]. Taking advantage of the optimal formulation of Yu and coworkers' study, we carried out the ES of amphiphilic NFs with the same ratio of PC and PVP (1:2 w/w) for HAE. As shown in Figure 4, the diameter of amphiphilic NFs in our study was much smaller than that obtained by Yu and coworkers (without HAE). Comparing to Yu and coworkers' study [8], our study involves some differences such as the grade of PVP (in our study K90), organic solvent, polymer concentration and air humidity, which could explain these differences. According to the literature, the changes in the abovementioned variables most likely affect (decrease) the viscosity of the ES solution and modify solvent evaporation, thus contributing a decrease in a fiber diameter [20,21].

3.3. Optical Microscopy of Self-Assembled Liposomes

The fate of the self-assembled liposomes in water was monitored by taking optical micrographs at regular intervals after exposing an amphiphilic nanofibrous template to the drop of purified water.

As shown in Figure 5, the liposomes were spontaneously formed (self-assembled) in water within few seconds. It was not possible to measure the size of the present self-assembled liposomes of soybean PC and HAE with optical microscopy due to their nanoscale size. The soybean PC releases from the amphiphilic nanofibrous PVP matrix (template) in contact with water and this results in the instant formation of the individual or co-aggregated vesicles (while PVP dissolves in water). Yu et al. [8] reported that PC molecules after releasing from the PVP nanofibrous matrix tend to co-aggregate in water, and the formation of liposomes is dependent on the location of original NFs in the matrix template. These are also in line with our findings. The optical microscopy images obtained in our study suggest that the molecular self-assembly strategy is applicable in the nanoformulation of a plant-origin alkaloid (HAE), and verify the formation of liposomes in water as intended.

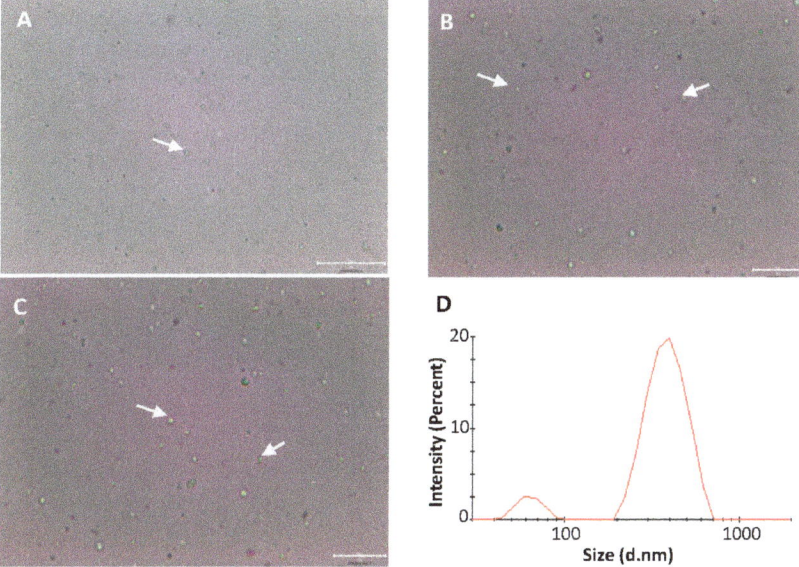

Figure 5. The optical microscopy images (**A–C**) and the PCS size and size distribution (**D**) of the self-assembled liposomes in purified water. The liposomes consisting of soybean PC and HAE are spontaneously dispersed from the electrospun amphiphilic nanofibrous template. Due to the limited magnification (50×) of an optical microscope, only the liposomes composed of large vesicles can be seen. Some selected clusters of liposomes are indicated by white arrows. Scale bar 20 µm with 20× (**A**), and 40× (**B,C**).

3.4. Particle Size Analysis of Self-Assembled Liposomes

To verify the molecular self-assembly process, the size and size distribution of the soybean PC and HAE containing liposomes was analyzed with PCS. The liposomes exhibited a bi-modal size distribution (Figure 5D). The average diameters of the self-assembled liposomes instantly formed from the hydrated amphiphilic nanofibrous templates of two populations were 63 ± 70 nm (10.3%) and 401 ± 64 nm (89.7%), respectively, with the polydispersity index (PDI) at 0.474. This suggests that in situ formation of liposomes occurred as intended. Yu et al. [8] investigated the hydrodynamic diameter and size distribution of the self-assembled liposomes by static and dynamic light scattering (SDLS), and the average vesicle size and PDI ranged from 64 nm to 369 nm and from 0.182 to 0.299, respectively. Our results with the present drug-loaded self-assembled liposomes are in good agreement with the results reported in the literature with non-drug-containing corresponding liposomes [8].

3.5. Physical Solid-State Properties

Physical solid-state analysis was conducted in order to verify potential process-induced solid-state transformations and molecular drug-polymer interactions on the course of the ES of amphiphilic NFs. The XRPD patterns, FTIR spectra and DSC thermograms of HAE (as a powder form) and HAE-loaded amphiphilic electrospun NFs are shown in Figure 6. The XRPD pattern of a pure active agent (HAE) exhibits numerous distinct reflections characteristics to its crystalline nature. The most predominant diffraction peaks of HAE are shown at 12.2, 12.6, 13.8, 16.1, 17.6, 19.6, 20.2, 21.1, 22.6, 23.8 and 27.8°2θ (Figure 6A). The XRPD pattern for the HAE-loaded electrospun NFs with two broad amorphous halos indicates most likely an amorphous state of the amphiphilic NFs (Figure 6A). However, the low drug loading in the NFs (approximately 4.5% *w/w*) challenges the interpretation of the present XRPD results on the solid state of HAE in the NFs. Since it is generally known that a high-energetic amorphous state fosters the dissolution of the material to water, this finding supports the molecular self-assemble strategy applied for the present nanoformulations of HAE. Our results are also in a good agreement with the findings reported by Yu at al. [8]. They found that the electrospun amphiphilic NFs of soybean PC and PVP (without HAE) are amorphous (XRD), but increasing the amount of PC in the NFs resulted in obvious phase separation (i.e., PC separates out from the PVP matrix template). The amorphous halos observed in the XRPD pattern of amphiphilic NFs are most likely contributed by PVP (Figure 6A).

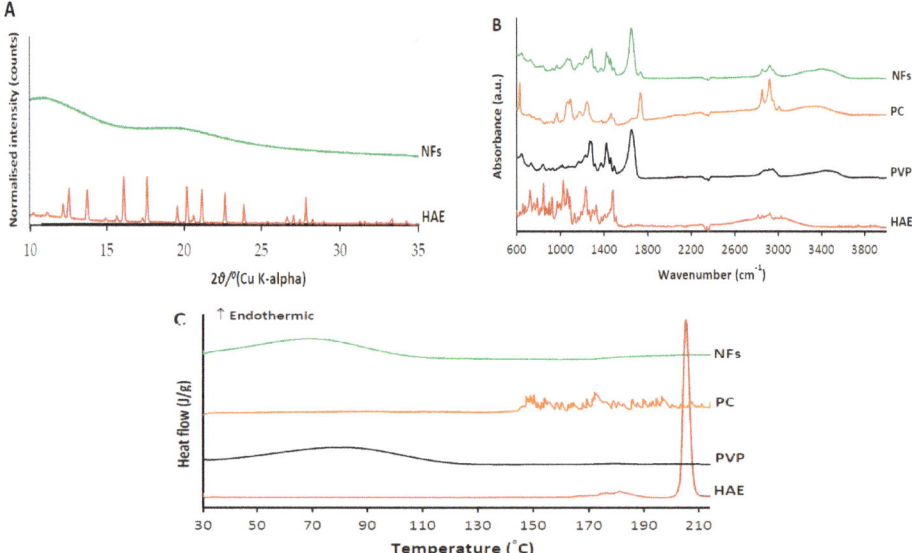

Figure 6. The XRPD patterns (**A**), FTIR spectra (**B**) and DSC thermographs (**C**) of HAE (as a powder form) and HAE-loaded amphiphilic electrospun NFs.

FTIR vibrational spectroscopy is a powerful tool for detecting the process-induced phase transitions and molecular drug-polymer interactions in the solvent-based manufacturing processes. Figure 6B shows the FTIR spectra of electrospun amphiphilic NFs loaded with HAE and pure materials (HAE, PC, PVP) in a powder form. The FTIR spectrum of HAE shows the distinct peaks in the region of C–H aromatic and aliphatic vibrations ranging from 3051 to 2810 cm^{-1} (Figure 6B). The peaks of the N–H, C–N and C–O groups of HAE were shown at 1475, 1225 and 1053 cm^{-1}. The FTIR spectrum of soybean PC shows four bands with corresponding distinct peaks at 2945, 2916, 2847 and 1450 cm^{-1}. This finding is also in a good agreement with Yu et al. [8], suggesting the presence of antisymmetric CH$_3$ stretching, antisymmetric CH$_2$, symmetric CH$_2$ and CH$_2$ scissoring, respectively. The characteristic band with a single peak at 961 cm^{-1} corresponds to the N$^+$ (CH$_3$)$_3$ stretching vibration (Figure 6B). The two distinct peaks at 1232 and 1056 cm^{-1} are in the region of the antisymmetric and symmetric PO_2^- stretching vibrations [22]. The FTIR spectrum for PVP shows distinct peaks at 2900, 1643 and 1261 cm^{-1}, representing antisymmetric CH_3 stretching, C=O amide stretching and C–N stretching vibration, respectively (Figure 6B).

Only small changes in the FTIR spectra of the HAE-loaded amphiphilic NFs compared to the spectra of pure materials were found (Figure 6B). The FTIR spectrum for the HAE-loaded NFs exhibited the weak absorbance bands characteristics to HAE and excipients (soybean PC, PVP), thus suggesting the absence of molecular interaction between the three materials used in a solvent-based ES. On the other hand, the concentration of HAE in the NFs is low, thus leading to some challenges to distinguish the characteristic peaks of the active agent.

DSC was used as a complementary method to verify the drug-excipient compatibility and interactions in the present amphiphilic NFs. The DSC thermogram of HAE showed a single sharp melting endotherm at 205.4 °C (Figure 6C). This is also in a good agreement with the characteristic melting point of HAE (206 °C) reported in the literature [23]. The DSC thermograms for PVP K90 and soybean PC showed a broad endotherm from 50 °C to 120 °C (due to dehydration) and multiple small endothermal events (peaks) ranging from 140 °C to 210 °C, respectively. These multiple fluctuating endothermal peaks for PC can be attributed to the heat-induced movement of polar moieties and the presence of unsaturated bonds, thus resulting in a phase transition from a gel state to a liquid crystal state [24,25]. The DSC thermogram of HAE-loaded amphiphilic NFs showed the characteristic endothermal curve of PVP (ranging from 40 °C to 110 °C), and the absence of the characteristic peak for the melting point of HAE (Figure 6C). Hence, the DSC results suggest that HAE is most likely in an amorphous form in the NFs. The excipients (PVP, PC), however, melt at lower temperatures, and consequently, HAE could dissolve in this melt, thus making it difficult to fully confirm the amorphous state of HAE. Moreover, there are no signs of significant interactions or incompatibilities between HAE and excipients, and the thermograms do not show any signs of chemical decomposition of HAE.

3.6. In Vitro Drug Release

The cumulative dissolution profiles of HAE as a powder and loaded in the amphiphilic electrospun NFs are shown in Figure 7. The theoretical amount of HAE in the solid nanofibers sample applied in the dissolution test was 0.89 mg (respective to 100% in the dissolution study). With HAE as a powder, approximately 50% of active ingredient dissolved within the first 2 h and over 80% of HAE dissolved within the next 16 h (after 18 h the dissolution reached the plateau). The release of HAE from the amphiphilic electrospun NFs and self-assembled liposomes occurred in three phases: More than 50% of HAE released within the first 2 h, approximately 80% released within the next 2 h, and the rest of the active agent (100%) released within 30 h (Figure 7). The initial burst release of the drug-loaded amphiphilic nanofibers could be attributed to the surface or near-surface distribution of HAE in the nanofibers and the physical solid state of HAE in the nanofibrous templates. The XRPD results (Figure 6A) suggested that HAE is distributed in an amorphous form in the electrospun nanofibers, thus showing the success of the strategy. In the last phase of the dissolution, a steady-state release pattern was observed obviously due to the drug release from the self-assembled liposomes. Khan and coworkers reported the disintegration and diffusion-controlled mechanism associated with the active release from the nanofibers loaded with oregano essential oil [26]. According to Yu and coworkers, when the amphiphilic NFs are exposed to water, the PC molecules (attached in the PVP chains) are hydrated and concentrated within the nanofibrous network [8]. This results in swelling of the nanofibrous template. The self-assembled liposomes are formed as hydrated PC molecules form co-aggregates, thus entrapping water inside the vesicles. In the final stage, the self-assembled liposomes are released in the dissolution medium [8]. Our dissolution study is only indicative to compare the dissolution properties of HAE and the present amphiphilic nanofibrous templates loaded with the active agent. More research is needed to gain an understanding of the self-assembly of liposomes in the aqueous media and actual release of the active agent from the formed liposomes.

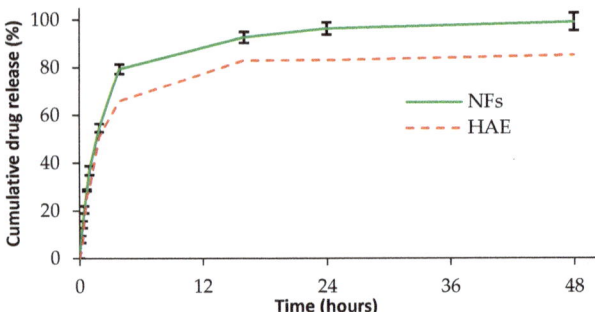

Figure 7. The in vitro dissolution profiles of HAE (as a powder form; a dotted red curve) and HAE-loaded amphiphilic electrospun NFs (a continuous green curve) ($n = 3$).

4. Conclusions

The therapeutic use of a plant-origin alkaloid, haemanthamine (HAE), is limited due to the formulation challenges associated with the complex molecular structure and physicochemical properties of the present active agent. We showed that HAE can be formulated to amphiphilic nanofibers (NFs) by solvent-based electrospinning (ES). The amphiphilic NFs provide a solid template for self-assembled liposomes intended to be spontaneously dispersed when the template is exposed to water. The spontaneous formation of self-assembled HAE containing liposomes in water can be proven. The present amphiphilic NFs loaded with HAE are an alternative approach for the formulation of a liposomal drug delivery system and for stabilization of the liposomes of the present alkaloid.

Author Contributions: Conceptualization, K.V.N., J.H., A.R. and H.T.N.; methodology, I.L., K.K., A.L. and A.M.; investigation, K.V.N., I.L., D.V.H., A.L. and A.M.; resources, A.R., J.H. and H.T.N.; writing—original draft preparation, K.V.N.; writing—review and editing, J.H., K.K., I.L., A.M., A.R., D.V.H and H.T.N.; visualization, K.V.N.; supervision, J.H., A.R. and H.T.N.; project administration, J.H., A.R. and H.T.N.; funding acquisition, J.H., A.R. and H.T.N.

Funding: This research was funded by the Erasmus Plus and Edushare Funding Programme. The research work was also funded by the national research projects in Estonia IUT34-18 and PUT1088.

Acknowledgments: J. Aruväli, University of Tartu, is kindly acknowledged for performing XRPD analyses. M. Külaviir, University of Tartu, is gratefully acknowledged for performing SEM experiments. Nhan Trong Le, Hue University of Medicine and Pharmacy, is gratefully acknowledged for collecting the plant material.

Conflicts of Interest: The authors declare no conflict of interest.

References

1. Yurteri, C.R.; Hartman, P.A.; Marijnissen, J.C.M. Producing pharmaceutical particles via electrospraying with an emphasis on nano and ano structured particles—A Review. *KONA Powder Part. J.* **2010**, *28*, 91–115. [CrossRef]
2. Havelek, R.S.; Kralovec, K.; Bruckova, L.; Cahlikova, L.; Rezacova, M.; Opletal, L.; Bilkova, Z. Effect of Amaryllidaceae alkaloids haemanthamine and haemanthidine on cell viability, apoptosis and cell cycle progression in human T-lymphoblast cell line. *FEBS J.* **2013**, *280*, 322–323.
3. Van Goietsenoven, G.; Andolfi, A.; Lallemand, B.; Cimmino, A.; Lamoral-Theys, D.; Gras, T.; Abou-Donia, A.; Dubois, J.; Lefranc, F.; Mathieu, V.; et al. Amaryllidaceae alkaloids belonging to different structural subgroups display activity against apoptosis-resistant cancer cells. *J. Nat. Prod.* **2010**, *73*, 1223–1227. [CrossRef] [PubMed]
4. Nair, J.J.; Bastida, J.; Viladomat, F.; van Staden, J. Cytotoxic agents of the crinane series of amaryllidaceae alkaloids. *Nat. Prod. Commun.* **2012**, *7*, 1677–1688. [CrossRef] [PubMed]

5. Weniger, B.; Italiano, L.; Beck, J.P.; Bastida, J.; Bergoñon, S.; Codina, C.; Lobstein, A.; Anton, R. Cytotoxic Activity of Amaryllidaceae alkaloids. *Planta Med.* **1995**, *61*, 77–79. [CrossRef]
6. Pellegrino, S.; Meyer, M.; Zorbas, C.; Bouchta, S.A.; Saraf, K.; Pelly, S.C.; Yusupova, G.; Evidente, A.; Mathieu, V.; Kornienko, A.; et al. The Amaryllidaceae alkaloid haemanthamine binds the eukaryotic ribosome to repress cancer cell growth. *Structure* **2018**, *26*, 416–425.e4. [CrossRef] [PubMed]
7. Torchilin, V.P. Recent advances with liposomes as pharmaceutical carriers. *Nat. Rev. Drug Discov.* **2005**, *4*, 145–160. [CrossRef]
8. Yu, D.G.; Branford-White, C.; Williams, G.R.; Bligh, S.A.; White, K.; Zhu, L.M.; Chatterton, N.P. Self-assembled liposomes from amphiphilic electrospun nanofibers. *J. Soft Matter* **2011**, *7*, 8239–8247. [CrossRef]
9. Sebe, I.; Szabó, P.; Kállai-Szabó, B.; Zelkó, R. Incorporating small molecules or biologics into nanofibers for optimized drug release: A Review. *Int. J. Pharm.* **2015**, *494*, 516–530. [CrossRef]
10. He, D.; Hu, B.; Yao, Q.F.; Wang, K.; Yu, S.H. Large-scale synthesis of flexible free-standing SERS substrates with high sensitivity: Electrospun PVA nanofibers embedded with controlled alignment of silver nanoparticles. *ACS Nano* **2009**, *3*, 3993–4002. [CrossRef]
11. Lu, X.; Wang, C.; Wei, Y. Synthesis by electrospinning and their applications. One-dimensional composite nanomaterials. *Small* **2009**, *5*, 2349–2370. [CrossRef] [PubMed]
12. Paaver, U.; Heinämäki, J.; Laidmäe, I.; Lust, A.; Kozlova, J.; Sillaste, E.; Kirsimäe, K.; Veski, P.; Kogermann, K. Electrospun nanofibers as a potential controlled-release solid dispersion system for poorly water-soluble drugs. *Int. J. Pharm.* **2015**, *479*, 252–260. [CrossRef] [PubMed]
13. Ho, H.N.; Laidmäe, I.; Kogermann, K.; Lust, A.; Meos, A.; Nguyen, C.N.; Heinämäki, J. Development of electrosprayed artesunate-loaded core-shell nanoparticles. *Drug Dev. Ind. Pharm.* **2017**, *43*, 1134–1142. [CrossRef] [PubMed]
14. Ingebrigtsen, L.; Brandl, M. Determination of the size distribution of liposomes by SEC fractionation, and PCS analysis and enzymatic assay of lipid content. *AAPS PharmSciTech* **2002**, *3*, 9–15. [CrossRef] [PubMed]
15. Lopez, S.; Bastida, J.; Viladomat, F.; Codina, C. Solid-phase extraction and reversed-phase high-performance liquid chromatography of the five major alkaloids in Narcissus confusus. *Phytochem. Anal.* **2002**, *13*, 311–315. [CrossRef] [PubMed]
16. Bastida, J.; Viladomat, F.; Llabres, J.M.; Codina, C.; Feliz, M.; Rubiralta, M. Alkaloids from Narcissus confuses. *Phytochemistry* **1987**, *26*, 1519–1524. [CrossRef]
17. Bohno, M.; Sugie, K.; Imase, H.; Yusof, Y.B.; Oishi, T.; Chida, N. Total synthesis of Amaryllidaceae alkaloids, (+)-vittatine and (+)-haemanthamine, starting from D-glucose. *Tetrahedron* **2007**, *63*, 6977–6989. [CrossRef]
18. Kogermann, K.; Penkina, A.; Predbannikova, K.; Jeeger, K.; Veski, P.; Rantanen, J.; Naelapää, K. Dissolution testing of amorphous solid dispersions. *Int. J. Pharm.* **2013**, *444*, 40–46. [CrossRef]
19. Shi, N.Q.; Yao, J.; Wu, Y.; Wang, X.L. Effect of polymers and media type on extending the dissolution of amorphous pioglitazone and inhibiting the recrystallization from a supersaturated state. *Drug Dev. Ind. Pharm.* **2014**, *40*, 1112–1122. [CrossRef]
20. Li, Z.; Wang, C. Effects of working parameters on electrospinning. In *One-Dimensional Nanostructures*; Springer: Berlin/Heidelberg, Germany, 2013; pp. 15–28.
21. Hu, X.; Liu, S.; Zhou, G.; Huang, Y.; Xie, Z.; Jing, X. Electrospinning of polymeric nanofibers for drug delivery applications. *J. Control. Release* **2014**, *185*, 12–21. [CrossRef]
22. Tantipolphan, R.; Rades, T.; McQuillan, A.J.; Medlicott, N.J. Adsorption of bovine serum albumin (BSA) onto lecithin studied by attenuated total reflectance Fourier transform infrared (ATR-FTIR) spectroscopy. *Int. J. Pharm.* **2007**, *337*, 40–47. [CrossRef] [PubMed]
23. PharmacyCodes. Haemanthamine [Online]. Available online: https://pharmacycode.com/Haemanthamine.html (accessed on 20 August 2019).
24. Maiti, K.; Mukherjee, K.; Gantait, A.; Saha, B.P.; Mukherjee, P.K. Curcumin-phospholipid complex: Preparation, therapeutic evaluation and pharmacokinetic study in rats. *Int. J. Pharm.* **2007**, *330*, 155–163. [CrossRef] [PubMed]

25. Koynova, R.; Caffrey, M. Phases and phase transitions of the phosphatidylcholines. *Biochim. Biophys. Acta* **1998**, *1376*, 91–145. [CrossRef]
26. Khan, A.U.R.; Nadeem, M.; Bhutto, M.A.; Yu, F.; Xie, X.; El-Hamshary, H.; El-Faham, A.; Ibrahim, U.A.; Mo, X. Physico-chemical and biological evaluation of PLCL/SF nanofibers loaded with oregano essential oil. *Pharmaceutics* **2019**, *11*, 386. [CrossRef] [PubMed]

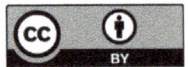

© 2019 by the authors. Licensee MDPI, Basel, Switzerland. This article is an open access article distributed under the terms and conditions of the Creative Commons Attribution (CC BY) license (http://creativecommons.org/licenses/by/4.0/).

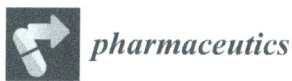

Communication

Design of a Novel Oxygen Therapeutic Using Polymeric Hydrogel Microcapsules Mimicking Red Blood Cells

Amanda Cherwin [1], Shelby Namen [1], Justyna Rapacz [1], Grace Kusik [1], Alexa Anderson [1], Yale Wang [2], Matey Kaltchev [1], Rebecca Schroeder [1], Kellen O'Connell [1], Sydney Stephens [1], Junhong Chen [2] and Wujie Zhang [1,*]

[1] BioMolecular Engineering Program, Physics and Chemistry Department, Milwaukee School of Engineering, Milwaukee, WI 53202, USA; cherwinae@msoe.edu (A.C.); namensl@msoe.edu (S.N.); rapaczj@msoe.edu (J.R.); kusikgo@msoe.edu (G.K.); andersonac@msoe.edu (A.A.); kaltchev@msoe.edu (M.K.); 13schrore@gmail.com (R.S.); kellen.d.oconnell@gmail.com (K.O.); sydneyjstephens@gmail.com (S.S.)
[2] Mechanical Engineering Department, University of Wisconsin-Milwaukee, Milwaukee, WI 53211, USA; yalewang@uwm.edu (Y.W.); jhchen@uwm.edu (J.C.)
* Correspondence: zhang@msoe.edu; Tel.: +1-414-277-7438

Received: 30 August 2019; Accepted: 5 November 2019; Published: 7 November 2019

Abstract: The goal of this research was to develop a novel oxygen therapeutic made from a pectin-based hydrogel microcapsule carrier mimicking red blood cells. The study focused on three main criteria for developing the oxygen therapeutic to mimic red blood cells: size (5–10 µm), morphology (biconcave shape), and functionality (encapsulation of oxygen carriers; e.g., hemoglobin (Hb)). The hydrogel carriers were generated via the electrospraying of the pectin-based solution into an oligochitosan crosslinking solution using an electrospinning setup. The pectin-based solution was investigated first to develop the simplest possible formulation for electrospray. Then, Design-Expert® software was used to optimize the production process of the hydrogel microcapsules. The optimal parameters were obtained through the analysis of a total of 17 trials and the microcapsule with the desired morphology and size was successfully prepared under the optimized condition. Fourier transform infrared spectroscopy (FTIR) was used to analyze the chemistry of the microcapsules. Moreover, the encapsulation of Hb into the microcapsule did not adversely affect the microcapsule preparation process, and the encapsulation efficiency was high (99.99%). The produced hydrogel microcapsule system shows great promise for creating a novel oxygen therapeutic.

Keywords: artificial red blood cells; electrospinning and electrospray; pectin; oligochitosan; hydrogel; microcapsules

1. Introduction

In the United States, approximately 36,000 units of red blood cells (RBCs) are needed every day, according to American Red Cross. However, less than 38 percent of the population is eligible to give blood or platelets [1]. Donated blood undergoes costly screenings before it can be used to test for infectious diseases, such as HIV and hepatitis B and C [2]. Factors including eligible donors, costly testing, and limited shelf-life also impact the available supply. While blood donations will always be necessary, an oxygen therapeutic has the potential to help alleviate a number of the complexities associated with blood supply and demand.

Different hemoglobin (Hb)-based oxygen therapeutics have been developed, but, unfortunately, no such product has been approved by the FDA for human use due to the toxicity of free hemoglobin, which can cause hypertension and cardiovascular dysfunction [3–6]. Nanoscale artificial oxygen transporter carriers, such as nanoparticles and liposomes, have been developed, showing promise in therapies such as wound healing and cancer treatment [7,8]. However, these carriers, even with PEGylation (which may lead to accelerated blood clearance (ABC)), tend to have a short circulation time compared with the 120 day circulation time of RBCs [6]. It is therefore critical to fully mimic the natural red blood cells, including their size and shape. Red-blood-cell-shaped carriers have been developed in recent years; for example, a polyelectrolyte microcapsule was produced using a red-blood-cell-shaped $Ca(OH)_2$ template [9]. However, low encapsulation efficiency (oxygen transporter molecules are encapsulated inside the carrier, not attached to the carrier surface) remains an issue [5,9–11].

The purpose of this research is to develop a polymeric microcapsule system which mimics red blood cells to encapsulate oxygen transporters for use as an oxygen therapeutic. In particular, this study focuses on three criteria for the development of the microcapsule oxygen therapeutic: size, morphology, and functionality. In our previous studies [5,12], micro-scale red-blood-cell-shaped hydrogel capsules, using pectin and oligochitosan, were successfully developed and were shown to be able to encapsulate macromolecules. However, it is challenging to produce microcapsules/particles of less than 100 μm using traditional methods/equipment [13]. The PRINT® technique has been used to fabricate red blood cell mimics but with a complex process [14]. The electrospinning setup for nanofiber production has been explored in order to generate microcapsules less than 10 μm in diameter through electrospray [15,16]. Electrospray offers such advantages as ease of upscaling and cost effectiveness. Very recently, electrospray based on an electrospinning setup has been successfully adopted to produce red-blood-cell-like microparticles [17,18]. As the electrospinning setup utilizes viscous liquids and a high voltage [19], pectin-based solution reformulation is necessary to increase the solution viscosity. The pectin-based solution and production process parameters were optimized through this research. Additionally, the impact of hemoglobin encapsulation on the key criteria and production process was explored. The result is a simplified and optimized production process of the pectin-based hydrogel microcapsules through formulation and parameter analysis. A pectin-based microcapsule encapsulating hemoglobin at the desired size and morphology was produced without adversely affecting the microcapsule preparation process.

2. Materials and Methods

2.1. Materials

Low methoxy (LM) pectin (20.4% esterification) was purchased from WillPowder (Miami Beach, FL, USA). Pharmaceutical grade oligochitosan (95% deacetylation) of 2 kD molecular weight was obtained from Zhejiang Golden-Shell Pharmaceutical Co. Ltd. (Yuhuan, Zhejiang, China). All other chemicals were purchased from Sigma-Aldrich (St. Louis, MO, USA) and used without additional purification.

2.2. Preparation of Hydrogel Microcapsules

Hydrogel microspheres were prepared through electrospray by using an electrospinning setup (Linari Engineering, Valpiana, Italy). A 6–10% (w/v) pectin solution was sprayed into a 5% (w/v) oligochitosan solution (gelation solution) for approximately 10–15 min. The hydrogel microspheres were formed by the formation of pectin-oligochitosan electrolyte complexes. To obtain hemoglobin-loaded hydrogel microcapsules, hemoglobin powder was dissolved in a small volume of deionized (DI) water and then mixed with the pectin solution gently before electrospray [5]. The mixture was then sprayed into the oligochitosan solution to form loaded hydrogel capsules.

2.3. Optimization of Hydrogel Microcapsule Preparation Process

Firstly, different concentrations of pectin were tested to determine the concentration to be used for the rest of the study. Moreover, preliminary testing was performed to select the parameters used for study as well as the working ranges for them (Table 1). Then, Design-Expert® (Version 11; Stat-Ease

Inc., Minneapolis, MN, USA) software was utilized to optimize the hydrogel microsphere preparation process. A Box–Behnken design (BBD) model was used. A total of 17 trials were run based on the design. Lastly, size and morphology were the responses for optimization. For the assessment of morphology, both size distribution and shape were considered and evaluated on a scale of 1–10. During optimization, the target size was between 5 and 10 µm with a morphology maximum rating of 10.

Table 1. Parameter optimization values. This table describes the optimized electrospray parameters determined using the Design-Expert® software.

Parameter	Range	Optimized Value
Voltage (kV)	20–25	25
Flow Rate [1]	5–15	15
Height (cm)	10–18	13

[1] The units of the flow rates shown are specific to the pump used.

2.4. Determination of Hemoglobin Encapsulation Efficiency

To determine the encapsulation efficiency, Hb-loaded microcapsules were prepared under the optimal condition. The encapsulation efficiency (EE) of hemoglobin within the capsules was determined by the difference between the initial amount of hemoglobin present and the unencapsulated hemoglobin in the supernatant:

$$EE = \frac{initial - unencapsulated}{initial} \times 100\% \quad (1)$$

A standard curve was generated, and hemoglobin concentrations were measured by using a UV–vis spectrophotometry (Evolution 60S; Thermo Fischer Scientific, Waltham, MA, USA) at 410 nm [5].

2.5. Characterization of the Hydrogel Microcapsules

Hydrogel microcapsules were dried in an oven and then Fourier transform infrared spectroscopy (FTIR; MIRacle 10, IR-Tracer 100; Shimadzu, Kyoto, Japan) was used to study the chemistry of the microcapsules.

3. Results and Discussion

3.1. Formulation of Hydrogel Microcapsules

In our previous studies [5,12], red-blood-cell-shaped microcapsules with diameters >300 µm, were successfully developed using a 3–4% (w/v) pectin solution through a vibration-based setup (minimum diameter of microcapsule/microbead which can be produced: 50 µm). Furthermore, a novel pectin-based nanofiber system was developed using an electrospinning setup. To reduce the microcapsule size, an electrospinning setup was chosen considering its capability to produce micro/nano-scale objects. Electrospinning, in general, involves a higher viscosity polymer solution and voltage compared with electrospray [19]. Both electrospray and electrospinning are based on similar principles. The major difference is the breaking of the jet, formed from the Taylor cone, into droplets during electrospray [19]. A pectin/PEO (viscosity enhancer)/glycerol (fluid modifier) mixture was tested and was able to produce red-blood-cell-shaped microcapsules less than 10 µm in size (data not shown). However, considering eventual industrial production and commercialization, a simple formulation is desired. To eliminate the viscosity enhancer and fluid modifier, 6–10% (w/v) pectin solutions were tested for their electrospray ability. When concentrations were lower than 7%, no biconcave-shaped microcapsules could be formed. On the other hand, the solution could not be sprayed when the concentration was higher than 9%. As a result, 8% was selected for formulating the hydrogel microcapsules.

3.2. Hydrogel Microcapsule Preparation Process Optimization

Based on the preliminary studies, voltage, flow rate, and height (from needle tip to the gelation solution (i.e., oligochitosan) surface) were found to have significant influences on the microcapsule preparation process and were chosen as the parameters for process optimization. As shown in Figure 1, the microcapsule morphology varied greatly when changing the process parameters. Table 1 describes the ranges of parameters explored to optimize the electrospray process and the Design-Expert® software was used to apply a Box–Behnken model to outline the 17 trials to be tested. Quadratic models were utilized to represent the data with the complete quadratic model shown in Equation (2). The software was then used to analyze the resulting diameter and morphology of at least 200 microcapsules per trial. The desired responses were a diameter of less than 10 µm and a maximum morphology rating of 10. The quadratic model basis for the 17 trials from the Design-Expert® software is shown below:

$$Y = \beta_0 + \sum_{i=1}^{k}(\beta_i X_i) + \sum_{i=1}^{k}(\beta_i X_i^2) + \sum_{i=1}^{k-1}\sum_{j>i}^{k}\beta_{ij}X_i X_j, \quad (2)$$

Y is the value of the response variable, β_0 is the intercept coefficient, the first β_i items are the linear coefficients, the second β_i items are the quadratic coefficients, and β_{ij} items are the coefficients of the interaction terms.

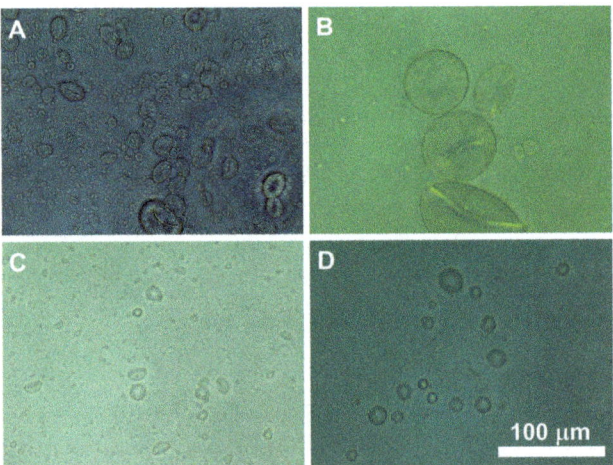

Figure 1. Representative images of microcapsules prepared during the optimization process. (**A**) Undesired shape and non-uniform size distribution; (**B**) Desired shape but large size; (**C**) Desired size but undesired shape; (**D**) Desired shape and size.

During the optimization process, the software returned the following equations based on the trial data input:

$$Y1 = -73.8429 + 3.3299A + 3.8211B + 3.4461C - 0.04478AB + 0.0199AC \\ - 0.1418BC - 0.1132A^2 - 0.0299B^2 - 0.0201C^2 \quad (3)$$

$$Y2 = 19.2689 + 1.6188A - 2.8900B - 0.4850C - 0.1125AB - 0.0438AC \\ + 7.0613E - 17\ BC + 0.0516A^2 + 0.1120\ B^2 + 0.0580C^2 \quad (4)$$

where Y1 and Y2 are size and morphology respectively, A, B, and C are the independent variables: height (cm), voltage (kV), and flow rate setting. Both models (Equations (3) and (4)) fit the model well, as the lack of fit is not significant with a p-value of 0.9913 and 0.1961, respectively.

As shown in Figure 1, images of microcapsules produced during the optimization experimentation were taken using an optical microscope (EVOS XL; Thermo Fisher Scientific, Waltham, MA, USA).

Figure 2 shows the surface response curves generated by Design-Expert® indicating the effects of two-factor interaction on capsule diameter and morphology. It was found that height (A) (p = 0.0328) produced a significant impact on microsphere size after model reduction by removing insignificant terms one at a time. The size of the droplet determines the size of the microcapsule. Under the same voltage, the electric field force decreases as the height increases [20,21]. However, the voltage had little effect on the microcapsule size, which might be due to the relatively narrow range of the voltage studied [22]. The significant terms found to impact the morphology are: B (p = 0.0095), AB (p = 0.0914) and C^2 (p = 0.0361). These findings indicated that the morphology of microcapsules produced during electrospray shares a linear relationship with voltage and a quadratic relationship with the flow rate. During electrospray, droplet formation is driven mainly by the interplay between surface tension, gravity, and electric field force. As the voltage increases, the microcapsule morphology improves. This could be explained by the formation of a stable jet leading to monodisperse droplets when electrostatic force rather than gravitational force dominates the pulling force against surface tension [20]. At the same time, increasing the flow rate leads to a more stable jet but larger droplets [13,23]. Moreover, both height and voltage affect the electric field strength, which explains the significant influence of the interaction term AB on microcapsule morphology [21].

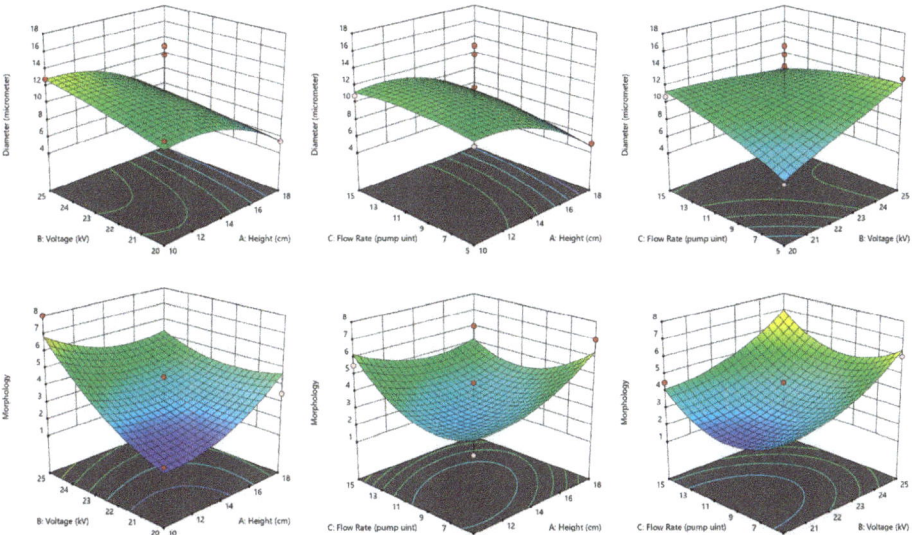

Figure 2. Response surface plots that show the effect of variables on the size (upper panel) and morphology (lower panel) before model reduction. The points which encompass the coordinates are displayed. Dark red dots: design points above predicted value; and pink dots: design points below predicted value.

Considering both responses, to achieve the highest morphology rating as well as a diameter of 5–10 µm, the optimized parameters were determined to be a height of 13 cm, a voltage of 25 kV, and flow rate setting of 15 (2.1 mL/hr) as shown in Table 1. All further experimentation was conducted using the optimal parameters, thereby improving the process.

3.3. Hemoglobin Encapsulation Efficiency

The encapsulation of Hb within the microcapsules was also investigated. It was confirmed that the hemoglobin could be successfully encapsulated within these capsules through a passive loading process with a very high encapsulation efficiency of 99.99 ± 0.06%. Hb-loaded microcapsules (Microencapsulated Hb) are shown in Figure 3. It can be noticed that the microcapsules show a biconcave shape with uniform size distribution. The encapsulation did not negatively impact the hydrogel microcapsule formation.

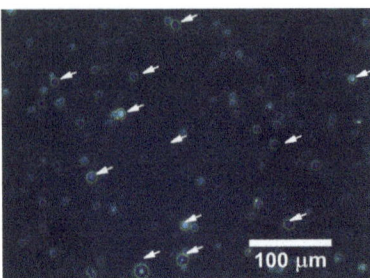

Figure 3. Image of hemoglobin (Hb)-loaded microcapsules (indicated by white arrows) prepared under the optimized condition.

FTIR spectroscopy was also used to confirm the successful encapsulation of hemoglobin within the microcapsules. As shown in Figure 4, the presence of Hb is clearly evidenced by the significant changes that occur in the Amide I and Amide II regions around 1530–1650 cm^{-1}. In particular, the peak around 1710 cm^{-1} becomes more pronounced due to the C=O stretching vibration of Hb [5,24]. This is also supported by the appearance of the strong peaks in the 1050–900 cm^{-1} region, which are typical for Hb [25].

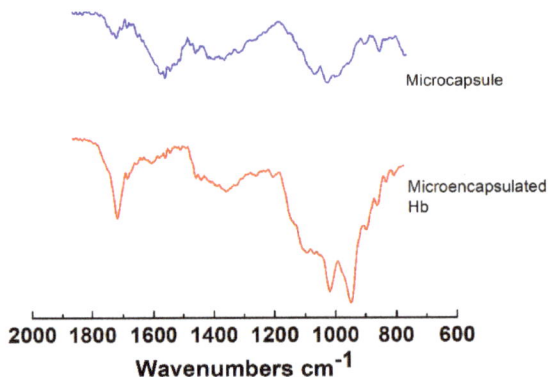

Figure 4. Fourier transform infrared (FTIR) spectra of hydrogel microcapsules and Hb-loaded microcapsules (microencapsulated Hb).

4. Conclusions

An 8% pectin solution, without a viscosity-modifier, was chosen as the formulation for the hydrogel microcapsule production. This formulation enables a simple and quick preparation, which is essential during future industrial-scale production. Furthermore, the removal of the viscosity-modifying chemicals allows for concentration of the sample via centrifugation, which was previously impossible. The optimized condition was determined by using the Design-Expert® software to produce microcapsules that are 5–10 µm in diameter and maintain a biconcave shape with a morphology resembling that of a natural red blood cell. Passive loading of hemoglobin into the microcapsules, confirmed by FTIR analysis, resulted in a high encapsulation efficiency of 99.99 ± 0.06%.

Future work includes stability testing of the hydrogel microcapsule carrier as well as oxygen transport property. Alternatives to hemoglobin such as a synthetic gas carrier will also be explored.

5. Patent

Polymeric red-blood-cell-like particles (Inventors: Wujie Zhang, Rebecca Schroeder, Sydney Stephens, Haley Stephens, Kellen O'Connell, Nataline Duerig, Devon McCune, Jung Lee, and Gene A. Wright; Publication number: 20190183982; Publication date: 20 June, 2019; U.S. Patent).

Author Contributions: A.C., S.N., J.R., G.K., A.A., Y.W., R.S., and S.S. performed the experiments; while K.O., M.K., and W.Z. performed data analysis. A.C., S.S., and W.Z. took the lead in the manuscript writing. W.Z. and J.C. supervised the project. All authors discussed the results and commented on the manuscript.

Funding: This work was funded by the Rader School of Business Seed Money Grant and the Faculty Summer Development Grant at the Milwaukee School of Engineering (MSOE).

Acknowledgments: The authors would like to recognize Krista Chamberlain, Mark Dunston, John Paul Carvalho, Katie Schuttenhelm, Bryson McCleary, Devon McCune, Nataline Duerig, and Haley Steiner for their technical assistance.

Conflicts of Interest: The authors declare no conflict of interest.

References

1. Facts about Blood Supply In The U.S. Available online: https://www.redcrossblood.org/donate-blood/how-to-donate/how-blood-donations-help/blood-needs-blood-supply.html (accessed on 14 August 2019).
2. World Health Organization. *Blood Donor Selection: Guidelines on Assessing Donor Suitability for Blood Donation*; World Health Organization: Geneva, Switzerland, 2012; Available online: https://apps.who.int/iris/handle/10665/76724 (accessed on 14 August 2019).
3. Chen, J.Y.; Scerbo, M.; Kramer, G. A review of blood substitutes: Examining the history, clinical trial results, and ethics of hemoglobin-based oxygen carriers. *Clinics (Sao Paulo)* **2009**, *64*, 803–813. [CrossRef]
4. Alayash, A.I. Blood substitutes: Why haven't we been more successful? *Trends Biotechnol* **2014**, *32*, 177–185. [CrossRef]
5. Zhang, W.; Bissen, M.J.; Savela, E.S.; Clausen, J.N.; Fredricks, S.J.; Guo, X.; Paquin, Z.R.; Dohn, R.P.; Pavelich, I.J.; Polovchak, A.L.; et al. Design of Artificial Red Blood Cells using Polymeric Hydrogel Microcapsules: Hydrogel Stability Improvement and Polymer Selection. *Int. J. Artif. Organs* **2016**, *39*, 518–523. [CrossRef]
6. Zhang, H.; Barralet, J.E. Mimicking oxygen delivery and waste removal functions of blood. *Adv. Drug Deliv. Rev.* **2017**, *122*, 84–104. [CrossRef]
7. Kawaguchi, A.T.; Okamoto, Y.; Kise, Y.; Takekoshi, S.; Murayama, C.; Makuuchi, H. Effects of liposome-encapsulated hemoglobin on gastric wound healing in the rat. *Artif. Organs* **2014**, *38*, 641–649. [CrossRef] [PubMed]
8. Murayama, C.; Kawaguchi, A.T.; Kamijo, A.; Naito, K.; Iwao, K.; Tsukamoto, H.; Yasuda, K.; Nagato, Y. Liposome-encapsulated hemoglobin enhances chemotherapy to suppress metastasis in mice. *Artif. Organs* **2014**, *38*, 656–661. [CrossRef]
9. She, S.; Li, Q.; Shan, B.; Tong, W.; Gao, C. Fabrication of red-blood-cell-like polyelectrolyte microcapsules and their deformation and recovery behavior through a microcapillary. *Adv. Mater.* **2013**, *25*, 5814–5818. [CrossRef] [PubMed]
10. Yadav, V.R.; Nag, O.; Awasthi, V. Biological evaluation of liposome-encapsulated hemoglobin surface-modified with a novel PEGylated nonphospholipid amphiphile. *Artif. Organs* **2014**, *38*, 625–633. [CrossRef]
11. Tao, Z.; Ghoroghchian, P.P. Microparticle, nanoparticle, and stem cell-based oxygen carriers as advanced blood substitutes. *Trends Biotechnol.* **2014**, *32*, 466–473. [CrossRef] [PubMed]
12. Crouse, J.Z.; Mahuta, K.M.; Mikulski, B.A.; Harvestine, J.N.; Guo, X.; Lee, J.C.; Kaltchev, M.G.; Midelfort, K.S.; Tritt, C.S.; Chen, J.; et al. Development of a Microscale Red Blood Cell-Shaped Pectin-Oligochitosan Hydrogel System Using an Electrospray-Vibration Method: Preparation and Characterization. *J. Appl. Biomater. Funct. Mater.* **2015**, *13*, 326–331. [CrossRef] [PubMed]

13. Zhang, W.; He, X. Encapsulation of Living Cells in Small (~100 μm) Alginate Microcapsules by Electrostatic Spraying: A Parametric Study. *J. Biomech. Eng.* **2009**, *131*, 074515. [CrossRef] [PubMed]
14. Merkel, T.J.; Jones, S.W.; Herlihy, K.P.; Kersey, F.R.; Shields, A.R.; Napier, M.; Luft, J.C.; Wu, H.; Zamboni, W.C.; Wang, A.Z.; et al. Using mechanobiological mimicry of red blood cells to extend circulation times of hydrogel microparticles. *Proc. Natl. Acad. Sci. USA* **2011**, *108*, 586. [CrossRef]
15. López-Rubio, A.; Sanchez, E.; Wilkanowicz, S.; Sanz, Y.; Lagaron, J.M. Electrospinning as a useful technique for the encapsulation of living bifidobacteria in food hydrocolloids. *Food Hydrocoll.* **2012**, *28*, 159–167. [CrossRef]
16. Mai, Z.; Chen, J.; He, T.; Hu, Y.; Dong, X.; Zhang, H.; Huang, W.; Ko, F.; Zhou, W. Electrospray biodegradable microcapsules loaded with curcumin for drug delivery systems with high bioactivity. *RSC Adv.* **2017**, *7*, 1724–1734. [CrossRef]
17. Hayashi, K.; Ono, K.; Suzuki, H.; Sawada, M.; Moriya, M.; Sakamoto, W.; Yogo, T. Electrosprayed synthesis of red-blood-cell-like particles with dual modality for magnetic resonance and fluorescence imaging. *Small* **2010**, *6*, 2384–2391. [CrossRef] [PubMed]
18. Hayashi, K.; Yamada, S.; Hayashi, H.; Sakamoto, W.; Yogo, T. Red blood cell-like particles with the ability to avoid lung and spleen accumulation for the treatment of liver fibrosis. *Biomaterials* **2018**, *156*, 45–55. [CrossRef] [PubMed]
19. Soares, R.M.D.; Siqueira, N.M.; Prabhakaram, M.P.; Ramakrishna, S. Electrospinning and electrospray of bio-based and natural polymers for biomaterials development. *Mater. Sci. Eng. C* **2018**, *92*, 969–982. [CrossRef]
20. Lai, W.-F.; Susha, A.S.; Rogach, A.L.; Wang, G.; Huang, M.; Hu, W.; Wong, W.-T. Electrospray-mediated preparation of compositionally homogeneous core–shell hydrogel microspheres for sustained drug release. *RSC Adv.* **2017**, *7*, 44482–44491. [CrossRef]
21. Moghaddam, M.K.; Mortazavi, S.M.; Khayamian, T. Preparation of calcium alginate microcapsules containing n-nonadecane by a melt coaxial electrospray method. *J. Electrost.* **2015**, *73*, 56–64. [CrossRef]
22. Bock, N.; Woodruff, M.A.; Hutmacher, D.W.; Dargaville, T.R. Electrospraying, a Reproducible Method for Production of Polymeric Microspheres for Biomedical Applications. *Polymers* **2011**, *3*, 131–149. [CrossRef]
23. Pathak, S.; Gupta, B.; Poudel, B.K.; Tran, T.H.; Regmi, S.; Pham, T.T.; Thapa, R.K.; Kim, M.-S.; Yong, C.S.; Kim, J.O.; et al. Preparation of High-Payload, Prolonged-Release Biodegradable Poly(lactic-*co*-glycolic acid)-Based Tacrolimus Microspheres Using the Single-Jet Electrospray Method. *Chem. Pharm. Bull.* **2016**, *64*, 171–178. [CrossRef] [PubMed]
24. Gao, W.; Sha, B.; Zou, W.; Liang, X.; Meng, X.; Xu, H.; Tang, J.; Wu, D.; Xu, L.; Zhang, H. Cationic amylose-encapsulated bovine hemoglobin as a nanosized oxygen carrier. *Biomaterials* **2011**, *32*, 9425–9433. [CrossRef] [PubMed]
25. Kuenstner, J.T.; Norris, K.H. Spectrophotometry of Human Hemoglobin in the near Infrared Region from 1000 to 2500 nm. *J. Near Infrared Spectrosc.* **1994**, *2*, 59–65. [CrossRef]

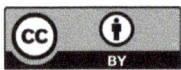

© 2019 by the authors. Licensee MDPI, Basel, Switzerland. This article is an open access article distributed under the terms and conditions of the Creative Commons Attribution (CC BY) license (http://creativecommons.org/licenses/by/4.0/).

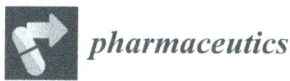

Article

Bi-Layered Polymer Carriers with Surface Modification by Electrospinning for Potential Wound Care Applications

Mirja Palo [1], Sophie Rönkönharju [1], Kairi Tiirik [2], Laura Viidik [2], Niklas Sandler [1] and Karin Kogermann [2,*]

[1] Pharmaceutical Sciences Laboratory, Åbo Akademi University, Tykistökatu 6A, FI-20520 Turku, Finland; mirja.palo@abo.fi (M.P.); sjer93@gmail.com (S.R.); niklas.sandler@abo.fi (N.S.)
[2] Institute of Pharmacy, University of Tartu, Nooruse 1, EE-50411 Tartu, Estonia; kairitiirik@hotmail.com (K.T.); laura.viidik@ut.ee (L.V.)
* Correspondence: karin.kogermann@ut.ee; Tel.: +372-737-5297

Received: 30 August 2019; Accepted: 10 December 2019; Published: 12 December 2019

Abstract: Polymeric wound dressings with advanced properties are highly preferred formulations to promote the tissue healing process in wound care. In this study, a combinational technique was investigated for the fabrication of bi-layered carriers from a blend of polyvinyl alcohol (PVA) and sodium alginate (SA). The bi-layered carriers were prepared by solvent casting in combination with two surface modification approaches: electrospinning or three-dimensional (3D) printing. The bi-layered carriers were characterized and evaluated in terms of physical, physicochemical, adhesive properties and for the safety and biological cell behavior. In addition, an initial inkjet printing trial for the incorporation of bioactive substances for drug delivery purposes was performed. The solvent cast (SC) film served as a robust base layer. The bi-layered carriers with electrospun nanofibers (NFs) as the surface layer showed improved physical durability and decreased adhesiveness compared to the SC film and bi-layered carriers with patterned 3D printed layer. Thus, these bi-layered carriers presented favorable properties for dermal use with minimal tissue damage. In addition, electrospun NFs on SC films (bi-layered SC/NF carrier) provided the best physical structure for the cell adhesion and proliferation as the highest cell viability was measured compared to the SC film and the carrier with patterned 3D printed layer (bi-layered SC/3D carrier). The surface properties of the bi-layered carriers with electrospun NFs showed great potential to be utilized in advanced technical approach with inkjet printing for the fabrication of bioactive wound dressings.

Keywords: electrospinning; wound dressings; solvent casting; 3D printing; polymeric carrier

1. Introduction

Wound dressings with different functionalities are widely used in medical applications to aid the healing process of acute and chronic wounds [1,2]. Typically, wound dressings are designed to contribute to the inhibition of bacterial contamination and infection development, and several other pharmacological and physical protection aspects of wound healing [1,2]. In modern preparations, the carriers are made from synthetic and natural polymers that have high biocompatibility and enable localized drug delivery with improved therapeutic efficacy [1,3]. Ideally, wound dressings should provide long-term functionality, maintain a moist healing environment, promote tissue regeneration, prevent any additional damage and cause minimal inconvenience to the patient [4]. On the other hand, mechanical and adhesive properties of wound dressings determine their producibility and durability upon storage and usage [1,4]. In addition, bioactive wound dressings with biologically active ingredients and/or active pharmaceutical ingredients (APIs), such as antibiotics, anti-inflammatory agents, vitamins and growth factors, are continuously being developed [3,5].

Wound dressings are produced by different methods depending on the desired structure and the materials used. In the current study, three commonly applied methods were exploited: solvent casting, extrusion-type three-dimensional (3D) printing and electrospinning. In solvent casting, polymeric films are prepared from drying of viscous solutions of polymer(s) with/without additives and active substances in a uniformly distributed layer [6,7]. Due to the simplicity of this method, solvent casting can be time-consuming, and the properties and stability of the films are dependent on the materials used [6,7]. Nevertheless, solvent cast (SC) polymer films are structurally more robust, and highly suitable to be exploited as base layer in multi-layered formulations.

Electrospinning is a versatile technology for the fabrication of polymeric fibers with good diffusion characteristics and high surface area to volume ratio, which are beneficial for wound care applications to hinder bleeding, absorb excessive wound fluid and promote tissue regeneration [4,8,9]. The stability, reproducibility and production yield of the electrospinning process is highly dependent on the compatibility of the materials: the polymer(s), the solvent(s) and other additives or active substances [10]. Furthermore, the concept of "green electrospinning", i.e., electrospinning of environmentally friendly and non-toxic polymeric materials and solvent systems, is gaining more attention especially in pharmaceutical and medical applications [11].

In general, 3D printing allows obtaining scaffolds with defined structures that could be exploited in various biomedical applications [12,13]. The extrusion-based 3D printing has been widely applied in bioprinting, i.e., printing of materials that contain living cells, and it is considered to be a gentle technique for manipulating semi-solid polymeric systems. This flexible method is used for tissue engineering, fabricating customized medical devices and drug delivery systems (DDSs) [14,15].

As wound dressings are expected to be actively contributing to the wound healing process, the utilization of multi-layered carriers could be beneficial. Previously, multi-layered drug-loaded formulations have been produced by electrospinning with a layer-by-layer approach [16–18], as well as by solvent casting [19]. Furthermore, integrated structures with improved mechanical strength can be obtained by electrospinning on top of 3D printed grid-like scaffolds [20]. A similar theoretical concept was recently presented by Maver et al. [21] for preparing a combination with carboxymethyl cellulose-based carriers manufactured by 3D printing and electrospinning for dual drug delivery from bi-layered wound dressings.

Inkjet printing is a technique, which has been used in pharmaceutical applications for the preparation of individualized DDSs [14,22]. It is a contactless method for precise deposition of liquids for tissue engineering [23] and pharmaceutical applications [24], as well as in fabrication of biosensors [25], ceramic [26] and electronic components [27], to name a few. Inkjet printing applies a drop-on-demand method for the signal-driven ejection of single droplets [28]. In DDSs, inkjet printing enables to control the precision of drug dosing and release behavior [29–31] and it has huge potential to be used as a method for preparing novel DDSs in combination with the polymeric carriers for wound healing applications.

Among various other materials, polyvinyl alcohol (PVA) is frequently used in polymeric carriers for medical applications due to its biocompatibility, solubility in water, non-toxicity, biodegradability, bioadhesiveness and processability [32,33]. In combination with other synthetic or natural polymers, the mechanical and physicochemical properties of PVA could be improved [34,35]. In addition, PVA-based formulations can be covalently crosslinked by different methods [36]. Sodium alginate (SA), a natural polymer extracted from brown algae, is widely used hydrophilic and biocompatible polymer in pharmaceutical applications [37]. A combination of PVA and SA is often used as a composite with improved liquid absorption, swelling, mechanical properties and thermal stability [32,38,39].

Considering the recent trends in the development of wound dressings, the utilization of combination fabrication approaches could be beneficial for preparing advanced wound dressings and novel DDSs. The aim of this study was to investigate a combinational technique for the fabrication of bi-layered carriers for the API delivery. The designed systems with modified surface layers were based on a polymer blend of PVA and SA. An electrospun layer was added onto the surface of solvent cast films of the same composition. The physicochemical, mechanical, adhesive properties of the carriers were characterized and compared with similar bi-layered carriers with 3D printed macroporous surface layer. Cell safety and viability testing was performed in order to understand the effect of different surface modifications on the cell behavior. Furthermore, a theoretical concept of inkjet printing of DDSs for the fabrication of bioactive wound dressings is presented.

2. Materials and Methods

2.1. Materials

Polyvinyl alcohol (PVA, Mowiol® 20–98, Mw 125,000 g/mol, 98.0–98.8 mol% hydrolysis, Sigma-Aldrich Chemie GmbH, Steinheim, Germany) and sodium alginate (SA, Sigma-Aldrich Chemie GmbH, Steinheim, Germany) were used as film forming agents. The polymer solutions were prepared separately and mixed to obtain final solutions. The PVA solutions were obtained by dissolving PVA in purified water at 85 °C under stirring. The SA solutions were obtained by dissolving SA in purified water at room temperature (RT, 20 ± 5 °C) under stirring. For solvent casting and electrospinning, a mixture of 12% PVA and 2% SA solutions in an 80:20 volume ratio (Solution A) was used. For three-dimensional (3D) printing, a mixture of 18% PVA and 3% SA solutions in an 80:20 ratio (Solution B) was used. Thus, the polymer weight ratio was kept constant throughout the system. A corresponding physical mixture (PM) of PVA and SA was prepared for reference.

2.2. Preparation of Carriers

2.2.1. Solvent Casting

Solvent cast (SC) films were cast from Solution A onto transparent copier film (Folex®IMAGING, X-10.0, Cologne, Germany) or aluminum foil with a film applicator (Multicator 411, ERICHSEN GmbH & Co. KG, Hemer, Germany) at a wet height of 500 μm. The SC films were lightly covered to prevent dusting and dried for 2 days at ambient conditions (RT and relative humidity (RH) of 35 ± 15%). The dried SC films were stored in the refrigerator (approximately 8 °C). The SC films were used as the base layer in the bi-layered carriers.

2.2.2. Electrospinning

The nanofiber (NF) mats were prepared from Solution A using the eS-robot© electrospinning machine (NanoNC, ESR-200Rseries, Seoul, Korea). The optimized single-spinneret electrospinning parameters were as follows: 23G needle, voltage of 11 ± 1 kV, flow rate of 0.3 mL/h and a distance of 15 cm between the needle tip and collector. The NF mats were collected onto a rotating metal collector (covered with aluminum foil) with a rotation speed of 25 rpm. The electrospinning was conducted at 25.4 ± 0.4 °C and RH of 17.5 ± 0.5%. A fiber mat of approximately 24 × 20 cm was obtained from 8 mL of Solution A. In the bi-layered solvent cast/nanofiber (SC/NF) carriers, the NFs were electrospun directly onto the SC films. Prepared NF mats and SC/NF carriers were stored in zip-lock bags in the refrigerator (approximately 8 °C) before further analysis.

2.2.3. 3D Printing

The patterned 3D printed (3D) mats were obtained from Solution B onto transparent copier film with semi-solid extrusion type Biobots 1 3D printer (BioBots Inc., Philadelphia, PA, USA, currently known as Allevi). The mats were printed as a single layer (wet height: 0.15 mm) in a 40% honeycomb infill pattern with 3 perimeters, creating a macroporous mat with an area of a 1.65 × 1.65 cm square. The 3D printing was performed with a 25G needle at a pressure of 60–70 psi with a printing speed of 4 mm/s. In the bi-layered solvent cast/3D printed (SC/3D) carriers, the patterned structure was 3D printed directly onto the SC films. The bi-layered SC/3D carriers were printed with a Biobots 1 3D printer and printer System 30M (Hyrel 3D, Norcross, GA, USA). Prepared 3D printed mats and SC/3D carriers were stored in zip-lock bags in the refrigerator (approximately 8 °C) before further analysis.

2.2.4. Crosslinking

A thermal crosslinking process was applied to make the carriers more stable in an aqueous environment. The thermal crosslinking was performed at 180 °C in an oven (Memmert, DIN 12880, Schwabach, Germany) for 10 min.

2.3. *Characterization Methods*

2.3.1. Visualization

Microscopic images of the carriers were obtained with an Evos XL Imaging System (InvitrogenTM, Thermo Fisher Scientific, Waltham, MA, USA), ProScope digital microscope (Bodelin Technologies, PSEDU-100, Oregon City, OR, USA) and scanning electron microscopes (SEM). The non-crosslinked electrospun NF mats were visualized with SEM (EVO MA 15, Zeiss®, Oberkochen, Germany) after magnetron-sputter coating with a 3 nm gold layer in an argon atmosphere. The crosslinked NF mats and bi-layered carriers were visualized with SEM (Leo Gemini 1530, Zeiss®, Oberkochen, Germany) that was equipped with secondary electron and In-Lens detectors. The bi-layered carriers were sputter-coated with carbon using a vacuum evaporator prior to imaging. The images were analyzed with ImageJ software (1.51j8, National Institute of Health, Bethesda, MD, USA).

2.3.2. Texture Analysis

The mechanical strength of the carriers was measured by a puncture test method using TA.XT*plus* Texture Analyzer (Stable Micro Systems, Surrey, UK) equipped with a film support rig and a spherical stainless steel probe ($\varnothing$ = 5 mm). The measurements settings were as follows: pre-test speed of 2 mm/s, test speed of 1 mm/s and a post-test speed of 10 mm/s. The maximum force (N) needed to break the carriers was recorded (burst strength).

A digital caliper (Mitutoyo, 500-171-21, CD-6", Kawasaki, Japan) was used to measure the thickness of the carriers.

2.3.3. Solid-State Characterization

The infrared (IR) spectra were collected from the carriers and the raw materials with a universal attenuated total reflectance Fourier transform IR spectroscope (ATR-FTIR, UATR Two, Perkin Elmer, Llantrisant, UK). The measurements were conducted in a spectral range from 450 to 4000 cm^{-1} with 4 scans per spectrum (n = 3). The data collection and the baseline correction of the IR spectra were performed with Spectrum 10.03 software (PerkinElmer, Llantrisant, UK).

The thermal properties of the SC films and electrospun NFs were measured by differential scanning calorimetry (DSC, Pyris Diamond, PerkinElmer, Waltham, MA, USA). Samples of 1–3 mg were analyzed in 30 µL aluminum pans with pierced lids. A heating rate of 10 °C/min was used in a measuring range of 25–250 °C. An N$_2$ purge gas was used with a flow rate of 40 mL/min. The DSC system was calibrated using indium (156.6 °C). Thermograms were baseline corrected prior to analysis.

2.3.4. Stability Study

A short-term stability study for one month was performed with non-crosslinked and thermally crosslinked SC films and electrospun NF mats. The samples were stored at two separate conditions: i) RT and low humidity (RH of 0%), and ii) accelerated conditions [40] at elevated temperature (40 °C) and humidity (RH of 75%). The solid-state properties of the samples were measured at three time points (24 h, 1 week, 1 month) by ATR-FTIR and DSC spectroscopy.

2.4. Behavior of Bi-Layered Carriers in Biorelevant Conditions and During DDSs Preparation

2.4.1. Swelling and Degradation in Aqueous Environment

The stability of the non-crosslinked and crosslinked carriers in aqueous environment was studied. The samples (1.65 × 1.65 cm squares) were weighed and immersed in 10 mL of pH 7.4 phosphate buffer saline (PBS) solution. The samples were mixed (30 rpm) at 37 °C for 24 h, 3 days and 7 days. The mass of the samples was recorded with a microbalance (d = 1 µg, MYA 2.4Y, Radwag Wagi Elektronicze, Radom, Poland).

The swelling degree was calculated as percentage of swelling ratio using Equation (1) [41]:

$$\text{Swelling degree (\%)} = (W_s - W_0 / W_0) \times 100, \tag{1}$$

where W_s is the swollen sample and W_0 is the initial sample weight. The swollen samples were weighed after excess fluid had been removed with filter paper immediately after taking the samples out of the PBS solution.

The degree of degradation was calculated as percentage of weight loss by Equation (2) [41]:

$$\text{Degradation degree (\%)} = (W_0 - W_1) / W_0 \times 100, \tag{2}$$

where W_0 is the initial weight of the sample and W_1 is the dry weight of the sample obtained after PBS immersion. The samples were dried for 7 days under a ventilated fume hood prior to weighing.

2.4.2. Simulated Bioadhesion Study

The adhesion of the non-crosslinked and thermally crosslinked carriers to artificial skin (VitroSkin® N-19, IMS Inc., Cape Coral, FL, USA) was tested with TA.XT*plus* Texture Analyser (Stable Micro Systems, Surrey, UK) equipped with a mucoadhesion rig and a cylinder delrin® probe (ø = 10 mm) at ambient conditions. A method developed by Tamm et al. [42] was used in a slightly modified format. Shortly, circular samples (ø = 11 mm) of the carriers were prepared and attached to the probe with an adhesive double-sided tape (Scotch™, 3M, Livonia, MI, USA). Simulated wound fluid (200 µL/sample) was pipetted on the artificial skin before the measurement. The simulated wound fluid contained 2% bovine serum albumin (Sigma-Aldrich, St Louis, MO, USA), 0.02 M $CaCl_2 \cdot 2H_2O$ (Merck, Darmstadt, Germany), 0.4 M NaCl (Sigma-Aldrich, St Louis, MO, USA), 0.08 M tris(hydroxymethyl)-aminomethane (Merck, Darmstadt, Germany) and purified water [43]. The testing conditions were set as follows: pre-test speed 0.5 mm/s, test speed 0.5 mm/s, post-test speed 5 mm/s, applied force 1 N, return distance 100 mm, contact time 60 s, and trigger force 0.05 N. Scotch™ adhesive double-sided tape and commercial wound dressing Aquacel™ (ConvaTec Inc., Reading, UK) were used as references.

2.4.3. Safety of Bi-Layered Carriers and the Effect of Surface Modification on Cell Viability

Safety studies of bi-layered crosslinked and non-crosslinked carriers were carried out using baby hamster kidney (BHK-21) fibroblast cells. Cells were grown in the Glasgow Minimal Essential Medium (GMEM) supplemented with 7.5% fetal bovine serum (FBS), 2% Tryptose Phosphate Broth Difco (TPB, Midland Scientific Inc., Omaha, NE, USA), 20 nM HEPES, 100 µg/mL penicillin and 100 µg/mL streptomycin. For the viability study, cells were placed into 24-well plates and grown 24 h at 37 °C in 5% CO_2 incubator. Samples with a size of 1 cm^2 were placed into the wells on top of the cells, media was changed and incubated for another 24 h. Safety was assessed qualitatively by optical microscopy and quantitatively by trypan blue exclusion (automated cell counter, Invitrogen, Thermo Fischer Scientific, Waltham, MA, USA), counting dead and live cells from which the viability (%) was calculated. The experiment was carried out in triplicate, whereas cells exposed only to the growth medium or placed on top of the glass plate in growth medium were used as healthy untreated controls.

To evaluate the viability of cells on bi-layered crosslinked carriers and crosslinked SC film, the MTS cell proliferation assay was performed. Samples were placed into 24-well plates using cell crown inserts (CellCrown®, Scaffdex Oy, Tampere, Finland). Size of the samples was 1.5 × 1.5 cm. 500 µL of BHK-21 cells were seeded on the samples, the number of cells per well was approximately 50,000. 700 µL of GMEM was added. After 24 h incubation the samples were removed from the inserts, washed with 1× PBS, then transferred to 500 µL Dulbecco's Modified Eagle medium (DMEM) without phenol red, and 80 µL of MTS reagent (K300-500, Biovision, Milpitas, CA, USA) was added. After 45 min of incubation at 37 °C in 5% CO_2 incubator the colored medium was pipetted onto a 96-well plate and absorbance was measured using plate reader at 490 nm. The experiment was carried out in triplicate together with appropriate controls. The graphs show the relative viable cell numbers whilst the substrates with the highest cell numbers obtained were considered as 100%.

2.4.4. Surface Behavior During Inkjet Printing

Inkjet printing was used to investigate the surface behavior of the bi-layered carriers upon contact with aqueous ink solution. A mixture of propylene glycol (PG, Sigma-Aldrich, St Louis, MO, USA) and purified water in 40:60 ratio with viscosity of 3.9 mPa·s and surface tension of 47.4 mN/m was used as the ink solution. Red food color (9%, Dr. Oetker Sverige AB, Gothenburg, Sweden) was included in the ink solution prior to printing for better visualization. The ink was deposited on the carriers with a piezoelectric inkjet printer (PixDro LP50, Meyer Burger Technology Ltd., Thun, Switzerland) equipped with a Spectra® SL-128AA printhead (Fujifilm, Valhalla, NY, USA) at a resolution of 100 dpi. The average droplet size of the ink during printing was approximately 45 pL.

A CAM 200 contact angle goniometer (KSV Instruments Ltd., Espoo, Finland, currently known as Biolin Scientific) paired with a camera (Basler, Ahrensburg, Germany) and OneAttension software (Theta1.4) was used for contact angle (sessile drop method) measurements. The shape of the 5 µL droplets was recorded at 24 ± 1 °C in the triplicate measurements.

2.5. Data Analysis

Results are expressed as a mean ± standard deviation (SD). Statistical analysis was performed by two-tailed Student's *t*-test assuming unequal variances with Microsoft Office Excel 365 ProPlus software ($p < 0.05$) where applicable.

3. Results and discussion

3.1. Characterization of Solvent Casted (SC) Films, Electrospun Nanofibers (NFs) and 3D Printed Mats

Before the preparation of bi-layered carriers, each layer was prepared separately and characterized. The SC films obtained were transparent with smooth surface (Supplementary Figure S1). After thermal cross-linking the films turned to yellowish, but no other structural changes nor cracking were observed (Supplementary Figure S1).

The SEM imaging showed the formation of well-defined nanofibrous structures by electrospinning (Figure 1). Electrospinning process was slow, but the solution was electrospinnable within those conditions after optimization. A low degree of merging of fibers was noted in non-crosslinked NF mats, possibly due to imperfect drying of the polymer solution. However, no visible changes were detected in the fiber morphology after crosslinking (Figure 1C). The diameter of the fibers followed a unimodal distribution trend in the nanometer-range (Figure 1). The average diameter increased slightly after crosslinking with a significant change in the distribution range of the fiber diameter.

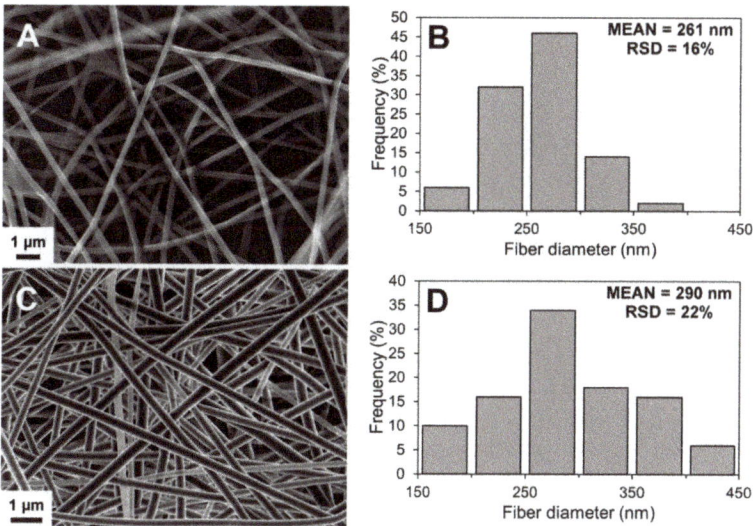

Figure 1. Scanning electron microscopy (SEM) image (**A**) and fiber diameter histogram (**B**) of non-crosslinked solvent cast/nanofiber (SC/NF) carriers, and SEM image (**C**) and fiber diameter histogram (**D**) of crosslinked SC/NF carriers with mean and relative standard deviation (RSD) values ($n = 50$).

The 3D printed mats were prepared by semi-solid extrusion 3D printing. Recently, this method was applied to prepare warfarin-loaded orodispersible films [44]. Here, the 3D printing of macroporous mats was performed onto a plastic support liner with a honeycomb infill pattern. The 3D printed pattern was clearly visible after printing (Supplementary Figure S2) and the dried mats remained intact after removal from the copier film. The 3D printed mats contained a patterned matrix with lemon-shaped pores with dimensions of approximately 990 × 1620 μm ($n = 8$).

3.2. Preparation and Structure of Bi-Layered Carriers

The bi-layered carriers were prepared through multi-step manufacturing processes (Figure 2). Adding a surface layer onto the SC film allows modifying the structure and functionality of wound dressings. In the bi-layered carriers, the use of same polymer composition enabled to create structures, where a thin layer of electrospun NFs adhered to the SC film base layer.

Preparing uniformly fibrous scaffolds for skin regeneration and wound healing requires a production of fiber mats that have the thickness and mechanical strength suitable for application handling. The production speed of electrospun fibers can be slow and varies considerably depending on the electrospinning setup and polymer system. The presented approach addresses these key aspects in the production of wound dressings. Adding a thin layer of electrospun fibers onto a strong polymer film could decrease the production time, improve cost-effectiveness, while still providing the unique properties, e.g., nanofibrous and porous structure together with the required adhesive and skin protective properties.

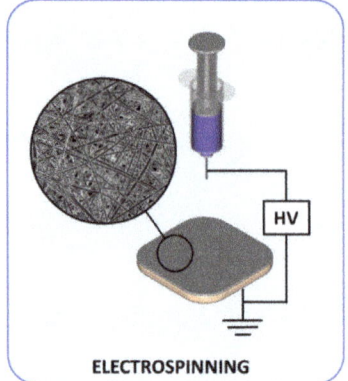 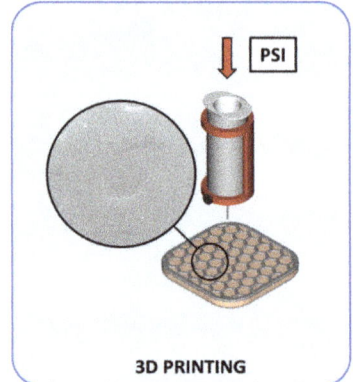

Figure 2. Preparation schematics of the designed bi-layered carriers for wound care. Key: HV—high voltage; 3D—three dimensional; PSI—pressure in pound per square inch.

Even though, the 3D printed mats could be used without any support layer, the bi-layered SC/3D carriers were prepared to investigate the differences presented by the additional surface layer onto the SC base layer. The patterned 3D printed mat covered 76 ± 4% ($n = 2$) of the sample area leaving a macroporous structure with small palpable cavities on the carrier surface. The shape of the design was not retained entirely, and the printing coverage was higher than the theoretical estimate (51%). This can be explained by the insufficient viscosity of the printed polymer solution, and the high shear forces applied in the needle tip during printing that further affected the viscosity of the solution.

In the bi-layered SC/NF and SC/3D carriers, the directly applied additional layer merged with the SC film and was non-removable. The structure of the carriers remained intact and the layers did not separate from each other (no lamination) during thermal crosslinking. In all formulations, the thermal treatment resulted in extensive crosslinking that caused a visible color change from white to yellowish as also previously reported [41,45]. In a study by Fuchs at al. [46], heat sealing was utilized to unite polycaprolactone (PCL)-based SC films and 3D structures obtained by melt electrospinning writing. This type of an extra step was not required in the setup presented here for the polymer blend with PVA and SA. It gives some supportive evidence that also drug-loaded systems (mats) can be produced using the same approach: the combination of the two techniques and using same ingredients.

3.3. Physical Properties

The physical properties of the SC films and the bi-layered carriers were measured to evaluate the effect of the additional layer to the SC base layer (Table 1). Expectedly, the thickness of the bi-layered carriers was increased compared to the SC film. The crosslinking affected the thickness of bi-layered SC/NF carriers, suggesting a notable thermal expansion in the fibrous structure. The thickness of both crosslinked bi-layered formulations was comparable to the copy paper (0.09 ± 0.01 mm).

Table 1. Physical properties of the solvent cast (SC) film, the electrospun nanofiber (NF) mat, the patterned 3D printed (3D) mat and the bi-layered carriers.

Sample Treatment	Thickness [a] (mm)	Puncture Test [a]		Swelling Degree [b] (%) After 24 h	Degradation Degree [b] (%) After 7 h
		Burst Strength (N)	Distance at Break (mm)		
Solvent Cast (SC) Film					
non-crosslinked	0.04 ± 0.01	40.2 ± 14.9	5.0 ± 2.1	NA	NA
crosslinked	0.03 ± 0.02	37.4 ± 30.2	3.1 ± 0.9	↑ 69 ± 19	↓ 1.2 ± 1.2
Electrospun Nanofiber (NF) Mat					
non-crosslinked	NA	NA	NA	NA	NA
crosslinked	NA	NA	NA	↑ 401 ± 52	↓ 4.9 ± 5.9 [c]
Patterned 3D Printed (3D) Mat					
non-crosslinked	0.04 ± 0.01	5.3 ± 1.1	2.9 ± 0.7	NA	NA
crosslinked	0.05 ± 0.01	5.3 ± 1.3	2.6 ± 0.4	↑ 75 ± 39	↓ 6.7 ± 0.7
Bi-Layered Solvent Cast/Nanofiber (SC/NF) Carrier					
non-crosslinked	0.05 ± 0.01	36.8 ± 5.7	6.4 ± 0.8	NA	NA
crosslinked	0.09 ± 0.02	45.5 ± 12.4	3.4 ± 0.8	↑ 338 ± 35	↓ 0.2 ± 0.3
Bi-Layered Solvent Cast /3D Printed (SC/3D) Carrier					
non-crosslinked	0.08 ± 0.03	38.4 ± 31.2	4.3 ± 1.8	NA	NA
crosslinked	0.11 ± 0.04	31.3 ± 10.9	2.4 ± 0.4	↑ 133 ± 20	↓ 2.8 ± 0.6

[a] mean ± standard deviation, $n = 10$; [b] mean ± standard deviation, $n = 3$; [c] after 24 h; NA—not applicable.

The puncture test revealed a high deviation in the burst strength of the carriers (Table 1). This can be contributed to the non-uniformity in the polymer films due to fluctuations in the drying conditions, volume of residual solvent [47] as well as other preparation related factors. The difference in the burst strength (N) between non-crosslinked and thermally crosslinked samples was shown to be statistically non-significant. However, the decrease in the distance at break (mm) in the crosslinked SC film and the bi-layered carriers suggests that the thermal treatment affected the elasticity of the formulation. On the other hand, the SC/NF carriers showed a slight increase in the average burst strength after crosslinking and longer distance to break (mm) compared to the SC/3D carriers. The addition of 3D printed layer seemed to decrease the elasticity of the crosslinked carriers, whereas this effect was not pronounced for the crosslinked carriers with electrospun NFs. Previously, it has been reported that NF mats from only PVA become brittle after thermal crosslinking [41]. In this study, the addition of SA to the mixture seemed to improve the integrity of the NF layer, and thus durable carriers with improved mechanical properties were obtained.

The effect of crosslinking was demonstrated in the stability study in an aqueous environment. The non-crosslinked samples disintegrated rapidly after immersion into the PBS solution (<24 h). The thermally treated samples remained visibly intact throughout the study period of 7 days. In an earlier study, crosslinked films of PVA and SA were investigated for 48 h with 10 subsequent cycles of dissolution and drying without any visible changes to their integrity [48]. Nevertheless, the swelling and degradation processes occurred simultaneously at a constantly changing ratio in all crosslinked formulations.

The crosslinked SC films and SC/NF carriers showed no significant weight loss after 7 days (Table 1). Whereas, the average degradation degree for SC/3D samples was 2.8% after 7 days, indicating that the additional 3D printed layer contributed to the interaction with the buffer solution due to increased surface area and/or decreased degree of crosslinking (thickness and volume of the carrier was higher compared to the SC film). As a comparison, the macroporous structure of the patterned 3D printed mats gave rise to an approximately 7% decrease in weight after immersion in the PBS solution for 7 days.

Due to the use of same materials, the combined layers in the bi-layered carriers showed high compatibility. No layer separation was detected in the bi-layered formulations after immersion in the PBS solution (Figure 3). Furthermore, the distinct surface structures remained visible after 7 days in aqueous environment. Notably, the surface of the SC/NF carriers was smoother due to the swelling and adhesion of the NFs to each other (Figure 3B).

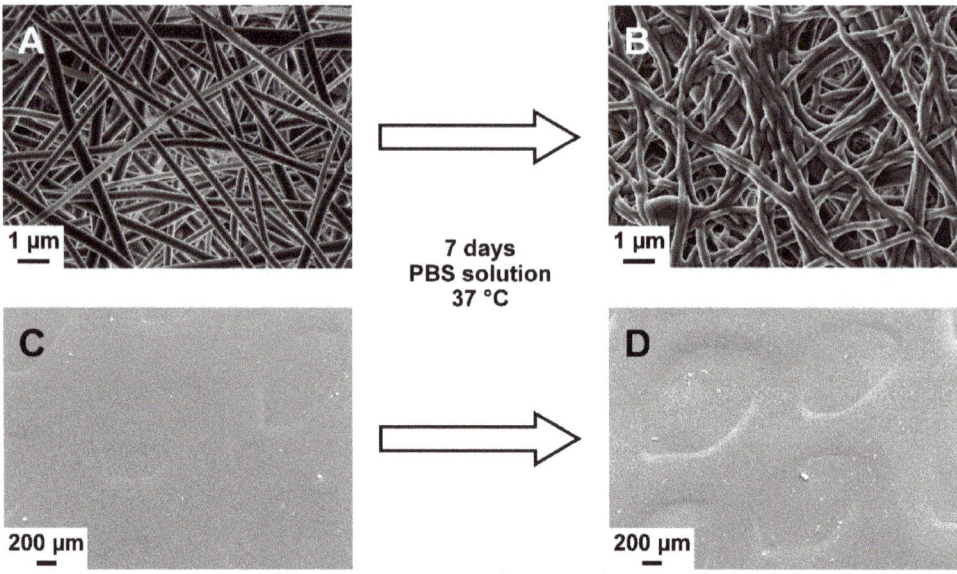

Figure 3. Scanning electron microscopy (SEM) images of crosslinked solvent cast/nanofiber (SC/NF) (**A**,**B**) and solvent cast/3D printed (SC/3D) (**C**,**D**) carriers before (**A**,**C**) and after (**B**,**D**) immersion in phosphate-buffered saline (PBS) solution at 37 °C for 7 days.

An initial burst in the uptake of water and/or salts from the buffer solution manifested within the first 24 h and declined later. The swelling degree was significantly higher for the SC/NF carriers compared to the SC/3D carriers (Table 1). The absorptive properties attributed to the NF structures promotes their applicability in wound care applications [9,49]. For example, manyfold higher absorption ratios have been reported for fibrous alginate wound dressings and other commercial gauzes using a different experimental setup [50]. In PVA/SA hydrogels, the water absorption and swelling capacity has shown to be dependent on the SA content [51]. Thus, the results suggest that in the preparation of bi-layered carriers the incorporation of NFs improves the degree of liquid uptake and usability as wound dressings. Furthermore, the liquid absorption degree would be improved by adjusting the polymer ratio in the formulations.

3.4. Stability and Solid-State Characterization

The stability and solid-state characteristics of SC films and electrospun NF mats were studied at two different conditions for one month. Spectroscopic analysis identified several absorbance bands characteristic to the raw materials (Figure 4). The spectrum of SA displayed absorbance bands in the fingerprint region for carboxylate group at 1598 and 1407 cm^{-1}, and skeletal C–O–C linkage at 1027 cm^{-1} [52,53]. The high degree of hydrolysis (98.0–98.8%) for pure PVA was seen by the low intensity of the absorption band in the 1700–1750 cm^{-1} region [54]. The preparation of aqueous solutions for electrospinning and 3D printing as well as the preparation processes themselves affected slightly the PVA hydrolysis degree in the prepared formulations. The intensity decrease of absorbance band at approximately 1715 cm^{-1} was observed in the spectra of the non-crosslinked/crosslinked SC films and electrospun NF mats compared to the spectrum of PVA and SA physical mixture (Figure 4). Interestingly, the crosslinking of the SC films and NF mats did not have an additional effect on the hydrolysis degree of PVA (based on the intensity of the absorbance band at 1715 cm^{-1}). Hence, the intensity of the band at 1715 cm^{-1} was similar with the intensity in the spectra of non-crosslinked samples (NF mats and SC films).

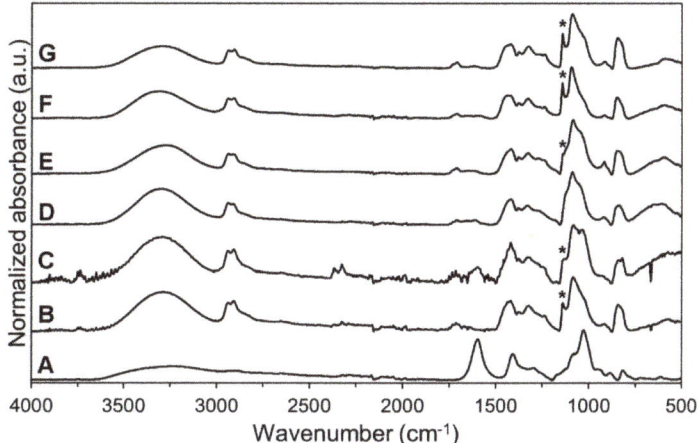

Figure 4. Attenuated total reflectance Fourier transform IR spectroscopy (ATR-FTIR) spectra (spectral range from 4000 to 500 cm^{-1}) of sodium alginate (SA) (**A**) and polyvinyl alcohol (PVA) powders (**B**); physical mixture of SA and PVA powders (**C**); non-crosslinked electrospun nanofiber (NF) mat (**D**); non-crosslinked solvent cast (SC) film (**E**); crosslinked electrospun NF mat (**F**) and crosslinked SC film (**G**). Asterisk (*) denotes the absorption band at 1141 cm^{-1} used to evaluate the crystallinity of PVA.

A broad absorbance band, attributed mainly to the hydroxyl groups in the molecules, was present in the range of 3600–3200 cm^{-1}. The broadening and intensity changes of the absorbance band for OH$^-$ groups were in correlation with the water content, degree of hydrolysis and the crystallization degree of the formulations. The ratio between the intensities of the absorbance bands at 3400–3200 cm^{-1} and 1420 cm^{-1} is related to the degree of chemical crosslinking [54]. The decreased ratio in the intensities refers to the higher degree of crosslinking. In the crosslinked SC films and electrospun NF mats it was seen that the ratio of the mentioned peaks was decreased. Thus, a relationship between thermal crosslinking and the presence of OH$^-$ groups was confirmed. These changes are most likely due to the decrease in the water content and hydrolysis. However, the presence of other crosslinking mechanisms cannot be confirmed.

The changes related to the absorption band at 1141 cm^{-1} (marked with an asterisk on Figures 4 and 5) were evaluated closely due to the strong relation between the peak intensity and the crystallinity of PVA [41,54,55]. All NF mats prepared by electrospinning were in an amorphous state, whereas the SC films showed to exhibit a semi-crystalline state (Figure 4). The amorphous state of the non-crosslinked NF mats was stable during storage at low humidity (Figure 5). However, the degree of crystallinity in the non-crosslinked NF mats increased at elevated storage conditions (40 °C and RH of 75%). The crystallinity in the non-crosslinked SC films increased over time at both storage conditions.

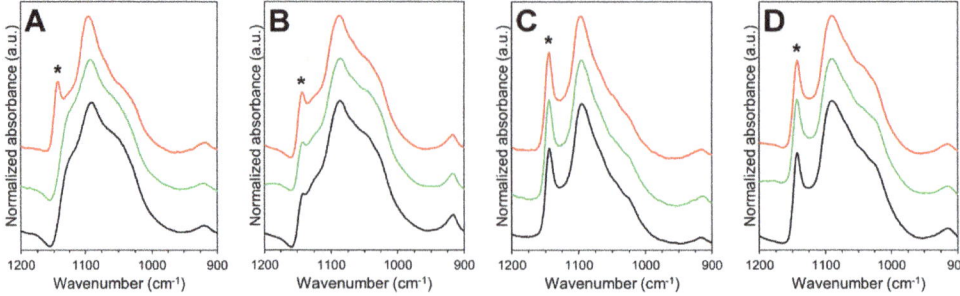

Figure 5. ATR-FTIR spectra (spectral range from 1200 to 900 cm^{-1}) from short-term stability study of non-crosslinked electrospun nanofiber (NF) mat (**A**) and solvent cast (SC) film (**B**); crosslinked electrospun NF mat (**C**) and SC film (**D**). Color legend: black—initial state, green—1 month at room temperature (RT) and relative humidity (RH) of 0%, red—1 month at 40 °C and RH of 75%. Asterisk (*) denotes the absorption band at 1141 cm^{-1} used to evaluate the crystallinity of polyvinyl alcohol (PVA).

Physical crosslinking of the SC films and electrospun NF mats resulted in the crystallization of the formulations. Similar findings have been previously reported by Miraftab et al. [41], where it was concluded that the degree of crystallinity is dependent on the temperature and heating time. The broadening of the absorption band for the hydroxyl group indicated that the crosslinking decreased the residual water content and/or inter- and intramolecular hydrogen bonding [56]. This phenomenon shows correlation with the physical properties of the carriers. During the stability study, no apparent changes in the solid-state properties of the crosslinked samples were detected at both storage conditions. On the other hand, the changes in the absorbance band for OH$^-$ groups indicated that the non-crosslinked SC films were more affected by the storage conditions than other formulations. The intensity of the absorbance band at 3400–3200 cm^{-1} increased about 70% after one month at elevated conditions (40 °C and RH of 75%) and decreased about 40% after storage at RT and RH of 0%.

The changes seen in the analysis of the infrared spectra are supported by the results from the thermal analysis by DSC. The semi-crystalline PVA exhibited a melting endotherm at 217 °C ($\Delta H \approx$ 75 J/g), which is in accordance with previous results [57]. SA is an amorphous material that decomposes in two steps—dehydration (approximately 100 °C) and exothermic decomposition (240–260 °C) [58]. The melting endotherm of non-crosslinked electrospun NFs (219 °C) increased slightly after incubation at elevated storage conditions due to changes caused by high humidity and temperature. As mentioned earlier, no changes were observed in the crosslinked electrospun NF mats at both storage conditions. The melting endotherm remained at approximately 214 °C with high enthalpy values ($\Delta H \approx$ 70 J/g) characteristic for formulations with crystalline PVA. The thermal analysis revealed no significant changes in the melting endotherm of SC films (217 °C) throughout the stability study. Interestingly, the SC samples exhibited some impurities and initial degradation above melting temperature, which was not apparent in the electrospun NF mats (data not shown).

A correlation between the solid-state properties and physical properties is obvious, and the properties of the carriers are highly affected by the thermal crosslinking. Therefore, the effect of time and storage-dependent solid-state changes on the physical properties of the carriers should be further investigated.

3.5. Bioadhesion within Simulated Wound Fluid

The force (N) and work (N·mm) required for the detachment of the carriers from the wetted artificial skin are presented in Figure 6. The effect of crosslinking on the adhesive properties is clearly visible for the samples. The NF mats and bi-layered carriers showed a statistically significant decrease in the detachment force (N) and the work of adhesion (N·mm) after crosslinking. However, the intact structure of the crosslinking patterned 3D printed mats seemed to increase their adhesion, while the polymer structure in the non-crosslinked samples dissolved fast upon contact with the simulated wound fluid.

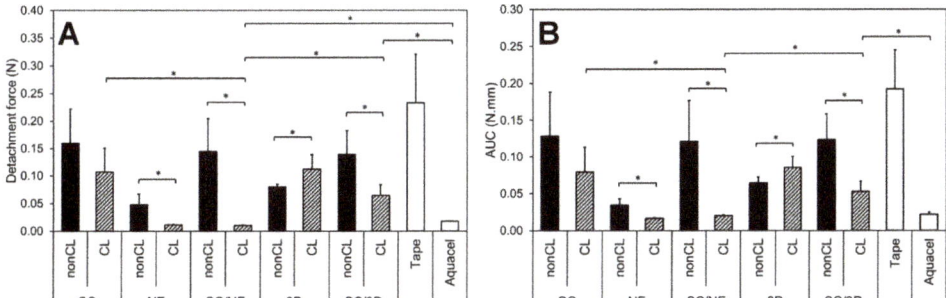

Figure 6. The detachment force (N) of adhesion (**A**) and work of adhesion as area under the curve (AUC, N.mm) (**B**) of non-crosslinked (nonCL) and crosslinked (CL) solvent cast (SC) film, electrospun nanofiber (NF) mat, bi-layered solvent cast/nanofiber (SC/NF) carrier, patterned 3D printed (3D) mat and solvent cast/3D printed (SC/3D) carrier as well as tape and Aquacel® wound dressing as reference (n = 5–8). Asterisk (*) denotes the statistical difference with $p < 0.05$.

In the bi-layered SC/NF carriers, the adhesiveness of the non-crosslinked formulations was comparable to the SC film base layer, indicating that the thin nanofibrous layer dissolved rapidly and did not contribute to the adhesion process. The relatively low adhesiveness of this formulation could be related to the low polymer concentration and viscosity of the in situ formed hydrogel [59].

The analysis revealed that in the crosslinked bi-layered SC/NF carriers the addition of electrospun NFs decreased the adhesiveness significantly compared to the SC film and SC/3D carriers (Figure 6). This indicates that bi-layered SC/NF carriers would be easily removable from damaged tissue and suitable for wound care applications. The intact crosslinked electrospun NF layer decreased the contact with the artificial skin surface most likely due to extensive swelling [60] with detachment values close to the detection limit. The SC/3D printed carriers behaved similarly to the SC film, suggesting that the macroporous surface structure is not enough to obtain favorable adhesive properties required for wound care.

An ideal wound dressing should be non-adherent and cause no additional injuries for the wound and pain to the patient during the removal [61]. However, in some cases the ability of wound dressings/skin adhesives to adhere on the skin or even on the damaged skin (e.g., hydrocolloid dressings) is crucial [62]. In the latter case, a good interaction between the dressing and the skin contributes to the absorption of excessive wound fluid and promotes healing by maintaining a moist environment [63]. Ideally, the wound dressings should be self-adhesive to the wound surface, yet easy and painless to remove [42]. Polymeric wound dressings are widely used; besides, if crosslinking is used to enhance their robustness, the adhesive properties of the formulations might be weakened [64,65], which was also apparent in the current study. Furthermore, the incorporation of APIs and/or use of polymer blends in the electrospun NF mats might significantly affect their bioadhesion, as it has been demonstrated with polyvinylpyrrolidone [42]. Thus, a balance between the mechanical and adhesive properties should be aimed for.

3.6. Safety of Bi-Layered Carriers and the Effect of Surface Modification on Cell Viability

Safety of all carriers were confirmed using BHK-21 fibroblast cells and direct viability testing method. All materials were biocompatible, and no statistically significant differences were observed between the carriers (non-crosslinked and thermally crosslinked) and untreated controls (Figure 7A and Supplementary Figure S3).

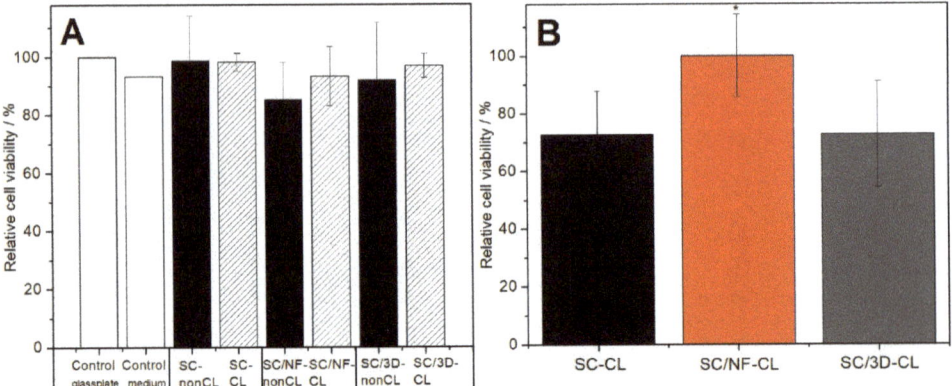

Figure 7. Cell viability assay results from trypan blue exclusion test (**A**) and MTS test (**B**) on different carriers: non-crosslinked (nonCL) and crosslinked (CL) solvent cast (SC) film, solvent cast/nanofiber (SC/NF) carrier and solvent cast/3D printed (SC/3D) carrier. Cells were incubated for 24 h and analyzed. Results presented as relative cell viability (%). In direct assay with trypan blue exclusion testing, the cell number of untreated BHK-21 fibroblasts on glass-plate was considered as a positive control providing 100% cell viability (other positive control was cells in plastic wells in growth medium). In MTS tests, the carrier with the highest cell viability (SC/NF-CL carrier) was considered as 100%. Data are expressed as mean ± standard deviation ($n = 3$). Asterisk (*) denotes the statistical difference with $p < 0.05$.

It was also confirmed that no changes in cell numbers were present due to the thermal crosslinking of the carriers. The latter nicely supports the findings observed in the solid-state characterization, as most likely no harmful substances (e.g., substances cytotoxic to fibroblast cells) were produced within the materials as a result of high temperature. Hence, such carriers, also stated as generally regarded as safe (GRAS) materials and approved within several medical devices by the U.S. Food and Drug Administration (FDA) [66], could be used for further wound dressing development.

Effect of surface modification on the cell viability was also determined. Crosslinked bi-layered SC/NF carrier enhanced the cell adhesion and proliferation as the highest cell viability (statistically significant, $p < 0.05$) was measured compared to other carriers, i.e., SC film and SC/3D carrier (Figure 7B). Interestingly, the cell viability on SC film and 3D/SC carriers was approximately the same (Figure 7B). Both materials (SA and PVA) are known to be biocompatible, biodegradable and good for the cells [67,68]. However, it is known that cells are able to sense the environment [69] and in addition to the material properties (internal chemical composition and the mechanical properties) [70], the material surface modification may change the behavior of the cells [71,72]. The overall idea of using surface modified structures is to stimulate the cells or their behavior. Usually the carriers used for the treatment of wounds are designed according to specific requirements and should provide a highly porous structure with interconnected pores [73]. These characteristics provide cells an appropriate environment for growth. Thus, carriers with such properties act as physical substrates for cell adhesion, proliferation, and differentiation, as well as for the integration to the host tissue in order to regenerate the defects, in case the mats are used as skin substrates. In the present study, it was also revealed that the porous electrospun surface layer provided the best surface for the cells. Interestingly, patterned 3D printed layer did not show superior cell viability values compared to the non-porous SC film. The latter most likely is due to the effect of too large pore size of the 3D printed layer. It is known that the best cell attachment for fibroblasts takes place between the pore size of 50–160 μm and nano-pored scaffolds with 1 μm pores improve the initial cell-surface interactions the most [74]. The pore size as well as geometry affect the successful regeneration of tissues [74].

3.7. Surface Properties During Inkjet Printing

Prior to inkjet printing, contact angle measurements were performed on the SC films and the bi-layered carriers (Figure 8). The contact angle of macroscale (5 μL) ink droplets on the non-crosslinked SC film was in the range of 31°–36°, which was significantly lower compared to the contact angle of purified water (70.8° ± 2.5°) on the same SC film.

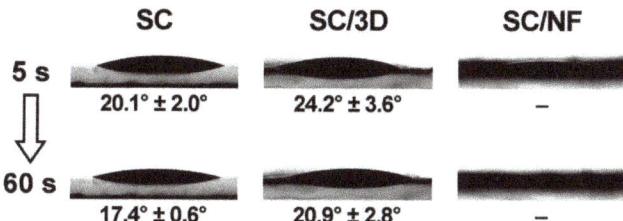

Figure 8. Contact angle (°) of the ink solution on crosslinked solvent cast (SC) film, bi-layered solvent cast/3D printed (SC/3D) carrier and solvent cast/nanofiber (SC/NF) carrier.

The crosslinking decreased the contact angle of the solution on the SC films (Figure 8). The ink droplets on the non-crosslinked and crosslinked SC/NF carriers spread out and absorbed the ink droplet quickly (<60 s). Thus, the contact angle could not be determined for these carriers. Whereas, the bi-layered SC/3D carriers behaved somewhat similarly to the SC films, which was expected. Although, the grid-like printed pattern on the SC/3D carriers caused higher variability in the contact angle values and irregularity in the droplet shape depending on the location of the deposition.

In general, the hydrophilicity of the carriers and the rheological properties of the ink solution contributed to the spreading and absorption of the solution into the surface layer of carriers. On the other hand, the carriers remained intact due to the thermal crosslinking.

Thereafter, inkjet printing was utilized to deposit microscale droplets of aqueous ink solution onto the bi-layered carriers to further investigate their surface characteristics. These measurements allowed revealing the behavior of the carriers and get an understanding about their use as DDSs for the wound healing application. The SEM images visualize clearly how the liquid adsorption differs on the surfaces of different carriers (Figures 9 and 10). The shape of the dried ink droplets is dependent on the liquid-carrier physical interaction, but also on the drying process. The higher contact angle between the liquid and the carrier surface allows obtaining deposited droplets with well-defined shape. Whereas, in the formulations that exhibit a lower contact angle the ink spreads out faster, and thus the shape of the droplet is uneven as the drying process is occurring simultaneously.

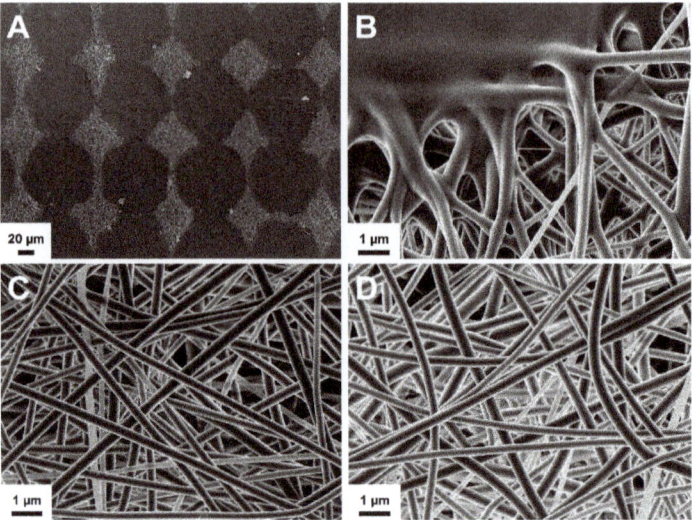

Figure 9. Scanning electron microscopy (SEM) images of non-crosslinked solvent cast/nanofiber (SC/NF) carrier after inkjet printing (**A**,**B**), and crosslinked SC/NF carrier before (**C**) and after (**D**) inkjet printing.

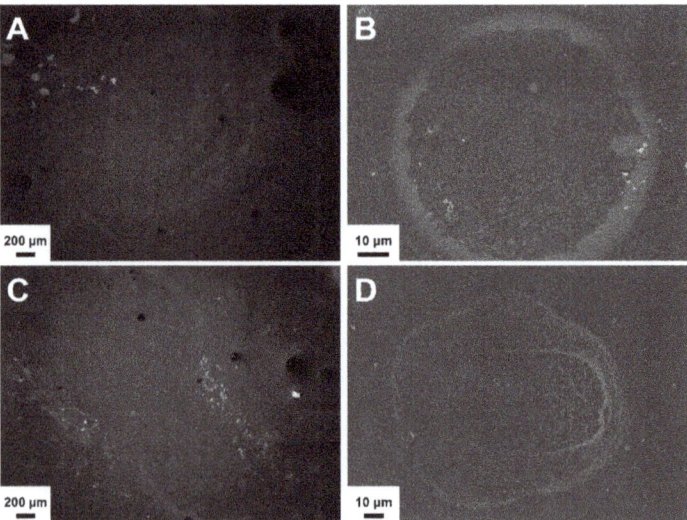

Figure 10. Scanning electron microscopy (SEM) images of non-crosslinked (**A**,**B**) and crosslinked (**C**,**D**) solvent cast/3D printed (SC/3D) carriers after inkjet printing.

On the SC/3D carriers, the ink droplets solidified mainly on the top layer and some sedimentation from the ink additives is visible on the droplet edges (Figure 10). The shape of the droplets indicates that the ink absorbed into the surface layer of the non-crosslinked SC/3D carrier, whereas on the crosslinked counterpart the ink dried in steps with minor penetration into the surface. In such formulations, the deposition of large liquid volumes would favor the droplets to merge within each other and result in an uneven coverage of the carrier.

The uniformity of ink deposition, which is a necessity to produce precision printed systems, was achieved for SC/NF carriers (Figure 9). In non-crosslinked SC/NF carriers, the ink solution dissolved the electrospun nanofibrous surface layer, resulting in a uniform liquid distribution. Besides that, the SC support film allowed for the carrier to remain intact and easy to handle. In crosslinked SC/NF carriers, separate ink droplets were not detectable by SEM, suggesting that the small amount of the solvent evaporated rapidly from the voids of the fibrous structure and any solid additives from the ink adhered to the surface of the NFs. The change in the light contrast (as difference in conductivity) of the SEM images obtained with the InLens detector could be related to this phenomenon (Figure 9).

Since the integrity of the nanofibrous system was maintained, the liquid absorption in the crosslinked SC/NF carriers is firstly dependent on the packing density of the NFs, and secondly on the swelling capacity of the crosslinked polymer(s). However, the defined liquid deposition is most likely dependent on the thickness of the NF layer. The hypothesis is that above a certain level, the higher liquid volume could result in an irregular spreading of the solution due to contact with the smooth SC base layer, as was noticed for the SC/3D samples.

The use of these polymeric bi-layered carriers could be beneficial for delivering APIs through the dermal or buccal administration ways. In these DDSs, the APIs can be incorporated by inkjet printing [29,75]. The precision of liquid dosing and location of solution deposition provided by inkjet printing could be highly beneficial for increasing the efficacy-dose ratio in antimicrobial preparations [30,76]. In the current study, the successful printing of a drug-free base solution demonstrates that bi-layered carriers with suitable nanofibrous surface layer could be useful components in the printed DDSs. The behavior of active ingredients in this type of printed DDSs is highly dependent on the drug properties and their physicochemical interactions with the polymer carriers. Thus, potential wound dressings with additional bioactive functionality should be studied case by case.

4. Conclusions

The utilization of bi-layered carriers allows adjusting the three main aspects of polymeric carriers: physical properties, bioadhesion properties and cell–carrier interactions. Crosslinked bi-layered carriers with a solvent cast (SC) base layer and an electrospun nanofibrous surface (SC/NF carrier) were prepared with good stability and physical properties. Adding a porous layer on the mechanically strong SC films improved their absorption capacity and suitability for wound care applications. The bi-layered carriers were non-adherent in the simulated bioadhesion study, presenting favorable properties for dermal use (non-adherent dressings) with minimized damage to the skin upon removal. All prepared carriers (non-crosslinked and crosslinked) were safe and exhibited good biocompatibility towards BHK-21 fibroblast cells. Surface modification by electrospinning (bi-layered SC/NF carrier) increased the cell viability compared to the SC film and carrier with pattern 3D printed layer (bi-layered SC/3D carrier). Hence, bi-layered SC/NF carriers are good physical substrates for the cells and provide help in skin regeneration during wound healing.

The inkjet printing trial demonstrated a uniform liquid absorption profile in the bi-layered carriers with electrospun nanofibers. Furthermore, the surface modification provides a platform for the fabrication of advanced drug delivery systems with active substances (e.g., pharmaceutical and/or bioactive substances) for enhanced wound healing or drug delivery through various administration routes.

Further investigation aims at developing multilayered wound dressings with bioactive substances and in more biorelevant conditions. The relationship between the properties of the carriers and the composition of the nanofibrous layer will be evaluated and the physical properties and stability of advanced drug delivery systems will be studied in depth. In addition, biodegradability and specific bioactivity behavior testing will be carried out to assess the applicability of bi-layered carriers with drug substances for clinical use.

Supplementary Materials: The following are available online at http://www.mdpi.com/1999-4923/11/12/678/s1, Figure S1: Photographic images of non-crosslinked (A) and crosslinked (B) solvent cast (SC) films, Figure S2: Optical microscopy images of non-crosslinked solvent cast (SC) film (A) and bi-layered solvent cast/3D printed (SC/3D) carrier (B), Figure S3: Optical microscopy images of baby hamster kidney (BHK-21) fibroblast cells after 24 h of incubation on top of crosslinked solvent cast (SC) film (A), bi-layered electrospun (SC/NF) carrier (C), 3D-printed (SC/3D) carrier (E) and non-crosslinked SC film (B), bi-layered electrospun (SC/NF) carrier (D), 3D-printed (SC/3D) carrier (F) together with positive healthy controls: pure medium with a glass-plate (G) and pure medium in plastic well (H).

Author Contributions: The research is part of the MSc thesis project of S.R.; project conceptualization, K.K., N.S., S.R. and M.P.; design and planning of electrospinning experiments, K.K. and S.R.; design and planning of 3D printing, M.P., S.R., L.V.; design and planning of 3D printing inkjet printing experiments, M.P., S.R., L.V.; electrospinning, S.R., K.K.; solvent casting, S.R., M.P., 3D printing S.R., L.V. and inkjet printing, S.R.; analyses in physical characterization (texture analyzer), stability study (ATR-FTIR spectroscopy, DSC), swelling and degradation study, simulated bioadhesion study (texture analyzer), S.R.; conceptualization, design and planning of biological cell studies, K.T., K.K.; conduction and formal analyses of biological cell studies K.T.; resources, K.K., N.S.; funding acquisition, K.K.; writing—original draft preparation, M.P.; writing—review and editing, M.P., S.R., K.T., L.V., N.S. and K.K.; data curation, M.P., K.K.; visualization, M.P.; S.R., K.T., K.K.; supervision, M.P., K.K.

Funding: This research was funded by the Estonian Research Council and Estonian Ministry of Education and Research for funding of PUT1088 project (K.K.). Erasmus Scholarships (S.R.).

Acknowledgments: Linus Silvander (Åbo Akademi University) is acknowledge for conducting the SEM imaging. Ermei Mäkilä (University of Turku) is thanked for the helping with the DSC measurements. Urve Paaver, Kristian Semjonov and Georg-Marten Lanno (University of Tartu) are thanked for SEM imaging.

Conflicts of Interest: The authors declare no conflict of interest.

References

1. Boateng, J.S.; Matthews, K.H.; Stevens, H.N.E.; Eccleston, G.M. Wound healing dressings and drug delivery systems: A review. *J. Pharm. Sci.* **2008**, *97*, 2892–2923. [CrossRef]
2. Percival, S.L.; Hill, K.E.; Williams, D.W.; Hooper, S.J.; Thomas, D.W.; Costerton, J.W. A review of the scientific evidence for biofilms in wounds. *Wound Repair Regen.* **2012**, *20*, 647–657. [CrossRef]
3. Rambhia, K.J.; Ma, P.X. Controlled drug release for tissue engineering. *J. Control. Release* **2015**, *219*, 119–128. [CrossRef]
4. Zahedi, P.; Rezaeian, I.; Ranaei-Siadat, S.-O.; Jafari, S.-H.; Supaphol, P. A review on wound dressings with an emphasis on electrospun nanofibrous polymeric bandages. *Polym. Adv. Technol.* **2010**, *21*, 77–95. [CrossRef]
5. Dwivedi, C.; Pandey, H.; Pandey, A.C.; Patil, S.; Ramteke, P.W.; Laux, P.; Luch, A.; Singh, A.V. In vivo biocompatibility of electrospun biodegradable dual carrier (antibiotic + growth factor) in a mouse model—Implications for rapid wound healing. *Pharmaceutics* **2019**, *11*, 180. [CrossRef]
6. Buanz, A.B.M.; Belaunde, C.C.; Soutari, N.; Tuleu, C.; Gul, O.; Gaisford, S. Ink-jet printing versus solvent casting to prepare oral films: Effect on mechanical properties and physical stability. *Int. J. Pharm.* **2015**, *494*, 611–618. [CrossRef]
7. Preis, M.; Knop, K.; Breitkreutz, J. Mechanical strength test for orodispersible and buccal films. *Int. J. Pharm.* **2014**, *461*, 22–29. [CrossRef]
8. Rodríguez-Tobías, H.; Morales, G.; Grande, D. Comprehensive review on electrospinning techniques as versatile approaches toward antimicrobial biopolymeric composite fibers. *Mater. Sci. Eng. C* **2019**, *101*, 306–322. [CrossRef]
9. Miguel, S.P.; Figueira, D.R.; Simões, D.; Ribeiro, M.P.; Coutinho, P.; Ferreira, P.; Correia, I.J. Electrospun polymeric nanofibres as wound dressings: A review. *Colloids Surf. B Biointerfaces* **2018**, *169*, 60–71. [CrossRef]
10. Agarwal, S.; Wendorff, J.H.; Greiner, A. Use of electrospinning technique for biomedical applications. *Polymer* **2008**, *49*, 5603–5621. [CrossRef]
11. Palo, M.; Özliseli, E.; Sen Karaman, D.; Kogermann, K. Electrospun biocomposite fibers for wound healing applications. In *Green Electrospinning*; Horzum, N., Demir, M.M., Muñoz-Espí, R., Crespy, D., Eds.; DeGruyter: Berlin, Germany; Boston, MA, USA, 2019; pp. 265–320.
12. Hölzl, K.; Lin, S.; Tytgat, L.; Van Vlierberghe, S.; Gu, L.; Ovsianikov, A. Bioink properties before, during and after 3D bioprinting. *Biofabrication* **2016**, *8*, 032002. [CrossRef] [PubMed]
13. Murphy, S.V.; Atala, A. 3D Bioprinting of tissues and organs. *Nat. Biotechnol.* **2014**, *32*, 773–785. [CrossRef] [PubMed]
14. Sandler, N.; Preis, M. Printed Drug-Delivery Systems for Improved Patient Treatment. *Trends Pharmacol. Sci.* **2016**, *37*, 1070–1080. [CrossRef] [PubMed]

15. Ventola, C.L. Medical applications for 3D Printing: Current and projected uses. *Pharm. Ther.* **2014**, *39*, 704–711.
16. Tort, S.; Acartürk, F.; Beşikci, A. Evaluation of three-layered doxycycline-collagen loaded nanofiber wound dressing. *Int. J. Pharm.* **2017**, *529*, 642–653. [CrossRef]
17. Tan, L.; Hu, J.; Zhao, H. Design of bilayered nanofibrous mats for wound dressing using an electrospinning technique. *Mater. Lett.* **2015**, *156*, 46–49. [CrossRef]
18. Alhusein, N.; de Bank, P.A.; Blagbrough, I.S.; Bolhuis, A. Killing bacteria within biofilms by sustained release of tetracycline from triple-layered electrospun micro/nanofibre matrices of polycaprolactone and poly(ethylene-co-vinyl acetate). *Drug Deliv. Transl. Res.* **2013**, *3*, 531–541. [CrossRef]
19. Thabet, Y.; Lunter, D.; Breitkreutz, J. Continuous manufacturing and analytical characterization of fixed-dose, multilayer orodispersible films. *Eur. J. Pharm. Sci.* **2018**, *117*, 236–244. [CrossRef]
20. Maurmann, N.; Pereira, D.P.; Burguez, D.; de S Pereira, F.D.A.; Inforcatti Neto, P.; Rezende, R.A.; Gamba, D.; da Silva, J.V.L.; Pranke, P. Mesenchymal stem cells cultivated on scaffolds formed by 3D printed PCL matrices, coated with PLGA electrospun nanofibers for use in tissue engineering. *Biomed. Phys. Eng. Express* **2017**, *3*, 1–15. [CrossRef]
21. Maver, T.; Smrke, D.M.; Kurečič, M.; Gradišnik, L.; Maver, U.; Kleinschek, K.S. Combining 3D printing and electrospinning for preparation of pain-relieving wound-dressing materials. *J. Sol-Gel Sci. Technol.* **2018**, *88*, 33–48. [CrossRef]
22. Scoutaris, N.; Ross, S.; Douroumis, D. Current trends on medical and pharmaceutical applications of inkjet printing technology. *Pharm. Res.* **2016**, *33*, 1799–1816. [CrossRef] [PubMed]
23. Zhu, W.; Ma, X.; Gou, M.; Mei, D.; Zhang, K.; Chen, S. 3D printing of functional biomaterials for tissue engineering. *Curr. Opin. Biotechnol.* **2016**, *40*, 103–112. [CrossRef] [PubMed]
24. Daly, R.; Harrington, T.S.; Martin, G.D.; Hutchings, I.M. Inkjet printing for pharmaceutics—A review of research and manufacturing. *Int. J. Pharm.* **2015**, *494*, 554–567. [CrossRef] [PubMed]
25. Setti, L.; Fraleoni-Morgera, A.; Ballarin, B.; Filippini, A.; Frascaro, D.; Piana, C. An amperometric glucose biosensor prototype fabricated by thermal inkjet printing. *Biosens. Bioelectron.* **2005**, *20*, 2019–2026. [CrossRef]
26. Derby, B. Additive manufacture of ceramics components by inkjet printing. *Engineering* **2015**, *1*, 113–123. [CrossRef]
27. Määttänen, A.; Ihalainen, P.; Pulkkinen, P.; Wang, S.; Tenhu, H.; Peltonen, J. Inkjet-printed gold electrodes on paper: Characterization and functionalization. *ACS Appl. Mater. Interfaces* **2012**, *4*, 955–964. [CrossRef]
28. Derby, B. Inkjet printing of functional and structural materials: Fluid property requirements, feature stability, and resolution. *Annu. Rev. Mater. Res.* **2010**, *40*, 395–414. [CrossRef]
29. Montenegro-Nicolini, M.; Reyes, P.E.; Jara, M.O.; Vuddanda, P.R.; Neira-Carrillo, A.; Butto, N.; Velaga, S.; Morales, J.O. The effect of inkjet printing over polymeric films as potential buccal biologics delivery systems. *AAPS PharmSciTech* **2018**, *19*, 3376–3387. [CrossRef]
30. Genina, N.; Fors, D.; Palo, M.; Peltonen, J.; Sandler, N. Behavior of printable formulations of loperamide and caffeine on different substrates—Effect of print density in inkjet printing. *Int. J. Pharm.* **2013**, *453*, 488–497. [CrossRef]
31. Genina, N.; Fors, D.; Vakili, H.; Ihalainen, P.; Pohjala, L.; Ehlers, H.; Kassamakov, I.; Haeggström, E.; Vuorela, P.; Peltonen, J.; et al. Tailoring Controlled-Release Oral Dosage Forms by Combining Inkjet and Flexographic Printing Techniques. *Eur. J. Pharm. Sci.* **2012**, *47*, 615–623. [CrossRef]
32. Kamoun, E.A.; Chen, X.; Mohy Eldin, M.S.; Kenawy, E.R.S. Crosslinked poly(vinyl alcohol) hydrogels for wound dressing applications: A review of remarkably blended polymers. *Arab. J. Chem.* **2015**, *8*, 1–14. [CrossRef]
33. DeMerlis, C.C.; Schoneker, D.R. Review of the oral toxicity of polyvinyl alcohol (PVA). *Food Chem. Toxicol.* **2003**, *41*, 319–326. [CrossRef]
34. Abdelgawad, A.M.; Hudson, S.M.; Rojas, O.J. Antimicrobial wound dressing nanofiber mats from multicomponent (chitosan/silver-NPs/polyvinyl alcohol) systems. *Carbohydr. Polym.* **2014**, *100*, 166–178. [CrossRef] [PubMed]
35. Charernsriwilaiwat, N.; Rojanarata, T.; Ngawhirunpat, T.; Opanasopit, P. Electrospun chitosan/polyvinyl alcohol nanofibre mats for wound healing. *Int. Wound J.* **2014**, *11*, 215–222. [CrossRef] [PubMed]
36. Bolto, B.; Tran, T.; Hoang, M.; Xie, Z. Crosslinked poly(vinyl alcohol) membranes. *Prog. Polym. Sci.* **2009**, *34*, 969–981. [CrossRef]

37. Shalumon, K.T.; Anulekha, K.H.; Nair, S.V.; Nair, S.V.; Chennazhi, K.P.; Jayakumar, R. Sodium alginate/poly(vinyl alcohol)/nano ZnO composite nanofibers for antibacterial wound dressings. *Int. J. Biol. Macromol.* **2011**, *49*, 247–254. [CrossRef]

38. Sobhanian, P.; Khorram, M.; Hashemi, S.S.; Mohammadi, A. Development of nanofibrous collagen-grafted poly (vinyl alcohol)/gelatin/alginate scaffolds as potential skin substitute. *Int. J. Biol. Macromol.* **2019**, *130*, 977–987. [CrossRef]

39. Kim, J.O.; Park, J.K.; Kim, J.H.; Jin, S.G.; Yong, C.S.; Li, D.X.; Choi, J.Y.; Woo, J.S.; Yoo, B.K.; Lyoo, W.S.; et al. Development of polyvinyl alcohol-sodium alginate gel-matrix-based wound dressing system containing nitrofurazone. *Int. J. Pharm.* **2008**, *359*, 79–86. [CrossRef]

40. European Medicines Agency. *Guideline on Stability Testing: Stability Testing of Existing Active Substances and Related Finished Products*; European Medicines Agency: London, UK, 2003; pp. 1–18.

41. Miraftab, M.; Saifullah, A.N.; Çay, A. Physical stabilisation of electrospun poly(vinyl alcohol) nanofibres: Comparative study on methanol and heat-based crosslinking. *J. Mater. Sci.* **2015**, *50*, 1943–1957. [CrossRef]

42. Tamm, I.; Heinämäki, J.; Laidmäe, I.; Rammo, L.; Paaver, U.; Ingebrigtsen, S.G.; Škalko-Basnet, N.; Halenius, A.; Yliruusi, J.; Pitkänen, P.; et al. Development of suberin fatty acids and chloramphenicol-loaded antimicrobial electrospun nanofibrous mats intended for wound therapy. *J. Pharm. Sci.* **2016**, *105*, 1239–1247. [CrossRef]

43. Huang, K.-T.; Fang, Y.-L.; Hsieh, P.-S.; Li, C.-C.; Dai, N.-T.; Huang, C.-J. Zwitterionic nanocomposite hydrogels as effective wound dressings. *J. Mater. Chem. B* **2016**, *4*, 4206–4215. [CrossRef]

44. Sjöholm, E.; Sandler, N. Additive manufacturing of personalized orodispersible warfarin films. *Int. J. Pharm.* **2019**, *564*, 117–123. [CrossRef] [PubMed]

45. Birck, C.; Degoutin, S.; Tabary, N.; Miri, V.; Bacquet, M. New crosslinked cast films based on poly(vinyl alcohol): Preparation and physico-chemical properties. *Express Polym. Lett.* **2014**, *8*, 941–952. [CrossRef]

46. Fuchs, S.; Hartmann, J.; Mazur, P.; Reschke, V.; Siemens, H.; Wehlage, D.; Ehrmann, A. Electrospinning of biopolymers and biopolymer blends. *J. Chem. Pharm. Sci.* **2017**, *974*, 2115.

47. Hansen, E.F.; Derrick, M.R.; Schilling, M.R.; Garcia, R. The effects of solution application on some mechanical and physical properties of thermoplastic amorphous polymers used in conservation: Poly(vinyl acetate)s. *J. Am. Inst. Conserv.* **1991**, *30*, 203–213. [CrossRef]

48. Stone, S.A.; Gosavi, P.; Athauda, T.J.; Ozer, R.R. In situ citric acid crosslinking of alginate/polyvinyl alcohol electrospun nanofibers. *Mater. Lett.* **2013**, *112*, 32–35. [CrossRef]

49. Morgado, P.I.; Lisboa, P.F.; Ribeiro, M.P.; Miguel, S.P.; Simões, P.C.; Correia, I.J.; Aguiar-Ricardo, A. Poly(vinyl alcohol)/chitosan asymmetrical membranes: Highly controlled morphology toward the ideal wound dressing. *J. Memb. Sci.* **2014**, *469*, 262–271. [CrossRef]

50. Qin, Y. Absorption characteristics of alginate wound dressings. *J. Appl. Polym. Sci.* **2004**, *91*, 953–957. [CrossRef]

51. El-Din, H.M.N.; Alla, S.G.A.; El-Naggar, A.W.M. Swelling, thermal and mechanical properties of poly(vinyl alcohol)/sodium alginate hydrogels synthesized by electron beam irradiation. *J. Macromol. Sci. Part A Pure Appl. Chem.* **2007**, *44*, 291–297. [CrossRef]

52. Safi, S.; Morshed, M.; Hosseini Ravandi, S.A.; Ghiaci, M. Study of electrospinning of sodium alginate, blended solutions of sodium alginate/poly(vinyl alcohol) and sodium alginate/poly(ethylene oxide). *J. Appl. Polym. Sci.* **2007**, *104*, 3245–3255. [CrossRef]

53. Lawrie, G.; Keen, I.; Drew, B.; Chandler-Temple, A.; Rintoul, L.; Fredericks, P.; Grøndahl, L. Interactions between alginate and chitosan biopolymers characterized using FTIR and XPS. *Biomacromolecules* **2007**, *8*, 2533–2541. [CrossRef] [PubMed]

54. Mansur, H.S.; Sadahira, C.M.; Souza, A.N.; Mansur, A.A.P. FTIR spectroscopy characterization of poly (vinyl alcohol) hydrogel with different hydrolysis degree and chemically crosslinked with glutaraldehyde. *Mater. Sci. Eng. C* **2008**, *28*, 539–548. [CrossRef]

55. Mallapragada, S.K.; Peppas, N.A. Dissolution mechanism of semicrystalline poly(vinyl alcohol) in water. *J. Polym. Sci. Part B Polym. Phys.* **1996**, *34*, 1339–1346. [CrossRef]

56. Gohil, J.M.; Bhattacharya, A.; Ray, P. Studies on the cross-linking of poly (vinyl alcohol). *J. Polym. Res.* **2006**, *13*, 161–169. [CrossRef]

57. El-Sayed, S.; Mahmoud, K.H.; Fatah, A.A.; Hassen, A. DSC, TGA and dielectric properties of carboxymethyl cellulose/polyvinyl alcohol blends. *Phys. B Condens. Matter* **2011**, *406*, 4068–4076. [CrossRef]

58. Soares, J.P.; Santos, J.E.; Chierice, G.O.; Cavalheiro, E.T.G. Thermal behavior of alginic acid and its sodium salt. *Eclet. Quim.* **2004**, *29*, 57–63. [CrossRef]
59. Carvalho, F.C.; Calixto, G.; Hatakeyama, I.N.; Luz, G.M.; Gremião, M.P.D.; Chorilli, M. Rheological, mechanical, and bioadhesive behavior of hydrogels to optimize skin delivery systems. *Drug Dev. Ind. Pharm.* **2013**, *39*, 1750–1757. [CrossRef]
60. Singh, S.; Jain, S.; Muthu, M.S.; Tiwari, S.; Tilak, R. Preparation and evaluation of buccal bioadhesive films containing clotrimazole. *AAPS PharmSciTech* **2008**, *9*, 660–667. [CrossRef]
61. Dhivya, S.; Padma, V.V.; Santhini, E. Wound dressings—A review. *BioMedicine* **2015**, *5*, 24–28. [CrossRef]
62. Rippon, M.; White, R.; Davies, P. Skin adhesives and their role in wound dressings. *Wounds UK* **2007**, *3*, 76–86.
63. Sood, A.; Granick, M.S.; Tomaselli, N.L. Wound dressings and comparative effectiveness data. *Adv. Wound Care* **2014**, *3*, 511–529. [CrossRef] [PubMed]
64. Horstmann, M.; Müller, W.; Asmussen, B. Principles of skin adhesion and methods for measuring adhesion of transdermal systems. In *Bioadhesive Drug Delivery Systems: Fundamentals, Novel Approaches, and Development*; Mathiowitz, E., Chickering, D.E., III, Lehr, C.-M., Eds.; Marcel Dekker, Inc.: New York, NY, USA, 1999; pp. 175–196.
65. Matos-Pérez, C.R.; White, J.D.; Wilker, J.J. Polymer composition and substrate influences on the adhesive bonding of a biomimetic, cross-linking polymer. *J. Am. Chem. Soc.* **2012**, *134*, 9498–9505. [CrossRef] [PubMed]
66. *Substances Generally Recognized as Safe, 21 C.F.R. § 182U.S.*; Food and Drug Administration; FDA: Silver Spring, MD, USA, 2019.
67. Orive, G.; Ponce, S.; Hernández, R.M.; Gascón, A.R.; Igartua, M.; Pedraz, J.L. Biocompatibility of microcapsules for cell immobilization elaborated with different type of alginates. *Biomaterials* **2002**, *23*, 3825–3831. [CrossRef]
68. Alexandre, N.; Ribeiro, J.; Gärtner, A.; Pereira, T.; Amorim, I.; Fragoso, J.; Lopes, A.; Fernandes, J.; Costa, E.; Santos-Silva, A.; et al. Biocompatibility and hemocompatibility of polyvinyl alcohol hydrogel used for vascular grafting—In vitro and in vivo studies. *J. Biomed. Mater. Res. Part A* **2014**, *102*, 4262–4275.
69. Ruprecht, V.; Monzo, P.; Ravasio, A.; Yue, Z.; Makhija, E.; Strale, P.O.; Gauthier, N.; Shivashankar, G.V.; Studer, V.; Albiges-Rizo, C.; et al. How cells respond to environmental cues—Insights from bio-functionalized substrates. *J. Cell Sci.* **2017**, *130*, 51–61. [CrossRef] [PubMed]
70. Evans, N.D.; Gentleman, E. The role of material structure and mechanical properties in cell–matrix interactions. *J. Mater. Chem. B* **2014**, *2*, 2345–2356. [CrossRef]
71. Richbourg, N.R.; Peppas, N.A.; Sikavitsas, V.I. Tuning the biomimetic behavior of scaffolds for regenerative medicine through surface modifications. *J. Tissue Eng. Regen. Med.* **2019**, *13*, 1275–1293. [CrossRef]
72. Amani, H.; Arzaghi, H.; Bayandori, M.; Dezfuli, A.S.; Pazoki-Toroudi, H.; Shafiee, A.; Moradi, L. Controlling cell behavior through the design of biomaterial surfaces: A focus on surface modification techniques. *Adv. Mater. Interfaces* **2019**, *6*, 1900572. [CrossRef]
73. O'Brien, F.J. Biomaterials & scaffolds for tissue engineering. *Mater. Today* **2011**, *14*, 88–95.
74. Bružauskaitė, I.; Bironaitė, D.; Bagdonas, E.; Bernotienė, E. Scaffolds and cells for tissue regeneration: Different scaffold pore sizes—Different cell effects. *Cytotechnology* **2016**, *68*, 355–369. [CrossRef]
75. Palo, M.; Kogermann, K.; Laidmäe, I.; Meos, A.; Preis, M.; Heinämäki, J.; Sandler, N. Development of oromucosal dosage forms by combining electrospinning and inkjet printing. *Mol. Pharm.* **2017**, *14*, 808–820. [CrossRef] [PubMed]
76. Palo, M.; Öhman, J.; Oja, T.; Sandler, N. Development of wound dressings for biofilm inhibition by means of inkjet printing. In Proceedings of the NIP32: International Conference on Digital Printing Technologies, Manchester, UK, 12–16 September 2016; pp. 1–3.

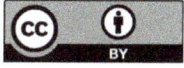

© 2019 by the authors. Licensee MDPI, Basel, Switzerland. This article is an open access article distributed under the terms and conditions of the Creative Commons Attribution (CC BY) license (http://creativecommons.org/licenses/by/4.0/).

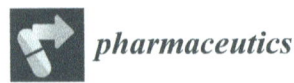

Article

Evaluation of Electrospun Poly(ε-Caprolactone)/Gelatin Nanofiber Mats Containing Clove Essential Oil for Antibacterial Wound Dressing

Irem Unalan [1], Stefan J. Endlein [1], Benedikt Slavik [2], Andrea Buettner [2], Wolfgang H. Goldmann [3], Rainer Detsch [1] and Aldo R. Boccaccini [1,*]

[1] Institute of Biomaterials, Department of Materials Science and Engineering, Friedrich-Alexander-University Erlangen-Nuremberg, Cauerstraße 6, 91058 Erlangen, Germany; irem.unalan@fau.de (I.U.); stefan.endlein@fau.de (S.J.E.); Rainer.Detsch@fau.de (R.D.)
[2] Chair of Aroma and Smell Research, Department of Chemistry and Pharmacy, Friedrich-Alexander-University Erlangen-Nuremberg, Henkestraße 9, 91054 Erlangen, Germany; benedikt.slavik@fau.de (B.S.); andrea.buettner@fau.de (A.B.)
[3] Institute of Biophysics, Department of Physics, Friedrich-Alexander-University Erlangen-Nuremberg, Henkestraße 91, 91052 Erlangen, Germany; wgoldmannh@aol.com
* Correspondence: aldo.boccaccini@ww.uni-erlangen.de; Tel.: +49-9131-8528601

Received: 16 October 2019; Accepted: 30 October 2019; Published: 1 November 2019

Abstract: The objective of this study was to produce antibacterial poly(ε-caprolactone) (PCL)-gelatin (GEL) electrospun nanofiber mats containing clove essential oil (CLV) using glacial acetic acid (GAA) as a "benign" (non-toxic) solvent. The addition of CLV increased the fiber diameter from 241 ± 96 to 305 ± 82 nm. Aside from this, the wettability of PCL-GEL nanofiber mats was increased by the addition of CLV. Fourier-transform infrared spectroscopy (FTIR) analysis confirmed the presence of CLV, and the actual content of CLV was determined by gas chromatography–mass spectrometry (GC-MS). Our investigations showed that CLV-loaded PCL-GEL nanofiber mats did not have cytotoxic effects on normal human dermal fibroblast (NHDF) cells. On the other hand, the fibers exhibited antibacterial activity against *Staphylococcus aureus* and *Escherichia coli*. Consequently, PCL-GEL/CLV nanofiber mats are potential candidates for antibiotic-free wound healing applications.

Keywords: electrospinning; PCL; gelatin; clove essential oil; antibacterial; biocompatibility

1. Introduction

Microorganisms can quickly enter and instantly grow in open wounds, causing exudate formation, delay in wound healing, and deformation of the skin [1]. Therefore, the most critical issue in the field of wound healing is preventing wound contamination. This drawback could be overcome by using antibacterial wound dressing that protects the area around the wound, providing a suitable moist environment and antibacterial properties [2]. More recently, there has been renewed interest in natural antibacterial agents such as phytotherapeutics for antibiotic-free wound healing applications [3,4]. In particular, essential oils are one of the most promising phytotherapeutics, aiming at the promotion of the wound healing process while minimizing bacterial infections [5–7].

Essential oils (EOs) are natural-based compounds that can provide antibacterial, anti-inflammatory, and antioxidation protection [8]. The antibacterial activity of EOs such as clove, cinnamon, oregano, and lemongrass essential oil depends on the chemical structure of their primary component and concentration [9]. Among these, clove essential oil (CLV) has been medicinally used for centuries for its therapeutic effects [10]. CLV is isolated from the aromatic flower buds of *Eugenia caryophyllata*, which is composed of eugenol (78%), β-caryophyllene (13%), and other compounds such as benzyl alcohol [11]. Its primary components have been widely used due to their medicinal properties such as antioxidant, anti-inflammatory, and antimicrobial activities [12]. Moreover, its antibacterial activity has been demonstrated to be particularly effective against bacterial strains such as *Escherichia coli*, *Staphylococcus aureus, Bacillus subtilis*, and *Pseudomonas fluorescens* [13]. On the other hand, the effective dose of CLV has enhanced cell viability [14,15]. According to our knowledge, a few studies related to EOs' influence on in vitro cell migration have been carried out. Aside from this, the application of CLV in wound dressing is limited due to its high volatility and sensitivity to degradation from exposure to oxygen, heat, and light [16]. In order to improve the applicability of CLV, different scaffold preparation methods have been used to develop polymer carriers for CLV, such as casting films [17,18], nanoparticles [19,20] and, more recently, electrospun fiber mats [21].

The electrospinning process is a convenient, versatile, and cost-effective method for fabricating homogeneous and porous macro- or nanofibers [22]. The nanostructure and high surface-area-to-volume ratio of electrospun nanofibers are attractive features to enhance the drug releasing capability for wound healing applications [23]. Poly(ε-caprolactone) (PCL), one of the promising synthetic polymers for wound healing applications, has an excellent processability, good biocompatibility and, compared to natural polymers, high mechanical properties, whereas the biodegradability, cell adhesion, and proliferation responses to PCL are limited [24]. On the other hand, the natural polymer gelatin (GEL) containing molecular components present in the extracellular matrix (ECM) promotes cell adhesion and proliferation properties [25]. Therefore, the combination of PCL and GEL in electrospun fibers should lead to improved mechanical and physical properties coupled with suitable biocompatibility [26]. There are only a limited number of studies reporting the incorporation of natural antimicrobial agents into PCL-GEL electrospun fibers for antibacterial wound dressing applications. For instance, Ramalingam et al. [27] fabricated PCL-GEL hybrid composite mats loaded with *Gymnema sylvestre* for wound dressing applications. Similarly, Fallah et al. [28] developed curcumin (CUR)-loaded electrospun PCL-GEL nanofibers. Their results indicated that the addition of CUR increased the antibacterial activity against both Gram-positive and Gram-negative bacteria [28].

Essential oil incorporated in electrospun fibers for wound dressings are a rather recent technology; therefore, there are no reports on the use of CLV and PCL-GEL for antibacterial wound dressing. In this study, PCL-GEL nanofiber mats containing various concentrations of CLV were fabricated using glacial acetic acid (GAA) as a "benign" (non-toxic) solvent for antibiotic-free wound healing applications. The use of benign solvents in so-called "green" electrospinning has special relevance when using natural products such as EOs [29,30] Here, we investigated the effect of various CLV concentrations (1.5%, 3%, and 6%, v/v) on morphology, average fiber diameter, contact angle (wettability), cell viability, cell morphology, rate of wound closure, and antibacterial activity. To the best of the authors' knowledge, the cell migration effect of CLV-loaded PCL-GEL nanofiber mats for wound healing applications has not been investigated before.

2. Materials and Methods

2.1. Materials

PCL (Mw = 80 kDa), GEL (~300 g Bloom, Type A), CLV (C8392, CAS number: 8000-34-8), standard eugenol (E51791, 99%), and fetal bovine serum (FBS; F2442) were purchased from Sigma Aldrich (Darmstadt, Germany). Glacial acetic acid (GAA; 87003-241) and dichloromethane (DCM; BDH1113-4LG) were obtained from VWR (Darmstadt, Germany). The microorganism strains of *S. aureus* (ATCC25923) and *E. coli* (ATCC25922) were used. Luria/Miller agar (X969.1) and lysogeny broth medium (Luria/Miller, 6673.1) were supplied by Carl Roth GmbH (Karlsruhe, Germany). Dulbecco's modified Eagle's medium (DMEM, 31885-023), penicillin/streptomycin (PS, 15140-122) and trypsin/EDTA (25200-056) were purchased from Thermo Scientific (Schwerte, Germany). The normal human dermal fibroblast (NHDF) cell line was obtained from Translation Research Center

(TRC) of Friedrich-Alexander-University Erlangen-Nuremberg. All reagents and solvents were of analytical grade.

2.2. Fabrication of PCL-GEL/CLV Nanofiber Mats

For the fabrication of PCL-GEL electrospun nanofiber mats, firstly GEL powder (4.8%, w/v) was dissolved in the GAA (90%, v/v) solvent at 45 °C for 4 hours. After the GEL was dissolved, PCL pellets (11.2%, w/v) were added to the solution and stirred overnight at room temperature. The total polymer concentration of GAA solution was fixed at 16% (w/v). For the preparation of CLV-incorporated solutions, PCL-GEL solution preparation was followed as explained above. After 30 min of addition of PCL pellets, different ratios of CLV (1.5%, 3%, and 6%, v/v) were separately added in a dropwise manner to the PCL-GEL solution and stirred overnight at room temperature. Then, each electrospinning solution was carried out under defined and constant ambient conditions (temperature (T): 25 °C and relative humidity (RH): 25%) using a commercially available electrospinning setup (IME's medical electrospinning machines, EC-16 CLI, IME Technologies, Netherlands). The solutions were loaded separately into a 3 mL plastic syringe equipped with a 23G needle and fed at 0.6 mL/h. The aluminum sheet wrapped around the rotating drum collector was placed at a distance of 12 cm from the needle tip to the collector. Electrospinning was conducted by applying a voltage of +19 kV in the needle and −1 kV to the target. Moreover, during the electrospinning process, the gas shield accessory with nitrogen flux was set at 8 mL/min for optimization of the Taylor cone. The samples were then stored at 4 °C in the dark until further analysis.

2.3. Characterization of Nanofiber Mats

The surface morphology of nanofiber mats was analyzed by scanning electron microscopy (SEM, ETH: 2 kV, Everhart-Thornley detector (SE2), AURIGA base 55, Carl Zeiss). The samples were coated with a thin layer of gold (Q150T Turbo-Pumped Sputter Coater/Carbon Coater, Quorum Technologies) before SEM analyses. The average fiber diameter of nanofiber mats was measured from the SEM images using the Image J analysis software (NIH, Bethesda, MD, USA). For calculation of the average fiber diameter and fiber distribution, 50 randomly selected different points were measured.

The contact angle meter (Drop Shape Analyzer, DSA 30, CA Measurement setup, Kruess GmbH, Hamburg, Germany) was used to investigate the wettability of nanofiber mats using a sessile drop method. Briefly, the samples were placed on a glass slide before the test and 8 µl of de-ionized water was dropped on the surface of the nanofiber mats. Four measurements were taken at different locations of the same mats and the average value was obtained.

The functional group of PCL-GEL and CLV-loaded PCL-GEL nanofiber mats PCL-GEL/CLV were analyzed by Fourier-transform infrared spectroscopy (FTIR, IRAffinity-1S, Shimadzu). The spectrum analysis was performed with wavenumbers ranging between 400 and 4000 cm^{-1} and at a spectral resolution of 4 cm^{-1}.

The investigation of the total CLV content in CLV-loaded PCL-GEL nanofiber mats was performed using gas chromatography–mass spectrometry (GC-MS, GC/MSD Systems, GC 7890A, MSD 5975C, Agilent Technologies, Waldbronn, Germany) equipped with a DB-FFAP (Durabond-Free Fatty Acid Phase) capillary column (GC Column, 30 m × 0.25 mm, film thickness 0.25 µm; Agilent Technologies, Santa Clara, CA). Briefly, the calibration curve of eugenol, that is, the main component in the volatile fraction of CLV, was prepared and the eugenol concentration was calculated using the peak area ($y = 77732x + 89964$, $R^2 = 0.9995$). On the other hand, the nanofiber mats (3 mg) were dispersed in DCM (20 mL) for 2 h. Subsequently, the solvent-assisted flavor evaporation technique (SAFE) [31] was used for the isolation of the CLV volatile fraction. The volatile fraction in DCM was dried over sodium sulfate and then filtered. The final volume (100 µL) was obtained using Vigreux and microdistillation at 50 °C [32]. Then, 1 µL of each sample was taken for the GC-MS measurements. The oven temperature was programmed at 40 °C for 2 min and then heated up at 8 °C/min to 240 °C and held for 5 min. Helium was used as carrier gas at a flow rate of 1 mL/min. Mass spectra were recorded in selected ion monitoring (SIM) mode (*m/z* ratio 164). Finally, the percentage of encapsulation efficiency was calculated as Equation (1):

$$\text{Encapsulation Efficiency (EE)}(\%) = \frac{M_a}{M_t} \times 100 \qquad (1)$$

where M_a and M_t are the actual and theoretical amounts of CLV in nanofiber mats, respectively.

2.4. Antibacterial Assay

The antibacterial activity of CLV-loaded PCL-GEL nanofiber mats was separately tested with *S. aureus* (Gram-positive) and *E. coli* (Gram-negative) bacteria. Initially, the bacterial suspensions were prepared for both bacteria stains in lysogeny broth medium at 37 °C for 24 h. Then, the optical density (OD) (600 nm, Thermo Scientific GENESYS 30, Germany) of the cultivated bacteria was arranged at 0.015. The nanofiber mats (~3 mg) were then cut and were sterilized by UV light irradiation for 30 min. The samples were immersed in lysogeny broth medium, and 20 µL of bacteria suspension was added. Finally, all the samples were incubated at 37 °C for 3, 6, and 24 h and then they were measured at each time interval at 600 nm OD. The relative viability of the bacteria was calculated according to Equation (2):

$$\text{Relative viability }(\%) = \frac{OD_{Sample}}{OD_{Control}} \times 100 \qquad (2)$$

The lysogeny broth medium and bacterial cell suspension in lysogeny broth medium were used as a blank and control (CNT), respectively. The experiments were performed three times.

2.5. In Vitro Assay

The cell viability, cell morphology, and wound closure rate of NHDF cells were analyzed to gain the first impression of the biological behavior of PCL-GEL, PCL-GEL/CLV1.5, PCL-GEL/CLV3, and PCL-GEL/CLV6 nanofiber mats.

2.5.1. Cell Culture

NHDF cells were cultured in DMEM supplemented with 10% FBS and 1% penicillin/streptomycin in 75 cm^2 cell culture flasks (Nunc, Denmark). Subsequently, NHDF cells were grown to confluency, and then the cells were detached by trypsinization and counted by trypan blue assay using a hemocytometer (Roth, Germany). Counted cells were seeded in 24-well plates at a density of 50.000 cell/well and incubated at 37 °C in a humidified incubator with 5% CO$_2$ for 24 h. Prior to cell culture experiments, the nanofiber mats were fixed on CellCrown 24 inserts (ScaffdexOy, Tampere, Finland) and sterilized by UV light irradiation for 30 min. After 24 h incubation, the medium of the cell was refreshed, and the samples were immersed in a 24-well plate without touching the cells. Finally, the cells were incubated with samples for a further 48 h.

2.5.2. Cell Viability

The viability of the cells was analyzed by a WST-8 cell counting assay kit (Sigma Aldrich). The basis of this assay is the reduction of yellow-colored tetrazolium salt in WST-8 to form orange formazan crystals by dehydrogenases enzymes secreted by mitochondria of metabolically active cells. The amount of these formazan crystals is directly proportional to the number of living cells. After culturing the cells for 48 h, they were washed with PBS to remove unattached cells and incubated with 5% WST-8 reagent in DMEM for a period of 2h at 37 °C. The absorbance of the dye was measured at 450 nm using a spectrophotometric plate reader (PHOmo, anthos Mikrosysteme GmbH, Germany). The percentage of cell viability was calculated as follows:

$$\text{Cell viability }(\%) = \frac{(\text{Absorbance of control} - \text{Absorbance of test sample})}{(\text{Absorbance of control} - \text{Absorbance of blank})} \times 100 \qquad (3)$$

All samples were measured in triplicate.

2.5.3. Hematoxylin and Eosin (H&E) Staining

Hematoxylin and eosin (H&E) staining methods were used for analyzing the cell density. Briefly, the cells were washed with PBS and fixed with Fluoro-Fix for 15 min. After that, the cells were stained with Hematoxylin for 20 min and washed with tap water followed by Scott's tap water for 5 min and then further rinsed with de-ionized water. After hematoxylin dying, the cells were stained with 0.4% eosin stain (in a saturated aqueous solution of 60% ethanol and 5% acetic acid) for 5 min. Cells were dehydrated with 95% and 100% ethanol, respectively, and air-dried in a fume hood. Finally, the cell density of the NHDF cells was examined using a light microscope (Primo Vert, Carl Zeiss).

2.5.4. In Vitro Wound Healing Assay (Scratch Test)

In vitro healing assay was performed according to the procedure described in [33]. The experimental set-up for the scratch test is schematically illustrated in Figure 1. Firstly, NHDF cells were seeded at 50,000 cell/well into 24-well plate and were incubated at 37 °C in 5% CO_2 for 24 h. Then, a vertical scratch was created using a 1000 mL sterile pipet tip in the middle of the NHDF monolayer. Subsequently, the nanofiber mats were fixed on CellCrown 24 inserts (ScaffdexOy, Tampere, Finland) and placed in the 24-well plate without touching the surface. Finally, the wound closure rate was monitored at different times (0 h, 4 h, 6 h, and 24 h) and photographed using a light microscope (Primo Vert, Carl Zeiss). The images were analyzed with Image J (NIH, Bethesda, MD, USA). The rate of wound closure was calculated using the following formula:

$$\text{Rate of wound closure (\%)} = \frac{(A_0 - A_t)}{A_0} \times 100 \tag{4}$$

where A_0 is the initial wound area and A_t is the wound area at the designated time.

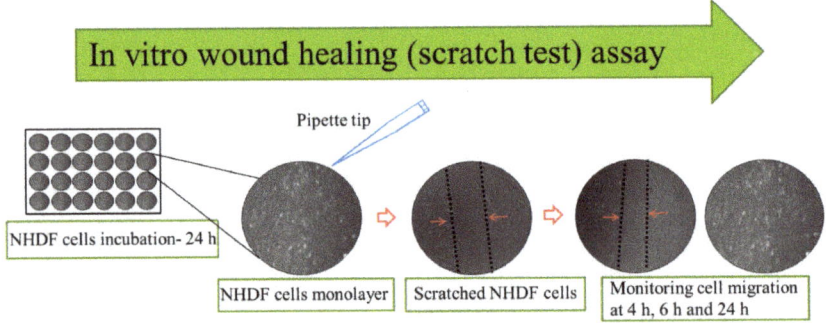

Figure 1. Schematic illustration of in vitro wound healing assay (scratch test) set-up for the study. NHDF: normal human dermal fibroblast.

2.6. Statistical Analysis

Data were analyzed by ANOVA and Bonferroni's test using the Origin (OriginLab, Northampton, MA, USA). The level of significance was determined as $p < 0.05$.

3. Results

3.1. Surface Morphology of PCL-GEL/CLV Nanofiber Mats

The morphology of PCL-GEL, PCL-GEL/CLV1.5, PCL-GEL/CLV3, and PCL-GEL/CLV6 nanofiber mats was investigated. The results revealed that all samples had a smooth, uniform, and bead-less morphology. Figure 2 and Table 1 show the fiber distribution and average fiber diameter, separately. The average fiber diameters were 241 ± 96, 285 ± 67, 300 ± 73, and 305 ± 82 nm for PCL-GEL, PCL-GEL/CLV1.5, PCL-GEL/CLV3, and PCL-GEL/CLV6, respectively. The results indicate that the fiber diameter had increased with the addition CLV compared to PCL-GEL.

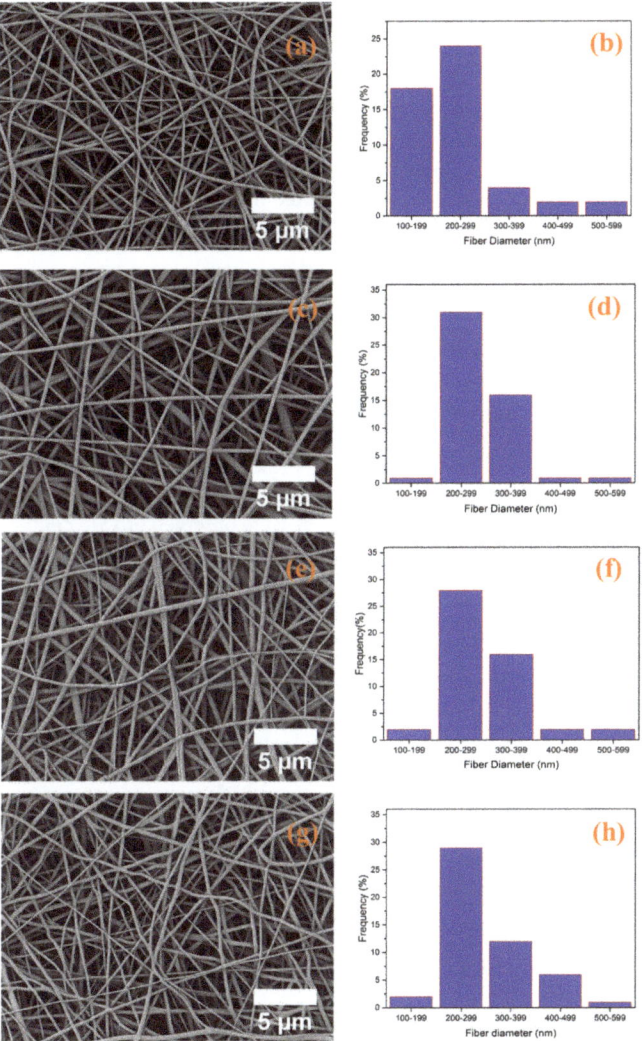

Figure 2. The morphology and fiber diameter distribution of poly(ε-caprolactone) gelatin (PCL-GEL) (**a,b**), PCL-GEL/clove essential oil (CLV)1.5 (**c,d**), PCL-GEL/CLV3 (**e,f**), and PCL-GEL/CLV6 (**g,h**) nanofiber mats, respectively.

Table 1. Sample composition, sample label, average fiber diameter, and loading efficiency of nanofiber mats.

Sample Code	PCL (w/v %)	GEL (w/v %)	CLV (v/v %)	Average Fiber Diameter (nm)	Contact Angle(°)	Encapsulation Efficiency (EE) (%)
PCL-GEL	11.2	4.8	-	241 ± 96	37 ± 8	-
PCL-GEL/CLV1.5	11.2	4.8	1.5	285 ± 67	18 ± 3	53 ± 4
PCL-GEL/CLV3	11.2	4.8	3	300 ± 73	21 ± 4	68 ± 11
PCL-GEL/CLV6	11.2	4.8	6	305 ± 82	27 ± 5	73 ± 3

3.2. Wettability

The wettability of the nanofiber mats was analyzed by the sessile drop method. The contact angle values of the samples are shown in Table 1. The incorporation of CLV within the PCL-GEL nanofiber mats resulted in a decreasing contact angle compared to the PCL-GEL nanofiber mats. The contact angle values were 37 ± 8°, 18 ± 3°, 21 ± 4°, and 27 ± 5° for PCL-GEL, PCL-GEL/CLV1.5, PCL-GEL/CLV3, and PCL-GEL/CLV6 nanofiber mats.

3.3. Fourier-Transform Infrared Spectroscopy Analysis

The presence of CLV within the nanofiber mats was analyzed by Fourier-transform infrared spectroscopy (FTIR) (Figure 3). The typical peaks of PCL were at 2942 and 2866 cm^{-1}, corresponding to the asymmetric and symmetric stretching of CH_2 bonds. Further peaks were at 1720, 1240, and 1168 cm^{-1} related to carbonyl stretching as well as both asymmetric and symmetric stretching of C–O–C bonds, respectively [30]. Characteristic GEL peaks were obtained at 1651 cm^{-1} for amide I and N–H deformation at around 1540 cm^{-1} for the amide II [34]. With the addition of CLV, a new peak appeared within the nanofiber mats. The CLV bands were observed at 1514 cm^{-1}, which corresponds to the main component of CLV—eugenol—attributed to the stretching vibration of C=C aromatic bonds [17].

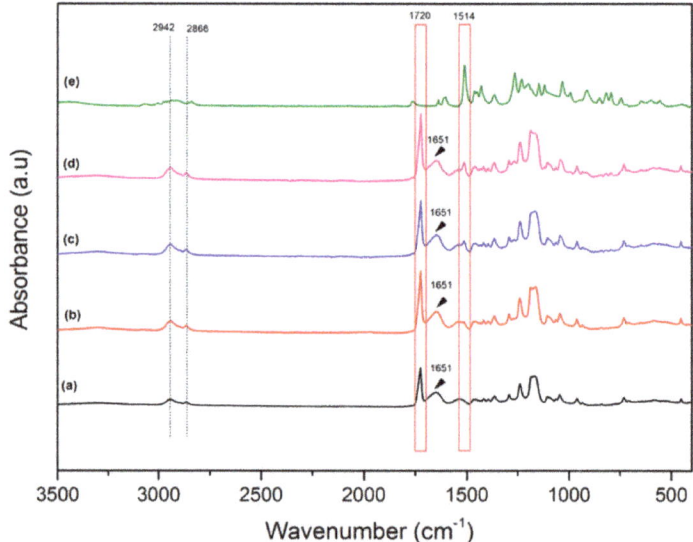

Figure 3. The Fourier-transform infrared spectroscopy (FTIR) spectra of PCL-GEL (**a**), PCL-GEL/CLV1.5 (**b**), PCL-GEL/CLV3 (**c**), and PCL-GEL/CLV6 (**d**) nanofiber mats and pure CLV (**e**).

3.4. CLV Content in PCL-GEL Nanofiber Mats

The encapsulation efficiency of CLV in PCL-GEL nanofiber mats was investigated by GC-MS. The effect of the different concentrations of CLV on the percentage of encapsulation efficiency is shown in Table 1. The encapsulation efficiency of PCL-GEL/CLV3 and PCL-GEL/CLV6 nanofiber mats were higher than the PCL-GEL/CLV1.5. However, there were no statistically significant differences between the PCL-GEL/CLV3 and PCL-GEL/CLV6.

3.5. Antibacterial Assay

The antibacterial activity of PCL-GEL, PCL-GEL/CLV1.5, PCL-GEL/CLV3, and PCL-GEL/CLV6 nanofiber mats was tested with *S. aureus* (Gram-positive) and *E. coli* (Gram-negative) bacteria. The bacterial viability against both bacteria strains is illustrated in Figure 4. CLV addition improved the antibacterial activity of nanofiber mats compared to PCL-GEL. The highest inhibition effect was observed at 6 h for *S. aureus*, whereas *E. coli* was active up to 24 h. However, there were no significant differences between the PCL-GEL/CLV1.5, PCL-GEL/CLV3, and PCL-GEL/CLV6 nanofiber mats. Moreover, after 24 h incubation, PCL-GEL/CLV3 and PCL-GEL/CLV6 showed lower *E. coli* bacteria viability than the control (CNT) and PCL-GEL. On the other hand, bacteria viability of *S. aureus* PCL-GEL/CLV1.5, PCL-GEL/CLV3, and PCL-GEL/CLV6 nanofiber mats were reduced compared to CNT at 6 h incubation.

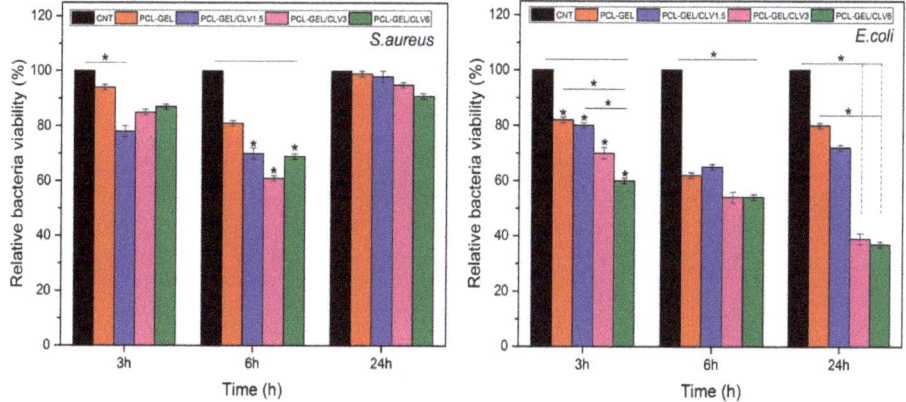

Figure 4. Antibacterial activity of PCL-GEL and CLV-loaded PCL-GEL nanofiber mats after 3, 6, and 24 h incubation with *S. aureus* (Gram-positive) and *E. coli* (Gram-negative) bacteria ($n = 3$, samples in triplicate,* $p < 0.05$).

3.6. In Vitro Assay

3.6.1. Cell Viability

The viability and growth of NHDF cells were determined to investigate the in vitro biocompatibility of PCL-GEL, PCL-GEL/CLV1.5, PCL-GEL/CLV3, and PCL-GEL/CLV6 nanofiber mats after 48 h of incubation, as shown in Figure 5. It is shown that there was no apparent difference between the nanofiber mats compared to the control (CNT). Furthermore, there was no significant change in NHDF cell viability with the increase of to CLV concentration in the nanofiber mats ($p < 0.05$). The results demonstrated that PCL-GEL and PCL-GEL/CLV nanofiber mats show no cytotoxicity on NHDF cells.

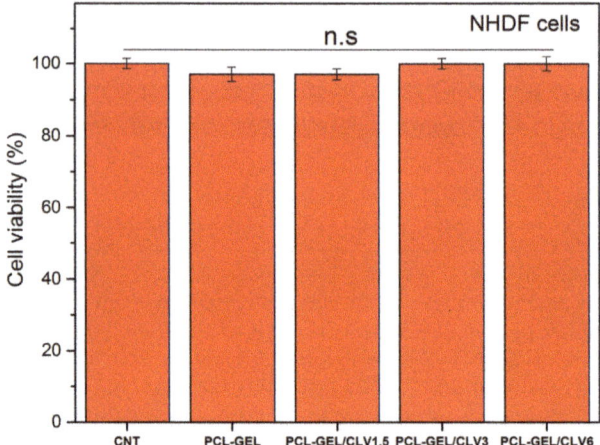

Figure 5. Cell viability percentage of PCL-GEL and CLV-loaded PCL-GEL nanofiber mats after 48 h incubation ($n = 6$, n.s: not significant).

3.6.2. Hematoxylin and Eosin (H&E) Staining

Light microscopy images of H&E-stained NHDF cells cultured with PCL-GEL, PCL-GEL/CLV1.5, PCL-GEL/CLV3, and PCL-GEL/CLV6 nanofiber mats after 48 h are shown in Figure 6. As evident from light microscope images, the cells exhibited phenotypical cell morphology and were firmly attached and well-spread on the well plate. Also, the addition and increasing the CLV did not affect the morphology and spreading of the NHDF cells. Moreover, the cell confluence obtained after each treatment was in agreement with cell viability measured by the WST-8 assay.

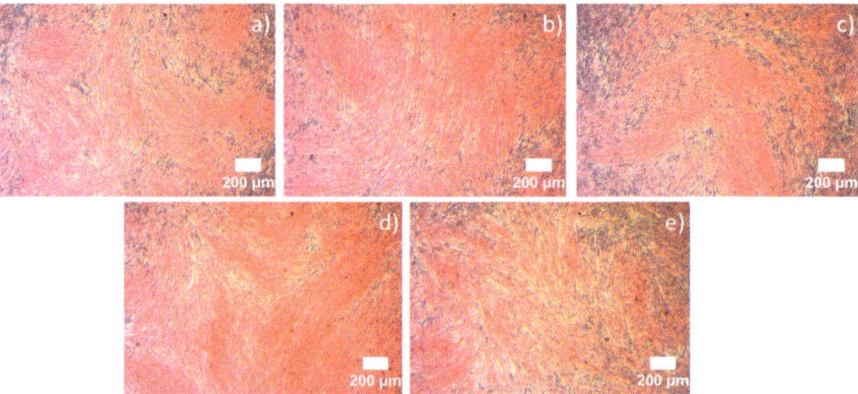

Figure 6. Light microscopy images of hematoxylin and eosin (H&E)-stained NHDF cells cultured with CNT (**a**), PCL-GEL (**b**), PCL-GEL/CLV1.5 (**c**), PCL-GEL/CLV3 (**d**), and PCL-GEL/CLV6 (**e**) nanofiber mats. The H&E staining highlighted the cell nuclei (blue) within the pink cytoplasm.

3.6.3. In Vitro Wound Healing Assay (Scratch Test)

The effect of CLV-loaded into PCL-GEL nanofiber mats to the wound healing activity of NHDF cells was assessed using the in vitro wound healing (scratch) assay. The cell migration into the wound areas and rate of wound closure are presented in Figures 7 and 8, respectively. After 6 h, the percentages of cells in the wound area for the control (CNT), PCL-GEL, PCL-GEL/CLV1.5, PCL-GEL/CLV3, and PCL-GEL/CLV6 nanofiber mats were 41 ± 1, 31 ± 1, 29 ± 3, 30 ± 2, and 16 ± 1%, respectively (Figure 8). However, after 24 h of treatment, in the CNT group complete closure was observed, whereas in PCL-GEL, PCL-GEL/CLV1.5, PCL-GEL/CLV3, and PCL-GEL/CLV6 nanofiber mats, this closure was 86 ± 1, 83 ± 3, 78 ± 2, and 68 ± 1%, respectively. Increasing CLV concentration inhibited NHDF cell migration and proliferation in a dose-dependent manner. On the other hand, there was no significant ($p < 0.05$) difference in wound closure rates between PCL-GEL and PCL-GEL/CLV1.5 at 4, 6, and 24 h.

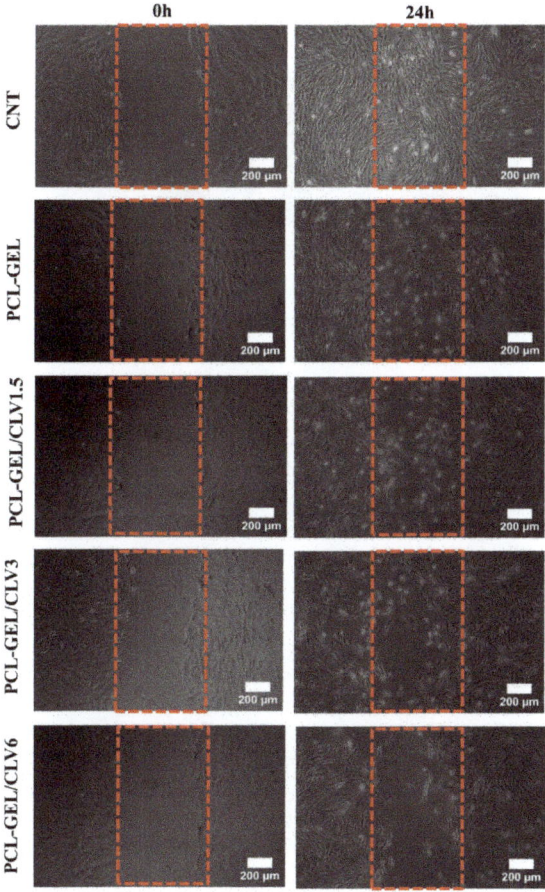

Figure 7. Illustrative micrographs of cell migrating into a scratch area over a 24 h period in CNT, PCL-GEL, PCL-GEL/CLV1.5, PCL-GEL/CLV3, and PCL-GEL/CLV6.

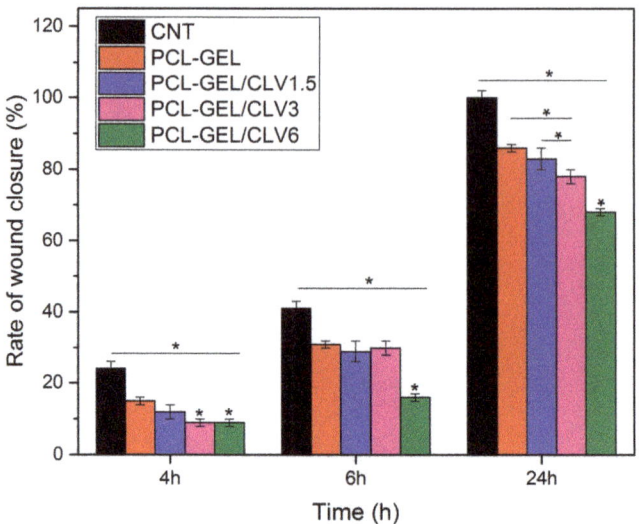

Figure 8. In vitro wound healing assay in the presence of CNT, PCL-GEL, PCL-GEL/CLV1.5, PCL-GEL/CLV3, and PCL-GEL/CLV6 in 24 h ($n = 3$, samples in triplicate, * $p < 0.05$).

4. Discussion

The usage of EOs for antibacterial wound dressing is attracting increasing interest due to their antibacterial, anti-inflammatory, and antioxidant properties. In this study, CLV-loaded PCL-GEL nanofiber mats were produced using benign solvents for antibacterial wound dressings. The concentrations used in the fabrication of nanofiber mats are shown in Table 1. SEM images of the obtained nanofiber mats with and without CLV are depicted in Figure 2. The results indicate that the incorporation of CLV did not affect the fiber formation. However, the average fiber diameter increased by the addition of CLV and increased the CLV amount from 1.5% to 6% (w/v). It is well known that the fabrication of uniform homogenous, smooth, and bead-free nanofiber morphology depends on electrospinning parameters such as polymer concentration, solution viscosity, electrical conductivity, temperature, and humidity [22]. The lower electrical conductivity of the solution affects the elongation of the jet by the electrical forces and can cause large fiber diameters [35]. The increment of the PCL-GEL/CLV nanofiber diameter could be attributed to the reduction of solution electric conductivity. Aside from this, increasing the solution viscosity led to increased average fiber diameter [36]. In the present study, the addition of CLV could reduce the solution viscosity due to the interaction between CLV and PCL-GEL. In a similar study, García-Moreno et al. [37] reported that the average fiber diameter of poly(vinyl alcohol) (PVA) nanofibers was increased with the encapsulation of fish oil. Mori et al. [38] showed similar results in that various concentrations of candeia essential oil addition increased the average fiber diameter of polylactic acid (PLA) nanostructured mats.

The contact angle measurement, which is a cost-effective and useful method used to investigate the effect of additives on surface properties, has been commonly used to demonstrate the wettability of biomaterials. Furthermore, the increment of the surface wettability enhances the absorption of excess wound exudates, which is important for wound healing applications [39]. In this study, the contact angle measurement was used to determine the effect of CLV on the PCL-GEL nanofiber mats (Table 1). Data obtained in this study indicated that the wettability of PCL-GEL nanofiber mats was increased with CLV addition. This result could be due to the chemical structure of CLV that presents polar phytochemicals and hydrophilic –OH groups. However, increasing the concentrations of CLV, the contact angle of PCL-GEL/CLV1.5, PCL-GEL/CLV3, and PCL-GEL/CLV6 nanofiber mats was slightly increased, which might be due to the loss of free functional groups (amino and hydroxyl groups) on the GEL. According to Liu et al. [40], cinnamon essential oil encapsulated chitosan nanoparticle incorporation in poly (lactic acid) (PLA) composite fibers, increasing the hydrophilic behavior. In another study, Anges Mary and Giri Dev [41] fabricated PCL electrospun matrices incorporated with aloe vera (AV). Their results revealed that the addition of AV decreased the contact angle value compared to pure PCL [41]. Similarly, findings of Ramalingam et al. [27] indicated that PCL/GEL hybrid composite mats comprising natural herbal extract (*Gymnema sylvestre*) had lower contact angle value.

FTIR analysis (Figure 3) revealed the presence of CLV loading in the PCL-GEL nanofiber mats, attributable to the characteristic peak of CLV.

The influence of different CLV ratios in PCL-GEL nanofiber mats on the encapsulation efficiency was examined (Table 1). On the basis of the findings in this study, increasing the CLV content from 1.5% to 3% (*v/v*) increased the encapsulation efficiency. However, the encapsulation efficiency of PCL-GEL/CLV3 and PCL-GEL/CLV6 nanofiber mats were not significantly different. This result could have been due to the capacity of nanofibers, which exhibited a maximum encapsulation efficiency of 73 ± 3%. Recently, clove oil (CO)/chitosan nanoparticles embedded gelatin nanofibers were produced by Cui et al. [20]. The encapsulation efficiency results revealed values that measured ranged from 21.1 ± 0.4% to 39.6 ± 0.8%. Similarly, Tampau et al. [42] reported the fabrication of starch or PCL-based matrices incorporated with carvacrol. The results showed that the encapsulation efficiency of carvacrol in starch or PCL-based matrices increased from 15% to 75% with increasing carvacrol ratios. Moreover, gelatin nanofiber mats encapsulated with orange essential oil were studied by Tavassoli-Kafrani et al. [43] They found that the increment of the orange essential oil ratio in the gelatin nanofibers increased the encapsulation efficiency from 35 ± 0.09% to 69.0 ± 0.22%.

The antibacterial properties of CLV have been investigated using various bacteria such as *E. coli*, *S. aureus*, *Bacillus subtilis*, and *Pseudomonas fluorescens* [13]. The present study investigated the antibacterial activity of CLV-loaded PCL-GEL nanofiber mats against *S. aureus* as Gram-positive bacteria and *E. coli* as Gram-negative bacteria for antibacterial wound dressings. The results indicated that the addition of CLV reduced the bacteria viability for both bacteria strains, as shown in Figure 4. The lowest bacterial viability was observed at 6 h for *S. aureus*, whereas bacterial viability of *E. coli* was reduced at 24 h. This result could have been due to different bacterial characteristics and morphology; for instance: Gram-negative bacteria have a thicker double layer cell membrane than the single membrane of Gram-positive bacteria [5,12]. In a similar study, Fallah et al. [28] reported that the incorporation with curcumin exhibited antibacterial activity against both Gram-positive and Gram-negative bacteria on PCL-GEL fiber mats. Similarly, Figueroa-Lopez et al. [44] produced GEL-coated PCL ultrathin fibers containing black pepper oleoresin (OR). Their results revealed that the viability of *S. aureus* was reduced with the addition of OR. In another study, Ramalingam et al. [27] evaluated the effect of the addition of *Gymnema sylvestre* as a natural herbal in PCL-GEL on the antibacterial performance of these nanofibrous mats. It was found that the antibacterial activity of the samples all increased with the addition of *Gymnema sylvestre*. Furthermore, our results revealed that the highest bacteria inhibition was observed in *E. coli* compared to *S. aureus*. According to Li et al. [45], eugenol loaded PCL-GEL fiber mats are more effective against *S. aureus* compared to *E.coli*; this is in contrast to our studies. The result might have been due to the chemical structure of CLV, which additionally consists of other components such as eugenyl acetate or beta-caryophyllene. In conclusion, the antibacterial activity of CLV-loaded PCL-GEL nanofiber mats confirms the present fibrous structures as promising materials for antibacterial wound dressing.

In the present study, the cell viability of PCL-GEL nanofiber mats with and without CLV was investigated with NHDF cells. The results indicated that there were no significant differences ($p < 0.05$) in cell viability and morphology of the nanofiber mats in comparison to control (Figures 5 and 6). Accordingly, the in vitro cell viability and morphology results demonstrated that PCL-GEL, PCL-GEL/CLV1.5, PCL-GEL/CLV3, and PCL-GEL/CLV6 nanofiber mats are biocompatible. In a related study, Tang et al. [46] produced peppermint and chamomile essential oil-loaded gelatin nanofibers.

Their cytotoxicity results indicated that incorporation of peppermint and chamomile essential oil into gelatin nanofibers did not change the NIH-3T3 fibroblast cell viability [46]. In another study, Hajiali et al. [47] investigated the antibacterial activity and biocompatibility of alginate–lavender nanofibers. The cell viability of lavender-incorporated alginate nanofibers was 91%. It was stated that the addition of lavender oil did not affect the cell viability of human foreskin fibroblast (HFF-1) cells compared to the control group [47]. Similarly, Balasubramanian and Kodam [48] assessed mouse fibroblasts (NIH-3T3) on polyacrylonitrile (PAN)/lavender oil nanofibrous mats. Lavender-loaded nanofibrous mats showed non-cytotoxic behavior for NIH-3T3, which is in agreement with our results [48].

Wound healing is a complex and multiphase process that can be categorized into wounding, hemostasis, inflammation, proliferation, and maturation [49]. During this process, the formation of new tissue and wound healing rate are also affected by external factors [50]. In our study, the potential effect of CLV on wound healing was investigated by an in vitro wound-healing assay. This assay revealed that increasing the CLV concentration reduced the NHDF cell migration and proliferation, whereas the same samples had no adverse effect on the NHDF cell viability. On the other hand, after 24 h measurements, PCL-GEL/CLV1.5 values were not significantly different when compared with PCL-GEL. In the literature, a few studies have been conducted to assess the cell migration effect of EOs. For instance, the dose-dependent wound healing effect of *Eugenia dysenterica* DC leaves were reported by da Silva et al. [51] In a similar study, Léguillier et al. studied keratinocyte cell migration ability at various concentrations of *Calophyllum inophyllum* oil (0.01%, 0.1%, and 1% diluted in olive oil) [52]. Their results proved that the effective dose of EO enhances cell migration [52]. To the best of the authors' knowledge, this is the first study on CLV-loaded PCL-GEL nanofiber mats using cultured NHDF cells to determine the wound closure rate. Therefore, the biological activity of CLV-loaded PCL-GEL nanofiber mats is promising and should be further investigated, quantifying in particular the time-dependent release of the EO and its effect on cell behavior.

5. Conclusions

We evaluated the antibacterial and biological activity of CLV-loaded PCL-GEL nanofiber mats on wound dressings. PCL-GEL and clove oil-loaded PCL-GEL nanofiber mats were successfully fabricated by electrospinning. Our results revealed that bead-free, uniform, and smooth fibers were obtained. However, the addition of CLV increased the average fiber diameter. The wettability study inferred that the addition of CLV decreased the contact angle value compared to PCL-GEL nanofiber mats. The FTIR spectrum suggested that the CLV component is loaded into the PCL-GEL nanofiber mats. Moreover, the cytotoxicity results revealed that the incorporation of CLV on the PCL-GEL nanofiber mats did not demonstrate a toxic effect on NHDF cell viability. Aside from this, the addition of CLV promoted the antibacterial properties against *S. aureus* and *E. coli*. In conclusion, CLV-loaded PCL-GEL nanofiber mats may have a potential in wound healing applications and can be considered as promising biomaterial for avoiding bacterial infections without using antibiotics.

Author Contributions: Conceptualization: I.U. and A.R.B., methodology: I.U. B.S., A.B., W.H.G. and R.D., formal analysis: I.U., S.J.E., B.S., A.B. and W.H.G., investigation: I.U., S.J.E. and A.R.B., resources: A.B. and A.R.B.; data curation: I.U., writing—original draft preparation: I.U., writing—review and editing: I.U., B.S., A.B., W.H.G., R.D. and A.R.B., visualization: I.U., supervision: A.R.B., project administration: A.R.B.

Funding: This research was partially funded by Deutscher Akademischer Austauschdienst (DAAD) [Research Grants—Doctoral Programs, Section ST21, 91652927].

Acknowledgments: The first author is funded by the Deutscher Akademischer Austauschdienst (DAAD) program of Research Grants – Doctoral Programs. The authors want to thank Raminder Singh from the Translational Research Center (TRC) Erlangen for the supply of normal human dermal fibroblasts.

Conflicts of Interest: The authors declare no conflict of interest.

References

1. Edwards, R.; Harding, K.G. Bacteria and wound healing. *Curr. Opin. Infect. Dis.* **2004**, *17*, 91–96. [CrossRef] [PubMed]
2. Macneil, S. Biomaterials for tissue engineering of skin. *Mater. Today* **2008**, *11*, 26–35. [CrossRef]
3. Ramos-e-Silva, M.; Ribeiro de Castro, D.C.M. New dressings, including tissue-engineered living skin. *Clin. Derm.* **2002**, *20*, 715–723. [CrossRef]
4. Dhivya, S.; Vijaya Padma, V.; Santhini, E. Wound dressings-a review. *BioMedicine* **2015**, *5*, 24–28. [CrossRef] [PubMed]
5. Silva, N.C.C.; Fernandes, J.A. Biological properties of medicinal plants: A review of their antimicrobial activity. *J. Venom Anim Toxins Incl. Trop. Dis.* **2010**, *16*, 402–413. [CrossRef]
6. Jaganathan, S.; Mani, M.; Polymers, A.K. Electrospun Combination of Peppermint Oil and Copper Sulphate with Conducive Physico-Chemical properties for Wound Dressing Applications. *Polymers* **2019**, *11*, 586. [CrossRef]
7. Sadri, M.; Arab-Sorkhi, S.; Vatani, H.; Bagheri-Pebdeni, A. New wound dressing polymeric nanofiber containing green tea extract prepared by electrospinning method. *Fibers Polym.* **2015**, *16*, 1742–1750. [CrossRef]
8. Bakkali, F.; Averbeck, S.; Averbeck, D.; Idaomar, M. Biological effects of essential oils – A review. *Food Chem. Toxicol.* **2008**, *46*, 446–475. [CrossRef]
9. Velluti, A.; Sanchis, V.; Ramos, A.J.; Egido, J.; Marın, S. Inhibitory effect of cinnamon, clove, lemongrass, oregano and palmarose essential oils on growth and fumonisin B1 production by Fusarium proliferatum in maize grain. *Int. J. Food Microbiol.* **2003**, *89*, 145–154. [CrossRef]
10. Prabuseenivasan, S.; Jayakumar, M.; Ignacimuthu, S. In vitro antibacterial activity of some plant essential oils. *Bmc Complement. Altern. Med.* **2006**, *6*, 39. [CrossRef]
11. Jirovetz, L.; Buchbauer, G.; Stoilova, I.; Stoyanova, A.; Krastanov, A.; Schmidt, E. Chemical composition and antioxidant properties of clove leaf essential oil. *J. Agric. Food Chem.* **2006**, *54*, 6303–6307. [CrossRef] [PubMed]
12. Teixeira, B.; Marques, A.; Ramos, C.; Neng, N.R.; Nogueira, J.M.F.; Saraiva, J.A.; Nunes, M.L. Chemical composition and antibacterial and antioxidant properties of commercial essential oils. *Ind. Crop. Prod.* **2013**, *43*, 587–595. [CrossRef]
13. Chaieb, K.; Hajlaoui, H.; Zmantar, T.; Kahla-Nakbi, A.B.; Rouabhia, M.; Mahdouani, K.; Bakhrouf, A. The chemical composition and biological activity of clove essential oil, Eugenia caryophyllata (Syzygium aromaticum L. Myrtaceae): A short review. *Phytother. Res.* **2007**, *21*, 501–506.
14. Khunkitti, W.; Veerapan, P.; Hahnvajanawong, C. In vitro bioactivities of clove buds oil (Eugenia caryophyllata) and its effect on dermal fibroblast. *Int. J. Pharm. Pharm. Sci.* **2012**, *4*, 556–560.
15. Prashar, A.; Locke, I.C.; Evans, C.S. Cytotoxicity of clove (Syzygium aromaticum) oil and its major components to human skin cells. *Cell Proliferation* **2006**, *39*, 241–248. [CrossRef]
16. Asbahani, A.; Miladi, K.; Badri, W.; Sala, M.; Addi, E.H.A.; Casabianca, H.; Mousadik, A.; Hartmann, D.; Jilale, A.; Renaud, F.N.R.; et al. Essential oils: From extraction to encapsulation. *Int. J. Pharma.* **2015**, *483*, 220–243. [CrossRef]
17. Wang, L.; Liu, F.; Jiang, Y.; Chai, Z.; Li, P.; Cheng, Y.; Jing, H.; Leng, X. Synergistic antimicrobial activities of natural essential oils with chitosan films. *J. Agric. Food Chem.* **2011**, *59*, 12411–12419. [CrossRef]
18. Pereira dos Santos, E.; Nicácio, P.H.M.; Coêlho Barbosa, F.; Nunes da Silva, H.; Andrade, A.L.S.; Lia Fook, M.V.; de Lima Silva, S.M.; Farias Leite, I. Chitosan/Essential Oils Formulations for Potential Use as Wound Dressing: Physical and Antimicrobial Properties. *Materials* **2019**, *12*, 2223. [CrossRef]
19. Alam, P.; Ansari, M.J.; Anwer, M.K.; Raish, M.; Kamal, Y.K.T.; Shakeel, F. Wound healing effects of nanoemulsion containing clove essential oil. *Artif. CellsNanomed. Biotechnol.* **2017**, *45*, 591–597. [CrossRef]
20. Cui, H.; Bai, M.; Rashed, M.M.A.; Lin, L. The antibacterial activity of clove oil/chitosan nanoparticles embedded gelatin nanofibers against *Escherichia coli* O157:H7 biofilms on cucumber. *Int. J. Food Microbiol.* **2018**, *266*, 69–78. [CrossRef]
21. Verma, C.; Rohit, P.S.; Anjum, S.; Gupta, B. Novel Approach for Nanobiocomposites by Nanoencapsulation of Lecithin-Clove oil within PVA Nanofibrous Web. *Mater. Today Proc.* **2019**, *15*, 183–187. [CrossRef]

22. Sill, T.; von Recum, H.A. Electrospinning: Applications in drug delivery and tissue engineering. *Biomaterials* **2008**, *29*, 1989–2006. [CrossRef] [PubMed]
23. Martins, A.; Reis, R.L.; Neves, N.M. Electrospinning: Processing technique for tissue engineering scaffolding. *Int. Mater. Rev.* **2008**, *53*, 257–274. [CrossRef]
24. Wang, L.; Abedalwafa, M.; Wang, F.; Li, C. Biodegradable poly-epsilon-caprolactone (PCL) for tissue engineering applications: A review. *Rev. Adv. Mater. Sci.* **2013**, *34*, 123–140.
25. Gaspar-Pintiliescu, A.; Stanciuc, A.-M.; Craciunescu, O. Natural composite dressings based on collagen, gelatin and plant bioactive compounds for wound healing: A review. *Int. J. Biol. Macromol.* **2019**, *138*, 854–865. [CrossRef]
26. Yao, R.; He, J.; Meng, G.; Jiang, B.; Wu, F. Electrospun PCL/Gelatin composite fibrous scaffolds: Mechanical properties and cellular responses. *J. Biomater. Sci. Polym. Ed.* **2016**, *27*, 824–838. [CrossRef]
27. Ramalingam, R.; Dhand, C.; Leung, C.M.; Ezhilarasu, H.; Prasannan, P.; Ong, S.T.; Subramanian, S.; Kamruddin, M.; Lakshminarayanan, R.; Ramakrishna, S.; et al. Poly-ε-caprolactone/gelatin hybrid electrospun composite nanofibrous mats containing ultrasound assisted herbal extract: Antimicrobial and cell proliferation study. *Nanomaterials* **2019**, *9*, 462. [CrossRef]
28. Fallah, M.; Bahrami, S.H.; Ranjbar-Mohammadi, M. Fabrication and characterization of PCL/gelatin/curcumin nanofibers and their antibacterial properties. *J. Ind. Text.* **2016**, *46*, 562–577. [CrossRef]
29. Chemat, F.; Vian, M. Green extraction of natural products: Concept and principles. *Int. J. Mol. Sci* **2012**, *13*, 8615–8627. [CrossRef]
30. Liverani, L.; Boccaccini, A.R. Versatile production of poly (epsilon-caprolactone) fibers by electrospinning using benign solvents. *Nanomaterials* **2016**, *6*, 75. [CrossRef]
31. Engel, W.; Bahr, W.; Schieberle, P. Solvent assisted flavour evaporation–a new and versatile technique for the careful and direct isolation of aroma compounds from complex food matrices. *Eur. Food Res. Technol.* **1999**, *209*, 237–241. [CrossRef]
32. Bemelmans, J.M.H. Review of Isolation and Concentration Techniques Progress in flavour research. *Appl. Sci.* **1976**, *8*, 79–98.
33. Liang, C.C.; Park, A.Y.; Guan, J.L. In vitro scratch assay: A convenient and inexpensive method for analysis of cell migration *in vitro*. *Nat. Protoc.* **2007**, *2*, 329. [CrossRef] [PubMed]
34. Ghasemi-Mobarakeh, L.; Prabhakaran, M.P.; Morshed, M.; Nasr-Esfahani, M.H.; Ramakrishna, S. Electrospun poly(ε-caprolactone)/gelatin nanofibrous scaffolds for nerve tissue engineering. *Biomaterials* **2008**, *29*, 4532–4539. [CrossRef] [PubMed]
35. Garg, K.; Bowlin, G.L. Electrospinning jets and nanofibrous structures. *Biomicrofluidics* **2011**, *5*, 013403. [CrossRef] [PubMed]
36. Cramariuc, B.; Cramariuc, R.; Scarlet, R.; Manea, L.R.; Lupu, I.G.; Cramariuc, O. Fiber diameter in electrospinning process. *J. Electrostat.* **2013**, *71*, 189–198. [CrossRef]
37. García-Moreno, P.J.; Guadix, A.; Guadix, E.M.; Jacobsen, C. Physical and oxidative stability of fish oil-in-water emulsions stabilized with fish protein hydrolysates. *Food Chem.* **2016**, *203*, 124–135. [CrossRef]
38. Mori, C.L.; Passos, N.A.D.; Oliveira, J.E.; Altoé, T.F.; Mori, F.A.; Mattoso, L.H.C.; Tonoli, G.H.D. Nanostructured polylactic acid/candeia essential oil mats obtained by electrospinning. *J. Nanomater.* **2015**, *16*, 33. [CrossRef]
39. Xu, L.C.; Siedlecki, C.A. Effects of surface wettability and contact time on protein adhesion to biomaterial surfaces. *Biomaterials* **2007**, *28*, 3273–3283. [CrossRef]
40. Liu, Y.; Wang, S.; Zhang, R.; Lan, W.; Qin, W. Development of poly(lactic acid)/chitosan fibers loaded with essential oil for antimicrobial applications. *Nanomaterials* **2017**, *7*, 194. [CrossRef]
41. Agnes Mary, S.; Giri Dev, V.R. Electrospun herbal nanofibrous wound dressings for skin tissue engineering. *J. Text. Inst.* **2015**, *106*, 886–895. [CrossRef]
42. Tampau, A.; González-Martinez, C.; Chiralt, A. Carvacrol encapsulation in starch or PCL based matrices by electrospinning. *J. Food Eng.* **2017**, *214*, 245–256. [CrossRef]
43. Tavassoli-Kafrani, E.; Goli, S.A.H.; Fathi, M. Encapsulation of Orange Essential Oil Using Cross-linked Electrospun Gelatin Nanofibers. *Food Bioprocess Technol.* **2018**, *11*, 427–434. [CrossRef]

44. Figueroa-Lopez, K.J.; Castro-Mayorga, J.L.; Andrade-Mahecha, M.M.; Cabedo, L.; Lagaron, J.M. Antibacterial and barrier properties of gelatin coated by electrospun polycaprolactone ultrathin fibers containing black pepper oleoresin of interest in active food biopackaging applications. *Nanomaterials* **2018**, *8*, 199. [CrossRef] [PubMed]
45. Li, Z.; Zhou, P.; Zhou, F.; Zhao, Y.; Ren, L.; Yuan, X. Antimicrobial eugenol-loaded electrospun membranes of poly(ε-caprolactone)/gelatin incorporated with REDV for vascular graft applications. *Colloids Surf B Biointerfaces* **2018**, *162*, 335–344. [CrossRef] [PubMed]
46. Tang, Y.; Zhou, Y.; Lan, X.; Huang, D.; Luo, T.; Ji, J.; Mafang, Z.; Miao, X.; Wang, H.; Wang, W. Electrospun Gelatin Nanofibers Encapsulated with Peppermint and Chamomile Essential Oils as Potential Edible Packaging. *J. Agric. Food Chem.* **2019**, *67*, 2227–2234. [CrossRef]
47. Hajiali, H.; Summa, M.; Russo, D.; Armirotti, A.; Brunetti, V.; Bertorelli, R.; Athanassiou, A.; Mele, E. Alginate-lavender nanofibers with antibacterial and anti-inflammatory activity to effectively promote burn healing. *J. Mater. Chem. B* **2016**, *4*, 1686–1695. [CrossRef]
48. Balasubramanian, K.; Kodam, K.M. Encapsulation of therapeutic lavender oil in an electrolyte assisted polyacrylonitrile nanofibres for antibacterial applications. *RSC Adv.* **2014**, *4*, 54892–54901. [CrossRef]
49. Rieger, K.A.; Birch, N.P.; Schiffman, J.D. Designing electrospun nanofiber mats to promote wound healing-a review. *J. Mater. Chem. B* **2013**, *1*, 4531–4541. [CrossRef]
50. Reinke, J.M.; Sorg, H. Wound repair and regeneration. *Eur. Surg. Res.* **2012**, *49*, 35–43. [CrossRef]
51. Da Silva, S.M.M.; Costa, C.R.R.; Gelfuso, G.M.; Guerra, E.N.S.; De Medeiros Nóbrega, Y.K.; Gomes, S.M.; Pic-Taylor, A.; Fonseca-Bazzo, Y.M.; Silveira, D.; De Oliveira Magalhães, P. Wound healing effect of essential oil extracted from eugenia dysenterica DC (Myrtaceae) leaves. *Molecules* **2019**, *24*, 2. [CrossRef]
52. Léguillier, T.; Lecsö-Bornet, M.; Lémus, C.; Rousseau-Ralliard, D.; Lebouvier, N.; Hnawia, E.; Nour, M.; Aalbersberg, W.; Ghazi, K.; Raharivelomanana, P.; et al. The wound healing and antibacterial activity of five ethnomedical Calophyllum inophyllum oils: An alternative therapeutic strategy to treat infected wounds. *PLoS ONE* **2015**, *10*, e0138602. [CrossRef]

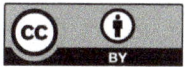

© 2019 by the authors. Licensee MDPI, Basel, Switzerland. This article is an open access article distributed under the terms and conditions of the Creative Commons Attribution (CC BY) license (http://creativecommons.org/licenses/by/4.0/).

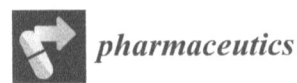

Article

In Vivo Biocompatibility of Electrospun Biodegradable Dual Carrier (Antibiotic + Growth Factor) in a Mouse Model—Implications for Rapid Wound Healing

Charu Dwivedi [1,2], Himanshu Pandey [2,3], Avinash C. Pandey [2], Sandip Patil [4], Pramod W. Ramteke [1,*], Peter Laux [5], Andreas Luch [5] and Ajay Vikram Singh [5,6,*]

1. Department of Biological Sciences, Sam Higginbottom University of Agriculture, Technology and Sciences, Allahabad 211007, India; charucas0505@gmail.com
2. Nanotechnology Application Centre, Faculty of Science, University of Allahabad, Allahabad 211002, India; himanshu.nac@gmail.com (H.P.); prof.avinashcpandey@gmail.com (A.C.P.)
3. Department of Pharmaceutical Sciences, Faculty of Health Sciences, Sam Higginbottom University of Agriculture, Technology & Sciences, Allahabad 211007, India
4. E-Spin Nanotech Pvt Ltd., Kanpur 208016, India; espinnanotech@gmail.com
5. Department of Chemical and Product Safety, German Federal Institute for Risk Assessment (BfR), Max-Dohrn-Strasse 8-10, 10589 Berlin, Germany; peter.laux@bfr.bund.de (P.L.); andreas.luch@bfr.bund.de (A.L.)
6. Physical Intelligence Department, Max Planck Institute for Intelligent Systems, 70569 Stuttgart, Germany
* Correspondence: avsingh@is.mpg.de or Ajay-Vikram.Singh@bfr.bund.de (A.V.S.); pwramteke@gmail.com (P.W.R.)

Received: 13 March 2019; Accepted: 11 April 2019; Published: 14 April 2019

Abstract: Tissue engineering technologies involving growth factors have produced one of the most advanced generations of diabetic wound healing solutions. Using this approach, a nanocomposite carrier was designed using Poly(D,L-lactide-co-glycolide) (PLGA)/Gelatin polymer solutions for the simultaneous release of recombinant human epidermal growth factor (rhEGF) and gentamicin sulfate at the wound site to hasten the process of diabetic wound healing and inactivation of bacterial growth. The physicochemical characterization of the fabricated scaffolds was carried out using scanning electron microscopy (SEM) and X-ay diffraction (XRD). The scaffolds were analyzed for thermal stability using thermogravimetric analysis and differential scanning calorimetry. The porosity, biodegradability, and swelling behavior of the scaffolds was also evaluated. Encapsulation efficiency, drug loading capacity, and in vitro drug release were also investigated. Further, the bacterial inhibition percentage and detailed in vivo biocompatibility for wound healing efficiency was performed on diabetic C57BL6 mice with dorsal wounds. The scaffolds exhibited excellent wound healing and continuous proliferation of cells for 12 days. These results support the applicability of such systems in rapid healing of diabetic wounds and ulcers.

Keywords: tissue engineering; growth factor; diabetic; wound healing; nanocomposite

1. Introduction

Wound healing or tissue repair is a complex multistep process comprising a multitude of cells, cytokines, extracellular matrix (ECM) molecules, blood cells, and a number of other factors [1]. Disturbances at proliferation or inflammation phases of wound healing lead to perturbations in the process [2]. Chronic wounds, such as those in diabetic patients, present worldwide health challenges as well as an economic burden. The existing therapies exhibit unsatisfactory results and despite treatment of these chronic wounds, which involves tight glucose control and meticulous wound care, the prognosis for their healing is quite poor and finally leads to morbidity [3,4]. Microorganisms are naturally present on the wound bed without any detrimental effects to the normal wound healing process since the number of bacteria is quite low. Since diabetes lowers the normal immunity of the body, such patients are more prone to infection in wounds [5]. Hence, chronic wounds, such as leg ulcers, foot ulcers, and pressure ulcers, are more prone to such microbial infections due to the presence of multiple microbial populations consisting of *S. aureus* [6], *P. aeruginosa* [7], coliform bacteria [8], *Streptococcus* spp., and *Enterococcus* spp. [9]. During injury, foreign bodies including pathogenic microbes can enter deep into the wounds causing chronic inflammatory responses and, thereby, delaying healing of the wounds. The patient may develop a more serious deep-wound infection, and require amputation due to the occurrence of anaerobic bacteria in diabetic foot ulcers and may also lead to abscess or granuloma formation [10,11].

Generally, the process of wound healing is driven by many cellular mediators including various growth factors which are proteinaceous molecules playing a key role in tissue repair and wound care [12]. One of the major obstacles in the treatment method involving growth factors is that the encapsulated growth factor tends to be released in a non-controllable manner due to its physical association with the drug reservoir systems [13]. Moreover, the growth factors are either easily degraded by proteinases or removed by exudate before reaching the wound bed. Until now, only platelet-derived growth factor-BB (PDGF-BB) has successfully passed clinical trials [1]. Epidermal growth factor (EGF) is a low-molecular-weight polypeptide and plays a significant role in wound healing as it stimulates proliferation, differentiation, and survival of cells [14]. Hence, recombinant human epidermal growth factor (rhEGF) was selected as the bioactive agent for immobilization on the nanofibrous scaffolds. It acts by binding with high affinity to epidermal growth factor receptor (EGFR) on the cell surface and stimulating the intrinsic protein-tyrosine kinase activity of the receptor. The tyrosine kinase activity, in turn, initiates a signal transduction cascade that results in a variety of biochemical changes within the cell—a rise in intracellular calcium levels, increased glycolysis and protein synthesis, and increases in the expression of certain genes including the gene for EGFR—that ultimately lead to DNA synthesis and cell proliferation [15].

In the recent scenario, due to their comprehensive assortment of implementations in the world of biomedicine, nanomaterials have emerged as potent tools for clinicians and researchers in different biomedical and allied fields of human life [16–18]. Nanomaterials possess notable virtues, such as high reactivity, large surface-to-mass ratio, and ultra-small size making them highly useful in biomedical applications [19,20].

In view of these strategies, current tissue engineering approaches are centered around the fabrication of three dimensional (3D) nanoscaffolds or ECM analogs that should conform to multifactorial requirements, for example, those associated with tissue repair [16]. Such scaffolds tune the biomimetic nature of the ECM, possess large surface area to volume ratio, are able to facilitate diffusion (as a result of high porosity), and have tunability of physical properties simultaneously providing a local release of different biomolecules to address successful tissue regeneration [21]. Numerous studies have been done to fabricate potentially applicable scaffold materials for tissue engineering and wound healing applications. Electrospun nanofibrous scaffolds have been successfully used in site-specific delivery of many bioactive molecules and for the treatment of various infections and cancers. Such scaffolds allow for the release of loaded biomolecules in therapeutic dosage and have a negligible influence on drug activity and possess well-controlled drug release rate [22,23]. One of the smart property of these scaffolds is that they possess physical resemblance with ECM and are easy to implement due to their superior mechanical durability, flexibility in surface functionalities, and interconnected and readily controlled secondary structures [24]. Polymers had been a choice material for the fabrication of nanofibrous scaffolds. Synthetic biodegradable polymers, such as poly(β-caprolactone), polyethylene oxide, poly(L-lactide-*co*-β-caprolactone) (PLCL), polylactic acid, poly(lactide-*co*-glycolide), and polyglycolic acid (PGA), Poly(vinyl alcohol (PVA), Polyvinyl chloride

(PVC), Poly-L-lactic acid (PLLA), nylon, gelatin, polyurethane, etc., have proven useful in the preparation of nanofibrous scaffolds. Researches have proved these scaffolds to be biocompatible and to enhance cell functions in vitro [25,26].

Cell functions include the growth, differentiation, and metabolism of cells via interaction with specific cell-surface receptors [27]. Polymers like Poly (D,L-lactide-co-glycolide) (PLGA) have been extensively used for application in drug-delivery, surgical implants, and tissue engineering scaffolds owing to their biodegradability and biocompatibility [28,29]. Further, it is imperative that the wound is free from infection-causing microbes and all factors which inhibit its natural healing process [30]. The addition of antibacterial agents into electrospun fibers has been a thrust area of research for clinicians especially as antibiotic-resistant bacteria strains increasingly emerge [31]. Gentamicin sulfate is a bactericidal aminoglycoside antibiotic that is widely used for the treatment of bacterial infections [32]. Electrospun nanofibers could increase the drug efficiency and drug solubility in aqueous solution due to their high surface-to-volume ratio. They could provide a controlled drug delivery to the site of action in the body in an optimal concentration-versus-time profile. A multitude of nanomaterials conjugated with vancomycin has been designed to enhance the pharmacokinetics and pharmacodynamics of the antibiotic molecule [31,33–36].

In this work, we fabricated a novel biomimetic drug and rhEGF delivery system by the electrospinning of PLGA/Gelatin solutions containing Gentamicin Sulfate (GS) and further immobilizing the scaffolds with rhEGF. The purpose of this work is to support diabetic wound healing and to eliminate microbial infections while releasing gentamicin and rhEGF in a controlled fashion. To our knowledge, synchronous release of drug and growth factor from electrospun scaffolds has not been investigated and we did not find any paper which discusses it. In the present scenario, controlled release of antibiotic and growth factor was achieved, and the dual delivery system allows for efficient and for the treatment of wounds in diabetic patients.

2. Experimental

2.1. Materials

Poly (D,L-lactide-co-glycolide) (LA/GA 85/15) (Gangwal Chemicals Pvt. Ltd., Mumbai, India), gentamicin sulfate (FDC India Ltd., Mumbai, India), streptozotocin (Sisco Research Laboratories Pvt. Ltd., Bhiwandi, India), nutrient broth and nutrient agar (Merck Specialities Pvt. Ltd. Mumbai, India), 2,2,2-trifluoroethanol, suberic acid bis(N-hydroxy-succinimide ester) (NHS), 1,6-diaminohexane and 2,2-dihydroxyindane-1,3-dione (ninhydrin) (Loba Chemie Pvt. Ltd. Mumbai, India) and rhEGF (Life Technologies India Pvt. Ltd., New Delhi, India). All other chemicals and reagents were of analytical grade as purchased.

2.2. Fabrication of GS-Loaded Composite PLGA/Gelatin Nanoscaffolds

Composite PLGA/Gelatin nanoscaffolds were fabricated as described in our previous study [21,37]. Schematic Figure 1 demonstrates the procedure for the fabrication of electrospun nanofibrous scaffolds, their immobilization with the growth factors (rhEGF and Gentamicin sulfate (GS)) and their application on wounds of diabetic mice for in vivo test. Poly (D,L-lactide-co-glycolide) was used with LA/GA in the ratio 85/15 due to the fact that it takes an average degradation time of 5 to 6 weeks [38]. Briefly, two different composite polymer solutions of 10% PLGA/Gelatin (wt. ratio 70:30 and 50:50, respectively) in 2,2,2-trifluoroethanol were prepared. Thereafter, 5 mg/mL gentamicin sulfate and 0.2 mL of PEG-400 was added to each of the prepared polymer solutions, and were electrospun into nanofibrous scaffolds using an electrospinning setup. The electrospinning was operated at the flow rate of 0.6 mL/h, and a high voltage (16 kV) was applied to the tip of the needle (0.9 mm inner hole diameter) attached to the syringe. The ultrafine aligned nanofibers were collected by a rotating the disc wrapped with a piece of aluminum foil with a horizontal distance of 10 cm from the needle tip. The obtained electrospun nanofibrous scaffolds were dried at room temperature under vacuum for 24 h to remove organic solvent and moisture. The scaffolds were stored at −20 °C for further analysis.

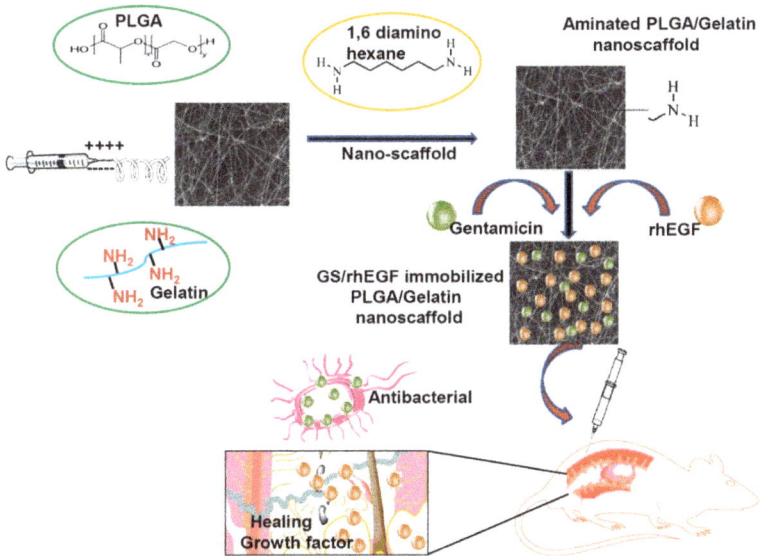

Figure 1. Process of fabrication of aminolyzed Poly(D,L-lactide-*co*-glycolide) (PLGA)/Gelatin nanoscaffolds and subsequent application on diabetic wounds.

2.3. Post-treatment of Composite Nanoscaffolds via Covalent Immobilization of rhEGF

The growth factor rhEGF was immobilized on the surface of the prepared nanoscaffolds by the covalent immobilization technique [21]. Before immobilization, the scaffolds were aminolyzed to introduce amine groups into the surface of the prepared scaffolds. Henceforth, the scaffold pieces (20 mm in diameter) were soaked into a 10% (*w/v*) solution of 1,6-hexanediamine prepared in isopropanol and were incubated at room temperature for 3 h and subsequently washed in PBS (phosphate-buffered saline, pH 7.4) five times. Then the scaffolds were rinsed with 70% ethanol and PBS. Thereafter, they were immersed in 10 mL PBS containing 0.08 mmol NHS with gentle agitation for 4 h at room temperature. The scaffolds were again rinsed gently five times with PBS to remove residual solvents and make sure that scaffolds are not removed from the substrate (Supplementary Material: Figure S1) five times with PBS. Finally, the activated scaffolds were soaked into 10 µg/mL rhEGF solutions in PBS with gentle shaking for 12 h at 4 °C. Then the rhEGF-immobilized composite nanoscaffolds were washed with PBS and freeze-dried.

2.4. Surface Topography and Properties

The surface topography and size of the composite nanofibrous scaffolds was examined by a Hitachi-4800 scanning electron microscope (SEM) (Hitachi India Pvt. Ltd, Mumbai, India). Before examination, the samples were adhered to SEM studs, and coated with 5 nm thin gold film using a sputter-coater (EMITECH K550X, EMITECH ENGINEERING (INDIA) PRIVATE LIMITED, Mumbai, India) for 4 min at 30 mA. The fibers were quantified using DiameterJ tool in imageJ (https://imagej.net/DiameterJ) and plot was generated into origin software.

2.5. Quantitative Analysis of rhEGF-Immobilized Composite Nanoscaffolds

The amine groups present on the surface of 1,6-hexanediamine treated nanoscaffolds (diameter 15 mm) were determined using ninhydrin assay [39,40]. Ninhydrin solution (1.0 M) was prepared in ethanol and each scaffold was immersed into this solution for 1 min. Then, the scaffolds were transferred to a glass vial that was heated for 15 min at 70 °C. The scaffolds were then dissolved in 2 mL tetrahydrofuron and isopropanol each and mixed with the solution. The absorbance was measured at 560 nm using a Lambda 25 UV–Vis spectrophotometer (Perkin-Elmer, New York, NY, USA). The amine groups on the scaffolds were quantified by plotting a standard curve of 1,6-hexanediamine solutions in isopropanol in the range of 5 to 25 µg/mL. To determine the amount of immobilized rhEGF, the fluorescence intensity of the tryptophan group of rhEGF immobilized on the nanofibrous scaffolds was measured. The rhEGF assay was performed using a fluorescence spectrophotometer (Perkin Elmer Model–LS 45, Perkin Elmer, New York, NY, USA) at 280 nm excitation and 342 nm emission wavelength as the intrinsic tryptophan fluorescence. The amount of immobilized rhEGF was determined by subtracting rhEGF residual intensity in solution at the end of the immobilization process from the initial amount of rhEGF in the solution.

2.6. Thermal Analysis

The thermal properties of composite nanoscaffolds were determined using thermogravimetric analysis (TGA) and differential scanning calorimetry (DSC). TGA was performed in an automatic thermal analyzer system Thermogravimetry/Differential Thermal Analysis (TG/DTA) (Diamond TG/DTA 8.0, Perkin-Elmer, Perkin Elmer India Ltd., Noida, India). Sealed samples were healed in an aluminum pan at 20.00 °C/min from 50.00 °C to 900.00 °C under a constant nitrogen flow rate of 150 mL/min through the sample chamber. The DSC measurements were carried out in an automatic thermal analyzer system (Diamond TG/DTA 8.0, Perkin-Elmer, New York, NY, USA) in the temperature range from −50 °C to 300 °C at a heating rate of 15 °C/min under a nitrogen atmosphere.

2.7. X-Ray Diffraction

The crystalline structure of composite nanoscaffolds was characterized by Spinner PW3064 XPERT-PRO diffraction (XRD) system using Cu Kα radiation with continuous scanning at 40 mA, 45 kV. The scan was performed from 5° to 60° (2θ). The plane spacing of different diffraction planes (d_{hkl}) can be calculated from the Bragg's Law (Equation (1)):

$$d_{hk} = \lambda/2 \sin\theta \hat{} \quad (1)$$

where λ is the wavelength of the copper anode source (λ = 1.54 Å), and θ stands for the diffraction angle of each indexed diffraction plane.

2.8. Degree of Swelling and Porosity.

The degree of swelling of nanoscaffolds was calculated by immersing them in phosphate buffer saline (pH 7.4) for 24 h at room temperature [21]. After 24 h, the nanoscaffolds were removed, and the excess buffer solution was wiped with filter paper and weighed. The weights were recorded, and the swelling index was calculated using Equation (2) as given below.

$$\text{Degree of swelling (\%)} = \frac{W - W_O}{W_O} \times 100 \quad (2)$$

where, W = weight of scaffolds after immersion and W_o = weight of scaffolds before immersion: The porosity of the composite nanoscaffolds was measured using the gravimetric method [21]. The thicknesses of the nanoscaffolds were measured using microcallipers, and then their apparent density ($\rho_{scaffold}$) and porosity(ε) were calculated according to the Equation (3).

$$\varepsilon = 1 - \frac{\rho_{scaffold}}{\rho_{material}} \quad (3)$$

where, $\rho_{scaffold}$ is the density of scaffold and $\rho_{material}$ is the density of bulk PLGA

2.9. Water Contact Angle Measurement

The water contact angle measurements were performed using an FTA1000 (First Ten Ångstroms Inc., Manchester, UK) instrument. An average obtained from at least five measurements of the contact angle was obtained with MilliQ water (volume ~3 nano-liters, FirstTenÅngstroms Inc., Noida, India) on different nanoscaffolds composite spots. For statistical validation of results, each measurement of a particular contact angle was recorded in 150 images taken within 5 s with a Pelco Model PCHM 575-4 camera (standard deviation ~2°, unless otherwise stated). Images analysis was performed by the FTA Windows Mode 4 software.

2.10. In Vitro Biodegradability Studies

To evaluate the in vitro biodegradability of composite nanoscaffolds, degradation studies were performed over a period of 14 days in phosphate buffer saline solution (PBS; pH 7.4) [21,41]. Degradation, as the percentage of weight loss (W_L) was calculated on 3rd, 7th, 10th, and 14th day using Equation (4).

$$W_L(\%) = \frac{W - W_O}{W_O} \times 100 \tag{4}$$

where W_O is initial weight and W is weight after degradation:

2.11. Drug-Polymer Profile

Drug assay was carried out to determine the drug entrapment efficiency of the composite nanoscaffolds as reported in our previous study [21]. Drug loaded nanoscaffolds were placed in phosphate buffer saline (pH 7.4) and centrifuged at 8000 rpm for 5 min. A 3 mL of ninhydrin reagent was added to the supernatant, and the absorbance was measured using a Lambda 25 UV–vis spectrophotometer (Perkin-Elmer, New York, NY, USA) at 566 nm. The amount of drug in the sample was calculated using the standard curve prepared from PBS. The drug entrapment efficiency was calculated by comparing the amount of drug used to prepare the scaffolds according to Equation (5).

$$\text{Drug entrapment efficiency (\%)} = \frac{M}{M_O} \times 100 \tag{5}$$

where, M = mass of entrapped drug and M_O = mass of drug used in the formulation. The drug loading capacity is the ratio of the mass of bound drug to the mass of the scaffold and was calculated using Equation (6).

$$\text{Drug loading capacity (\%)} = \frac{F}{W} \times 100 \tag{6}$$

2.12. In Vitro Drug Release Studies

The release of gentamicin sulfate from composite nanoscaffolds was studied at different pH values. It is well known that the pH values have a significant impact on the assembly and organization of nanoscaffolds by affecting the surface charge density of weak electrolytes. It also has an effect on the degree of ionization of weak polyelectrolytes [42]. The membrane diffusion technique was used for the in-vitro release studies of gentamicin sulfate from composite nanoscaffolds, as described in our previous study [21,41]. The studies were conducted within a temperature controlled incubator (37 ± 0.5 °C) using PBS (150 mM, pH 7.4) under gentle mixing.

The nanoscaffolds were incubated in 5 mL of aqueous buffer solution with pH 3, 7.4, and 9, respectively. Aliquots of 1.0 mL of the diffusion medium were withdrawn at certain incubation time points and were replaced with an equal quantity of a fresh diffusion medium. Samples were quantitatively analyzed using Systronics 10 UV–Vis spectrophotometer at 566.0 nm, after treatment with ninhydrin reagent against the mixture of diffusion medium and ninhydrin reagent as blank.

2.13. In Vitro Antibacterial Activity Testing

Antibacterial activity of composite nanoscaffolds was evaluated against *Staphylococcus aureus*, a Gram-positive bacteria in liquid medium [21,24]. *Staphylococcus aureus* was obtained from the Microbiology department, Sam Higginbottom Institute of Agriculture, Technology and Sciences, Allahabad. The bacterial culture was grown in nutrient broth, and when the absorbance reached 0.1 to 0.2 at 625 nm, 5 mL of the culture was taken in test tubes, and the drug loaded nanoscaffolds were submerged in them. GS powder was taken as a positive control while the tube without scaffold was taken as negative control. Another tube with cotton gauze was set as another negative control. The samples were incubated on a shaker at 200 rpm for 24 h at 37 °C. After that, the absorbance at 625 nm was monitored using UV–vis spectroscopy. All experiments were performed in triplicate, and only the average values were reported. The percentage of bacterial inhibition was calculated from Equation (7).

$$\text{Bacterial inhibition}(\%) = \frac{I_C - I_S}{I_C} \times 100 \qquad (7)$$

where Ic and Is are the average absorbance readings of the control group and the experimental group, respectively.

The assessment was conducted based on the disc agar diffusion method [21,24]. Nutrient agar plates were prepared by autoclaving the nutrient agar media and pouring onto petri dishes and air-dried. A 100 µL aliquot of bacteria reconstituted in nutrient broth and previously subcultured was spread onto an agar plate. The GS-free and GS-containing nanoscaffolds were cut into circular discs (15 mm in diameter) and placed on the top of the agar plate. The plates were incubated at 37 °C for 24 h. If inhibitory concentrations were reached, there would be no growth of the bacteria, which could be seen as a clear zone around the scaffold specimens. The zone was then recorded as an indication of inhibition against the bacterial species.

2.14. In Vivo Wound Healing Studies in Diabetic Mice

In vivo studies were performed in accordance with the Institutional Animal Ethics Committee (IAEC) constituted as per directions of the Committee for the Purpose of Control and Supervision of Experiments on Animals (CPCSEA), under the Ministry of Animal Welfare Division, Government of India, New Delhi. The approval from the Institutional Animal Ethical Committee of Bundelkhand University, Jhansi, was taken before the experimental work (BU/Pharm/IAEC/13/29). Five groups of Female C57BL/6 mice weighing (14–15 g) were selected, each group having 6 mice. All animals were allowed to adapt to cages for 3 days, after which they were fasted overnight. Streptozotocin (STZ) was freshly dissolved in (0.1 M, pH 4.5) citrate buffer and non-insulin-dependent diabetes mellitus was induced in overnight fasted mice by a single intraperitoneal injection of Streptozotocin (40 mg/kg bodyweight). Blood glucose levels were measured 4 days after STZ injection, and only mice with fasting blood glucose levels greater than 200 mg/dL were considered to be diabetic and were used in the experiment. Wounds in the diabetic mice were created by following the excision wound model, whereby their dorsal hairs were shaven, and an excision made with scissors and tweezer on the back of the animal. The wound areas were sterilized with povidone iodide. All treatments started 4 days after STZ injection. For determination of wound healing activity, the following treatments were applied after creating wounds on five groups—Group 1 (C)—no treatment (negative control), Group 2 (G)—pure GS solution (positive control), Group 3 (P)—PLGA/Gelatin 70:30 scaffold without GS and rhEGF, Group 4 (PG)—PLGA/Gelatin 70:30 scaffold loaded with GS and rhEGF both and Group 5 (PG)—PLGA/Gelatin 70:30 scaffold loaded with GS only. The treatments were applied to aseptically treated wounds to determine the therapeutic effects on the wounds. After each treatment interval, the scaffolds were removed with tweezers. The wounds were photographed on day 1 and the treatment regime repeated on day 4, 8, and 12. The percentage reduction of the wound area was calculated using Equation (8) below.

$$\text{Wound area (\%)} = \frac{A}{A_i} \times 100 \tag{8}$$

where, A_i is the initial wound area, and A is the wound area after a fixed time interval.

2.15. Statistical Analysis

Data are expressed as means ± standard deviation. For the statistical validation of data, three independent experiments (n = 3) were performed in triplicates. Statistical analysis was conducted using a paired *t*-test or an unpaired, two-tailed Student's *t*-test. A *p*-value of <0.05 was considered to be statistically significant.

3. Results and Discussion

3.1. Surface Topography and Properties of Composite Nanoscaffolds

The morphologies of the PLGA/Gelatin 70:30 and PLGA/Gelatin 50:50 nanofibrous scaffolds as depicted by SEM micrographs are shown in Figure 2A,B, respectively.

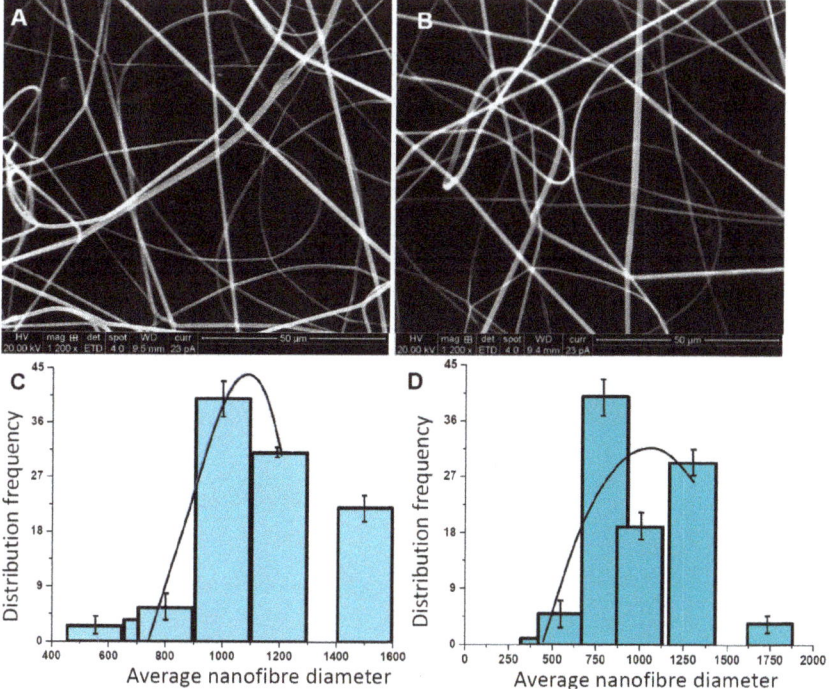

Figure 2. Physical Characterization. Scanning electron microscopy (SEM) micrographs of (**A**) PLGA/Gelatin 70:30 (**B**) PLGA/Gelatin 50:50 nanofibrous scaffolds and (**C**) Average fiber size distribution in PLGA/Gelatin 70:30 and (**D**) PLGA/Gelatin 50:50 nanofibrous scaffolds. The results are expressed as the median ± standard deviation obtained from analysis of 20 to 25 images for each electrospun polymer film (the black curve is drawn to shows the Gaussian distribution of frequency).

The corresponding average fiber diameters are shown as a bar plot in Figure 2C,D, respectively. The graph indicates that there is a random distribution of fibers in both, PLGA/Gelatin 70:30 and 50:50 nanoscaffolds. The average fiber diameter in PLGA/Gelatin 70:30 is slightly higher than 50:50 (~750 nm to 900 nm). The fibers exhibit ECM like interconnectivity, and no bead formation was observed. As gelatin adds viscosity to the solution, both types of fibers were smooth and without any breakage. The probability of fiber breakage increases with increasing gelatin content since an increase in gelatin content decreases the viscosity of the polymeric solution. The calculated average diameters of PLGA/Gelatin 70:30 and PLGA/Gelatin 50:50 nanofibers were 589.6 nm and 566.0 nm, respectively. As the concentration of gelatin increased, the diameter of the nanofibers decreased. This may be attributed to the fact that on increasing the gelatin content, the viscosity of the composite solution decreased, and the amino acids of the gelatin improved the self-repulsion and stretching force due to the increasing charge density of the jet during the electrospinning process. This resulted in the smaller fiber diameter [43]. The overall structure of the fibers mimics that of the ECM.

3.2. Quantitative Analysis of rhEGF-Immobilized Nanoscaffolds

The number of amine groups (µg per scaffold) on scaffolds treated with ninhydrin was quantified using the standard curve, and the results are shown in Figure 3A. It can be inferred from the graph that the quantified amount of amine groups were 25 µg and 30 µg per scaffold in PLGA/Gelatin 70:30 and PLGA/Gelatin 50:50 nanoscaffolds, respectively. The presence of amine groups in both the scaffolds clearly indicates the success of aminolysis. The results obtained from fluorescence spectrophotometry confirmed the presence of rhEGF on the surface of the nanofibrous scaffolds. The rhEGF-conjugated PLGA/Gelatin 50:50 and PLGA/Gelatin 70:30 nanoscaffolds had 7.46 µg and 2.92 µg of rhEGF, respectively, per scaffold when 10 µg of rhEGF was employed for a chemical reaction. Thus, the rhEGF immobilization efficiencies reached 74.6% and 29.2% for PLGA/Gelatin 50:50 and PLGA/Gelatin 70:30 nanofibrous scaffolds, respectively. It could be attributed to the fact that since the number of amine groups per scaffold was higher in PLGA/Gelatin 50:50 scaffolds, they were able to immobilize a greater amount of rhEGF than the PLGA/Gelatin 70:30 nanofibrous scaffolds.

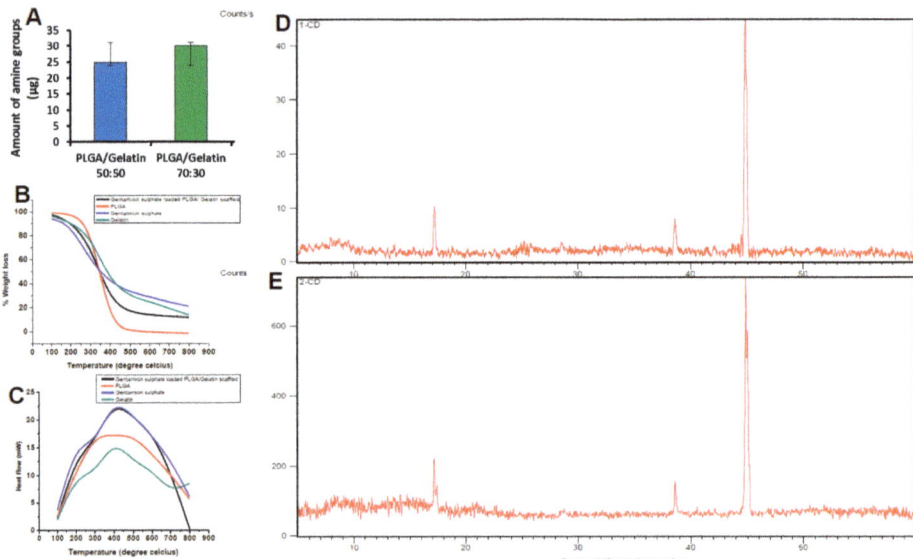

Figure 3. Biochemical characterization. (**A**) 2,2-dihydroxyindane-1,3-dione (ninhydrin) assay applied to 1,6 hexanediamine treated nanofibrous scaffolds (the results are expressed as the median ± standard deviation). (**B**) Thermogravimetric analysis (TGA) curves of PLGA, Gentamicin sulfate loaded PLGA 70:30 nanofibrous scaffolds, Gentamicin sulfate and Gelatin. (**C**) Differential scanning calorimetry (DSC) curves of PLGA, Gentamicin sulfate loaded PLGA nanofibrous scaffolds, Gentamicin sulfate and Gelatin. (**D**) X-Ray diffraction (XRD) spectra of (**A**) PLGA/gelatin 70:30 and (**E**) PLGA/gelatin 50:50 nanofibrous scaffolds.

3.3. Thermal Analysis

The thermal properties of composite nanoscaffolds and other supplements were characterized using TGA and DSC. TGA curves are shown in Figure 3B. The results from the TGA showed two significant weight losses for the gentamicin sulfate at 220 °C and 330 °C. The TGA curves of raw PLGA showed weight losses at 210 °C and 400 °C. In contrast, the TGA curve of gentamicin loaded PLGA/gelatin 70:30 nanofibrous scaffolds showed single significant weight loss at about 260 °C, respectively. As the weight loss of gentamicin sulfate and pure PLGA started at lower temperature compared to the gentamicin sulfate loaded scaffolds, it showed better thermal stability of the composite scaffolds in comparison to gentamicin sulfate or pure polymer alone. Due to the formation of covalent bonds between gentamicin and PLGA/gelatin scaffolds, the labile oxygen containing functional group availability was decreased. Less than 2% weight loss occurred below 200 °C. In addition, the slow weight loss of about 40% below 260 to 350 °C that may be due to the loss of residual functional group on the gentamicin-loaded scaffolds. These observations were missing in the negative control without the gentamicin.

The DSC thermograms of PLGA/Gelatin 70:30 nanofibrous scaffolds are shown in Figure 3C. A peak was observed at the temperature of 210 °C on the DSC thermogram of pure gentamicin sulfate powder, corresponding to the melting point of 210 °C. Another peak was seen at 410 °C, which was due to the reaction between the gentamicin sulfate structures, i.e., degradation of gentamicin sulfate. In the pure PLGA polymer, no sharp peak was observed which may be attributed to the amorphous nature of the PLGA. Whereas, the DSC curve of gelatin showed a peak at 405 °C. In contrast, in the DSC curves of gentamicin loaded PLGA/gelatin 70:30 nanofibrous scaffolds, the peak occurred at 430 °C. This clearly demonstrates that the stability of the drug is enhanced due to encapsulation of the drug between polymeric chains.

3.4. X-Ray Diffraction Analysis

The nanofibrous scaffolds are able to form a stable colloidal layered structure in aqueous solution, that facilitates drug encapsulation. The encapsulation of drug within the PLGA/Gelatin interlayer space may result in a change in the interlayer distance, that can be determined by XRD technology. The XRD patterns of the PLGA/gelatin 70:30 and PLGA/gelatin 50:50 scaffolds after gentamicin sulfate encapsulation are shown in Figure 3D,E, respectively. All the three types of nanofibrous scaffolds displayed patterns lacking any distinct peaks indicating that they are fully amorphous materials. In amorphous materials, X-rays will be scattered in many directions leading to a large bump distributed in a wide range (2 Theta) instead of high intensity narrower peaks. Appearance of the broad peaks in the $2\theta = 5$–$40°$ region was attributed to the amorphous nature of the PLGA. The absence of any distinct peaks of crystalline gentamicin sulfate in the XRD spectra indicates that the drug is no longer present as crystalline material, but had been totally converted to an amorphous state. The XRD data suggested that the incorporation of gentamicin sulfate within polymers is primarily via the drug intercalation within the polymer interlayer space.

It is also possible that a small portion of gentamicin sulfate can be adsorbed onto the polymer surface via hydrogen bonding or other weak forces. The XRD spectrum of the scaffolds displayed two peaks at 19.3° and 23.5° which were located at the same position with the PEG 400. The sharp XRD peaks indicate the crystallization of PEG in the scaffolds.

3.5. Degree of Swelling and Porosity Analysis

The gentamicin sulfate loaded PLGA/Gelatin 70:30 and PLGA/ Gelatin 50:50 nanofibrous scaffolds were analyzed to determine the swelling behavior by incubating them in PBS (pH 7.4) for 24 h at 37 °C. The results are represented graphically in Figure 4A. The swelling ratios of the PLGA/Gelatin 70:30 and PLGA/ Gelatin 50:50 nanofibrous scaffolds were 421.33 ± 8.22% and 445.33 ± 4.99%, respectively. The swelling index of cotton gauze was only 280.00 ± 8.64%. It can be inferred from these results that the higher swelling index of PLGA/ Gelatin 50:50 scaffolds was due to more concentration of gelatin as compared to the PLGA/Gelatin 70:30 scaffolds, as gelatin improves the hydrophilicity of the scaffold. This may be due to the amine and carboxylic functional groups present in the gelatin structure [44]. The obtained swelling index enables the prepared scaffolds to be used as wound dressings for absorbing excess exudates even from deep wounds with high amounts of exudates [44,45].

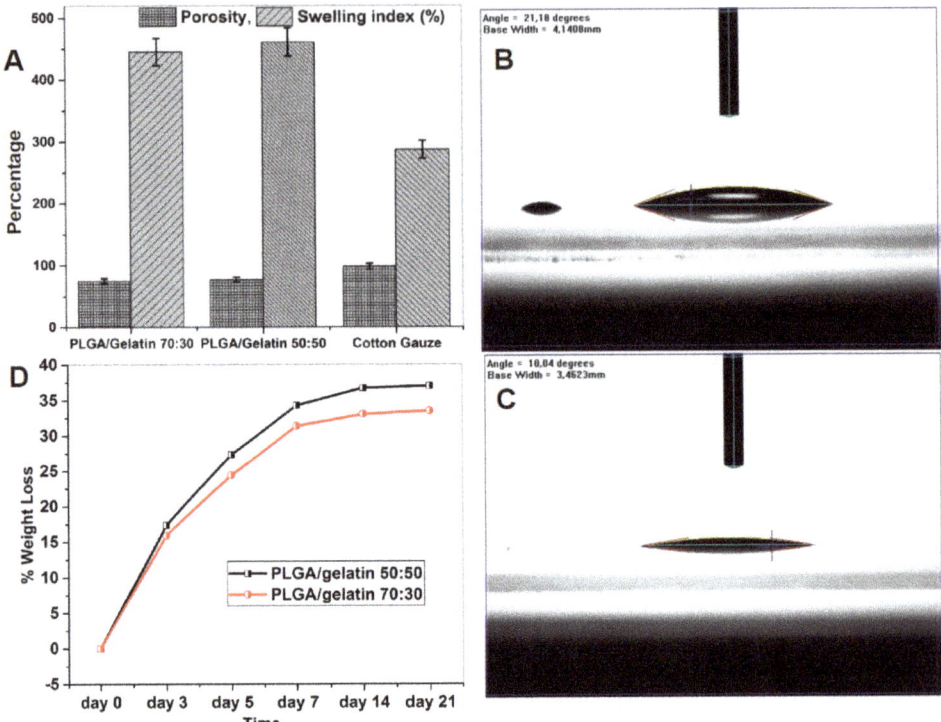

Figure 4. Scaffold stability and wettability analysis. (**A**) Comparison of swelling index and porosities of electrospun PLGA/gelatin 70:30 and 50:50 nanofibrous scaffolds (the results are expressed as the median ± standard deviation from five samples). (**B**) Water Contact Angle Value for PLGA/Gelatin 50:50 Nanofibrous Scaffold. (**C**) Water Contact Angle Value for PLGA/Gelatin 70:30 Nanofibrous Scaffold. (**D**) Biodegradability characteristics of PLGA/gelatin 50:50 and PLGA/gelatin 70:30 nanofibrous scaffolds.

Porosity is a very important criteria for the application of nanofibrous scaffolds in tissue engineering and wound healing practices because the microscale and nanoscale porous structure are most suitable for convenient passage and exchange of nutrients and gases, that are important for cellular growth and tissue regeneration [46]. Porosity should be in the range of 60 to 90% for cellular penetration and efficient tissue regeneration [47]. In the present work, porosity was calculated by the gravimetric method and the results are represented graphically in Figure 4A. The porosities of PLGA/Gelatin 50:50 and PLGA/Gelatin 70:30 nanofibrous scaffolds were 74.1% and 77%, respectively. In contrast, the porosity of cotton gauze was 102%. The possible reason could be that the increased gelatin content decreased the fiber diameter, which caused the decreased porosity of scaffolds.

3.6. Water Contact Angle Measurements

Generally, if the water contact angle is smaller than 90°, the solid surface is considered hydrophilic and wettable, and if the water contact angle is larger than 90°, the solid surface is considered hydrophobic and not wettable. Figure 4B,C, respectively show that the water contact angle values for PLGA/Gelatin 70:30 and PLGA/Gelatin 50:50 nanofibrous scaffolds were 10.04° and 21.18°, respectively. Hence, it could be concluded that the water contact angles of both the scaffolds was much lesser than 90°. Therefore, the surface of the scaffolds could be considered highly hydrophilic. Moreover, the water contact angle of PLGA/Gelatin 50:50 nanofibrous scaffolds were lower than that of PLGA/Gelatin 70:30 nanofibrous scaffolds due to more amount of Gelatin on the former as compared to the latter.

3.7. In Vitro Biodegradability Studies

The in vitro biodegradation studies of the PLGA/Gelatin 70:30 and PLGA/Gelatin 50:50 nanofibrous scaffolds were performed in Phosphate Buffer Saline (PBS; pH 7.4). The scaffolds were placed in a 24-well plate containing 1 mL of PBS in each well and were incubated in vitro at 37 °C for different periods of time (3, 5, 7, 14 days). Figure 4D shows the percent weight losses. A rapid 27.33 ± 1.15% and 24.4 ± 1.82% mass loss was observed in electrospun PLGA/gelatin 50:50 and PLGA/gelatin 70:30 nanofibrous scaffolds, respectively, in first 5 days. After 7 days, the degradability of both scaffolds was decreased which was due to more PLGA in the remaining composition of scaffolds. Since gelatin easily dissolves in water at a temperature of 40 °C, and, hence, by increasing the content of gelatin, the biodegradability of the PLGA/gelatin 50:50 scaffolds was greater as compared to PLGA/gelatin 70:30 scaffolds. In contrast, PLGA nanofibrous scaffolds and cotton gauze used as control did not exhibit any weight loss during the 14 days of incubation.

3.8. Drug Loading Capacity and Drug Entrapment Efficiency

Drug loading capacity is the ratio of the mass of bound drug to the mass of the scaffold, whereas, the drug entrapment efficiency is the ratio of the mass of drug released to the mass of total drug added. The mass of gentamicin sulfate loaded per 20 mg of the scaffolds was investigated by UV-Vis spectrophotometry. The results are summarized in Table 1. It was found to be 174.24 μg and 161.68 μg for PLGA/Gelatin 70:30 and PLGA/Gelatin 50:50 nanofibrous scaffolds, respectively. On the other hand, the entrapment efficiency was found to be 87.12% and 80.26% for PLGA/Gelatin 70:30 and PLGA/Gelatin 50:50 nanofibrous scaffolds, respectively. The comparatively higher entrapment efficiency may be due to the fact that PLGA, being a high molecular weight polymer, and the molecular weight further supplemented by gelatin, is able to absorb a comparatively greater amount of active substances. As shown herein, more than 80% entrapment efficiency ensures more than 150 μg of gentamicin sulfate delivered to the wound site for in-situ release. These results are in line with therapeutically used dosages of gentamicin sulfate 100 μg or more, immobilized on the synthetic carrier for successful treatment of infection in mouse model [48].

Table 1. Drug loading capacity and drug entrapment efficiency of nanofibrous scaffolds.

Nanofibrous Scaffold	Drug Loading Capacity (μg)	Drug Entrapment Efficiency (%)
PLGA/Gelatin 50:50	161.68 ± 13.2	80.26 ± 6.9
PLGA/Gelatin 70:30	174.24 ± 19	87.12 ± 8.1

3.9. In Vitro Drug Release Studies

The gentamicin sulfate release curves from PLGA/Gelatin 70:30 and PLGA/Gelatin 50:50 nanofibrous scaffolds were studied at different pH values, and the release curves are illustrated in Figure 5A,B. The studies from each type of scaffolds revealed constant drug release and no burst effect was observed. It indicates that the drug was homogeneously dispersed in the polymeric matrix and there was no significant amount of drug adsorbed onto the surface of nanofibers. Figure 5A shows the release of gentamicin sulfate from PLGA/Gelatin 70:30 nanofibrous scaffold. At pH 7.4, gentamicin sulfate was released slowly from the PLGA/Gelatin 70:30 nanofibrous scaffold and only 36.64 ± 0.51% of the total bound gentamicin sulfate was released in 12 h. However, 91.46 ± 0.61% and 75.43 ± 0.82%

of the drug was released in acidic and basic conditions, respectively, after 12 h. Figure 5B illustrates the release of gentamicin sulfate from PLGA/Gelatin 50:50 nanofibrous scaffold. At pH 7.4, gentamicin sulfate was released slowly from the PLGA/gelatin 50:50 nanofibrous scaffold and only 44.97 ± 0.14% of the total bound gentamicin sulfate was released in 12 h. However, 93.33 ± 0.82% and 76.03 ± 0.75% of the drug was released in acidic and basic conditions, respectively, after 12 h. The release at pH 3 and pH 9 is much higher than that released at pH 7.4. This is so because the hydrogen bonding interaction between gentamicin sulfate and the nanofibrous scaffolds is strongest at the neutral pH. Whereas, at pH 3 and 9, there is a comparatively weaker hydrogen bonding interaction, so the higher amount of gentamicin sulfate was released at pH 3 and 9. There was a higher percentage release of gentamicin sulfate at pH 3 compared to pH 9 because the hydrogen bonding interaction formed under basic conditions was stronger than that under acidic conditions.

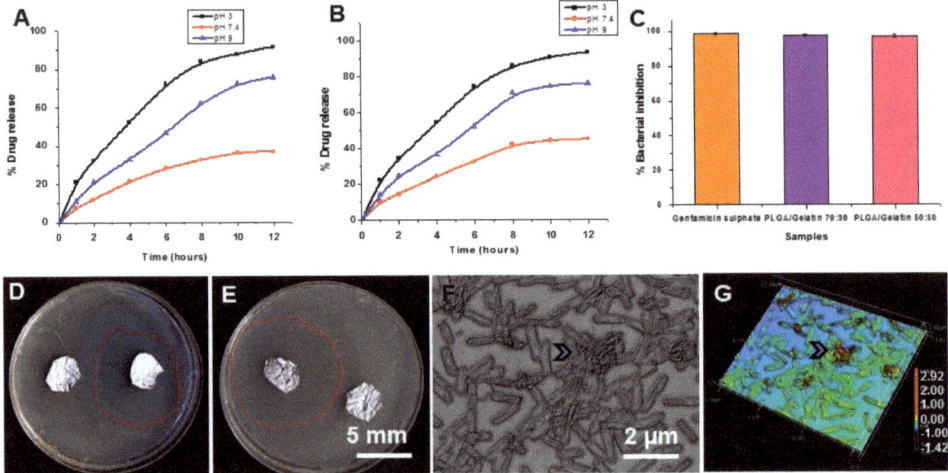

Figure 5. In vitro antibacterial assay. (**A,B**) Release profile of gentamicin sulfate on PLGA/Gelatin 70:30 (A) and 50:50 (B) nanofibrous scaffolds at three different pH values. (**C**) Growth inhibition of *Staphylococcus aureus* after treatment with PLGA/Gelatin 70:30, PLGA/Gelatin 50:50 nanofibrous scaffolds and Gentamicin sulfate powder in aqueous media. The results are expressed as the median ± standard deviation from five independent experiments performed in triplicate (n = 5). (**D**) Antibacterial activity of gentamicin sulfate loaded PLGA/ Gelatin 70:30 nanofibrous scaffolds against *Staphylococcus aureus* on LB Agar semisolid media. (**E**) Antibacterial activity of gentamicin sulfate loaded PLGA/Gelatin 50:50 nanofibrous scaffolds against *Staphylococcus aureus* (dotted red line show zone of inhibitions-ZOI around test sample, next to control). (**F,G**) Optical and laser scanning micrograph from bacterial cells seeded on Gentamicin Sulfate (GS)/PLGA/Gelatin (50:50) surfaces show sunken morphology of bacterial cells trapped in a network of nanofibers scaffolds (arrow heads).

3.10. In Vitro Antibacterial Activity

The in vitro antibacterial activity of the gentamicin sulfate loaded PLGA/Gelatin 70:30 and PLGA/Gelatin 50:50 nanofibrous scaffolds were explored against *Staphylococcus aureus* M 0092 in aqueous medium. *S. aureus* bacteria are commonly found in diabetic wounds and used as a pathogenic bacterial model for in vitro antibacterial efficacy [49]. Figure 5C illustrates the results of the antibacterial activity assays. The negative control, which was the tube with cotton gauze, completely failed to inhibit bacterial growth. Gentamicin sulfate powder, which was used as the positive control exhibited 98.73 ± 0.68% inhibition of the bacterial growth at the concentration of 5 mg/mL. The PLGA/Gelatin 70:30 and PLGA/Gelatin 50:50 nanofibrous scaffolds showed 97.39 ± 0.62% and 97.20 ± 0.99% inhibition of bacterial growth, respectively. This may be attributed to the active diffusion of the drug molecules from the scaffolds into the liquid medium, thus, inhibiting the growth of bacteria. These results are promising, since the antibacterial activity of the PLGA/Gelatin 70:30 and PLGA/Gelatin 50:50 nanofibrous scaffolds are comparable to that of the pure gentamicin powder, which presents them as a perfect drug releasing vehicle. Thus, the developed nanofibrous scaffolds could be used as a potential wound dressing material that would successfully eliminate infections, thereby, accelerating wound healing.

The antibacterial activity of the PLGA/Gelatin 70:30 and PLGA/Gelatin 50:50 nanofibrous scaffolds was also analyzed over a solid medium. Figure 5C,D shows the digital photographs of the zone of inhibition on nutrient agar plates. The gentamicin sulfate loaded PLGA/Gelatin 50:50 and PLGA/Gelatin 70:30 nanofibrous scaffolds had "zone of inhibition" values of 40 mm (Figure 5B) and 41 mm (Figure 5C), respectively. These results suggested that each nanofibrous scaffold had a good bacterial inhibition efficacy under the studied conditions. In contrast, PLGA/Gelatin nanofibrous scaffolds without gentamicin sulfate encapsulation did not inhibit the bacterial growth, suggesting that the bacterial inhibition effect is solely related to the encapsulated Gentamicin sulfate drug. Hence, the gentamicin sulfate loaded nanofibrous scaffolds were bactericidal to the testing microorganism due to the strong antibacterial ability of gentamicin sulfate. The results indicate that gentamicin sulfate loaded scaffolds possess efficient antibacterial property and can be effectively used in the treatment of wound healing or dermal bacterial infections, thereby, proving a potential application for use as a drug delivery and as a wound dressing agent [50].

We also studied the morphologies and biovolume of bacterial cells seeded on two nanofibrous scaffold supplemented with GS using laser scanning microscope to quantify surface and biovolume (Figure 5F–G and Supplementary Figure S2A–E). As seen in optical and 3D height profile images, the bacterial cells are entangled into fibers, which affect bacterial cells surface into sunken morphology, reducing their biovolume compare with untreated control cells showing flagella and normal morphology (arrow, Figure 5F–G and Figure S1C).

3.11. In Vivo Wound Healing Activity on Diabetic Mice and Organ Toxicity Evaluation

Animals with induced diabetes were confirmed with diabetic symptoms and were subjected to wound healing treatments with the gentamicin-rhEGF-nanofibrous scaffolds and controls. The wound area was measured daily from day 0 to 12 and wounds were monitored qualitatively (Figure 6A), and quantitatively (Figure 6B) for the wound closure to assess the efficacy of therapeutics designed. The results revealed that rhEGF immobilized nanofibrous scaffolds significantly increased the wound closure rates compared to other treatments. The representative images at 1, 4, 8, and 12 days after treatment with rhEGF-PLGA/Gelatin 70:30 nanofibrous scaffold, PLGA/gelatin 70:30 nanofibrous scaffold with gentamicin sulfate, PLGA/gelatin 70:30 nanofibrous scaffold without rhEGF, untreated wound and gentamicin sulfate are shown in Figure 6A. Specifically, the animals with PLGA/Gelatin 70:30 nanofibrous scaffolds with rhEGF and gentamicin sulfate showed 19.13 ± 5.68% open wound area on the 4th day (Figure 6A), 12.99 ± 1.17% open wound area on the 8th day (Figure 6An), and 3.25 ± 2.95% open wound area on the 12th day (Figure 6As), which were much less than other treatments. The data represented the mean ± S.D. for six mice per group.

We also took samples from different organs of mice treated with GS/PLGA/gelatin 50:50 after day 12 and compared with the controls group without any treatment. As shown in Figure 7, histopathological examination results showed that there was no apparent change in different organs morphology and no other abnormal changes in the mice tissue in control versus experimental group. This confirms that the nanofibrous scaffolds, thus, prepared are biocompatible and do not cause any side effects. These results open new opportunities for rapid wound healing in different vascular lesions as advance therapeutics, which is sought as a major challenge in current nanomedicine in vascular biology [51,52].

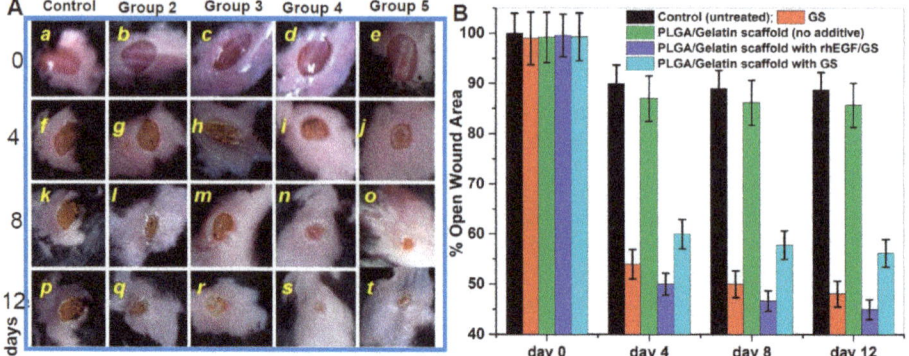

Figure 6. In vivo wound healing assay in mouse model. (**A**) Wound Healing in Diabetic C57/BL6 Mice after Treatment with Various Electrospun Nanofibrous Scaffolds (Batch 1) [a–t represent the extent of wound healing during 12 days period] Group 1—No treatment (negative control); Group 2—0.1% gentamicin sulfate ointment (positive control); Group 3—PLGA/Gelatin 70:30 scaffold without gentamicin sulfate and rhEGF; Group 4—PLGA/Gelatin 70:30 scaffold with gentamicin sulfate and rhEGF; Group 5—PLGA/Gelatin 70:30 scaffold with gentamicin sulfate and without rhEGF. (**B**) Open wound area (% of initial area) over 12 days for each treatment group from control and three experimental groups performed from five different wound healing assays. The results are expressed as the median ± standard deviation from five independent experiments performed in triplicate (n = 5).

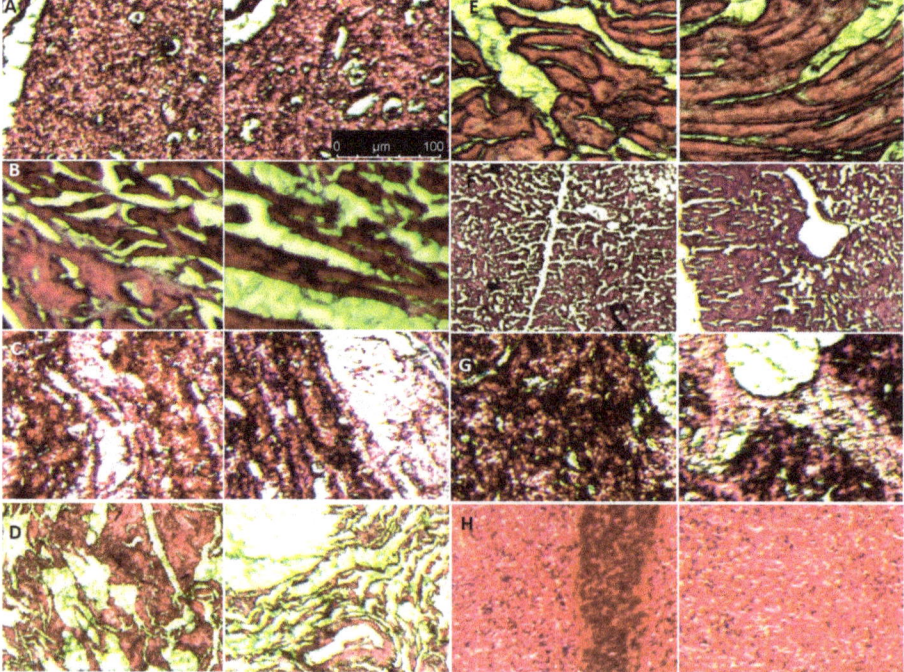

Figure 7. Histological evaluation of In vivo *organ* toxicity with histopathological staining on organ sections. (**A**) Brain (**B**) Heart (**C**) Kidney (**D**) Lung (**E**) Muscle (**F**) Liver (**G**) Pancreases (**H**) Spleen. Each image from **A**–**H** has control (left panel) and scaffold applied (right panel) sample section with Hematoxylin and Eosin (**H,E**) staining.

4. Conclusions

In summary, a novel nanocomposite carrier device composed of PLGA/Gelatin 70:30 and PLGA/Gelatin 50:50 nanofibrous scaffolds loaded with gentamicin sulfate and immobilized with rhEGF was developed for diabetic wound healing applications. The developed nanofibrous scaffolds resembled the morphology and architecture of the native extracellular matrix (ECM), which makes them useful as a suitable wound-healing scaffold. The gentamicin sulfate stability and bactericidal properties were not affected by the encapsulation process and release. The rhEGF accelerated wound-healing rates at the initial stage of the healing process. The results obtained are promising, since the simultaneous delivery of antibiotic and bioactive molecule from a nanocarrier material to inactivate bacteria in diabetic wounds and hasten the wound healing at the same time was clearly demonstrated. The nanocomposite has the potential to synergistically improve the impaired wound healing in diabetic patients via combined antibacterial activity and rhEGF supply.

Supplementary Materials: The following are available online at http://www.mdpi.com/1999-4923/11/4/180/s1, Figure S1: The SEM of nanofibrous scaffolds after gentle rinsing and dehydration. Figure S2: Quantitative analysis of bacterial biovolume on nanofibrous scaffolds. (A-B) 3D height map and optical micrograph of control bacterial cells showing normal morphology and flagella (C). (D-E) Example of extracting individual bacterial biovolume from the optical images (cells shown in dotted red line in D as an example) to quantify the biovolume of bacteria on different surfaces.

Author Contributions: Conceptualization, C.D., A.V.S. and P.W.R.; methodology, C.D., A.V.S., S.P.; software H.P., A.C.P.; validation A.V.S., P.L., A.L., and H.P.; formal analysis, C.D., A.V.S.; investigation, H.P., A.V.S., C.D.; resources, A.C.P., A.L., P.L., P.W.R.; data curation, C.D., A.V.S.; writing—original draft preparation, C.D., A.V.S.; writing—review and editing, A.V.S., C.D., P.W.R., A.L., P.L.; visualization, A.C.P., P.W.R.; supervision, A.V.S., P.W.R.; project administration, P.W.R., A.V.S.; funding acquisition, A.V.S., P.W.R.

Funding: This research was funded by Max Planck Society Grassroots fund for the year 2017 (M10335) and 2018 (M10338).

Acknowledgments: Charu Dwivedi acknowledges Council of Scientific and Industrial Research (CSIR), Ministry of HRD, Government of India for CSIR-SRF Fellowship support and National Centre of Laboratory Animal Sciences (National Institute of Nutrition-ICMR), Hyderabad, (NCLAS/ASC/2015/B.U./F-278) for providing C57/BL6 mice.

Conflicts of Interest: The authors declare no competing financial interest. The funders had no role in the design of the study; in the collection, analyses, or interpretation of data; in the writing of the manuscript, or in the decision to publish the results.

References

1. Xie, Z.; Paras, C.B.; Weng, H.; Punnakitikashem, P.; Su, L.-C.; Vu, K.; Tang, L.; Yang, J.; Nguyen, K.T. Dual growth factor releasing multi-functional nanofibers for wound healing. *Acta Biomater.* **2013**, *9*, 9351–9359. [CrossRef] [PubMed]
2. Singh, A.V.; Subhashree, L.; Milani, P.; Gemmati, D.; Zamboni, P. Interplay of iron metallobiology, metalloproteinases, and fxiii, and role of their gene variants in venous leg ulcer. *Int. J. Low. Extrem. Wounds* **2010**, *9*, 166–179. [CrossRef]
3. Gandhimathi, C.; Venugopal, J.R.; Bhaarathy, V.; Ramakrishna, S.; Kumar, S.D. Biocomposite nanofibrous strategies for the controlled release of biomolecules for skin tissue regeneration. *Int. J. Nanomed.* **2014**, *9*, 4709.
4. Sandhya, S.; Kumar, S.; Vinod, K.; Banji, D.; Kumar, K. Plant as potent anti diabetic and wound healing agent—A review. *Hygeia J. Drugs Med.* **2011**, *3*, 11–19.
5. Tiaka, E.K.; Papanas, N.; Manolakis, A.C.; Maltezos, E. The role of nerve growth factor in the prophylaxis and treatment of diabetic foot ulcers. *Int. J. Burn. Trauma* **2011**, *1*, 68.
6. Djahmi, N.; Messad, N.; Nedjai, S.; Moussaoui, A.; Mazouz, D.; Richard, J.-L.; Sotto, A.; Lavigne, J.-P. Molecular epidemiology of staphylococcus aureus strains isolated from inpatients with infected diabetic foot ulcers in an algerian university hospital. *Clin. Microbiol. Infect.* **2013**, *19*, E398–E404. [CrossRef] [PubMed]
7. Kamtikar, R.; Mitra, N. Clinico microbiological profile of pseudomonas aeruginosa isolated from diabetic foot ulcer. *J. Sci. Innov. Res.* **2014**, *3*, 478–481.
8. Bowen, K. Managing foot infections in patients with diabetes. *Aust. Prescr.* **2007**, *30*, 21–24. [CrossRef]

9. Lipsky, B.A.; Berendt, A.R.; Deery, H.G.; Embil, J.M.; Joseph, W.S.; Karchmer, A.W.; LeFrock, J.L.; Lew, D.P.; Mader, J.T.; Norden, C. Diagnosis and treatment of diabetic foot infections. *Clin. Infect. Dis.* **2004**, *39*, 885–910. [CrossRef] [PubMed]
10. Spichler, A.; Hurwitz, B.L.; Armstrong, D.G.; Lipsky, B.A. Microbiology of diabetic foot infections: From louis pasteur to 'crime scene investigation'. *BMC Med.* **2015**, *13*, 2. [CrossRef]
11. Trivedi, U.; Parameswaran, S.; Armstrong, A.; Burgueno-Vega, D.; Griswold, J.; Dissanaike, S.; Rumbaugh, K.P. Prevalence of multiple antibiotic resistant infections in diabetic versus nondiabetic wounds. *J. Pathog.* **2014**, *2014*, 173053. [CrossRef] [PubMed]
12. Dwivedi, C.; Pandey, H.; Pandey, A.C.; Ramteke, P.W. Nanofiber based smart pharmaceutical scaffolds for wound repair and regenerations. *Curr. Pharm. Des.* **2016**, *22*, 1460–1471. [CrossRef] [PubMed]
13. Choi, J.S.; Leong, K.W.; Yoo, H.S. In vivo wound healing of diabetic ulcers using electrospun nanofibers immobilized with human epidermal growth factor (EGF). *Biomaterials* **2008**, *29*, 587–596. [CrossRef] [PubMed]
14. Herbst, R.S. Review of epidermal growth factor receptor biology. *Int. J. Radiat. Oncol. Biol. Phys.* **2004**, *59*, S21–S26. [CrossRef]
15. Fallon, J.H.; Seroogy, K.B.; Loughlin, S.E.; Morrison, R.S.; Bradshaw, R.A.; Knaver, D.; Cunningham, D.D. Epidermal growth factor immunoreactive material in the central nervous system: Location and development. *Science* **1984**, *224*, 1107–1109. [CrossRef] [PubMed]
16. Vikram Singh, A.; Hasan Dad Ansari, M.; Wang, S.; Laux, P.; Luch, A.; Kumar, A.; Patil, R.; Nussberger, S. The adoption of three-dimensional additive manufacturing from biomedical material design to 3d organ printing. *Appl. Sci.* **2019**, *9*, 811. [CrossRef]
17. Singh, V.; Kashyap, S.; Yadav, U.; Srivastava, A.; Singh, A.V.; Singh, R.K.; Singh, S.K.; Saxena, P.S. Nitrogen doped carbon quantum dots demonstrate no toxicity under in vitro conditions in a cervical cell line and in vivo in swiss albino mice. *Toxicol. Res.* **2019**. [CrossRef]
18. Dwivedi, C.; Pandey, I.; Misra, V.; Giulbudagian, M.; Jungnickel, H.; Laux, P.; Luch, A.; Ramteke, P.W.; Singh, A.V. The prospective role of nanobiotechnology in food and food packaging products. *Integr. Food Nutr. Metab. (IFNM)* **2018**. [CrossRef]
19. Abdel-Wahhab, M.A.; Márquez, F. Nanomaterials in biomedicine. *Soft Nanosci. Lett.* **2015**, *5*, 53–54. [CrossRef]
20. Singh, A.V.; Laux, P.; Luch, A.; Sudrik, C.; Wiehr, S.; Wild, A.-M.; Santomauro, G.; Bill, J.; Sitti, M. Review of emerging concepts in nanotoxicology: Opportunities and challenges for safer nanomaterial design. *Toxicol. Mech. Methods* **2019**, 1–10. [CrossRef]
21. Dwivedi, C.; Pandey, I.; Pandey, H.; Patil, S.; Mishra, S.B.; Pandey, A.C.; Zamboni, P.; Ramteke, P.W.; Singh, A.V. In vivo diabetic wound healing with nanofibrous scaffolds modified with gentamicin and recombinant human epidermal growth factor. *J. Biomed. Mater. Res. Part A* **2018**, *106*, 641–651. [CrossRef] [PubMed]
22. Gupta, K.C.; Haider, A.; Choi, Y.-R.; Kang, I.-K. Nanofibrous scaffolds in biomedical applications. *Biomater. Res.* **2014**, *18*, 5. [CrossRef] [PubMed]
23. Venugopal, J.; Ramakrishna, S. Applications of polymer nanofibers in biomedicine and biotechnology. *Appl. Biochem. Biotechnol.* **2005**, *125*, 147–157. [CrossRef]
24. Wang, S.; Zheng, F.; Huang, Y.; Fang, Y.; Shen, M.; Zhu, M.; Shi, X. Encapsulation of amoxicillin within laponite-doped poly (lactic-co-glycolic acid) nanofibers: Preparation, characterization, and antibacterial activity. *ACS Appl. Mater. Interfaces* **2012**, *4*, 6393–6401. [CrossRef]
25. Hajiali, H.; Shahgasempour, S.; Naimi-Jamal, M.R.; Peirovi, H. Electrospun pga/gelatin nanofibrous scaffolds and their potential application in vascular tissue engineering. *Int. J. Nanomed.* **2011**, *6*, 2133. [CrossRef] [PubMed]
26. Nigam, R.; Mahanta, B. An overview of various biomimetic scaffolds: Challenges and applications in tissue engineering. *J. Tissue Sci. Eng.* **2014**, *5*, 1.
27. Steed, D.L. The role of growth factors in wound healing. *Surg. Clin. N. Am.* **1997**, *77*, 575–586. [CrossRef]
28. Fouad, H.; Elsarnagawy, T.; Almajhdi, F.N.; Khalil, K.A. Preparation and in vitro thermo-mechanical characterization of electrospun plga nanofibers for soft and hard tissue replacement. *Int. J. Electrochem. Sci.* **2013**, *8*, 2293–2304.

29. Ansary, R.H.; Awang, M.B.; Rahman, M.M. Biodegradable poly (D,L-lactic-co-glycolic acid)-based micro/nanoparticles for sustained release of protein drugs-a review. *Trop. J. Pharm. Res.* **2014**, *13*, 1179–1190. [CrossRef]
30. Dwivedi, C.; Pandey, H.; Pandey, A.C.; Ramteke, P.W. Novel gentamicin loaded electrospun nanofibrous scaffolds for wound healing: An in-vitro study. *Int. J. Pharm. Sci. Res.* **2013**, *4*, 2224–2227.
31. Singh, A.V.; Aditi, A.S.; Gade, W.N.; Vats, T.; Lenardi, C.; Milani, P. Nanomaterials: New generation therapeutics in wound healing and tissue repair. *Curr. Nanosci.* **2010**, *6*, 577–586. [CrossRef]
32. Singh, D.; Saraf, S.; Dixit, V.K.; Saraf, S. Formulation optimization of gentamicin loaded eudragit rs100 microspheres using factorial design study. *Biol. Pharm. Bull.* **2008**, *31*, 662–667. [CrossRef]
33. Deng, A.; Yang, Y.; Du, S.; Yang, S. Electrospinning of in situ crosslinked recombinant human collagen peptide/chitosan nanofibers for wound healing. *Biomater. Sci.* **2018**, *6*, 2197–2208. [CrossRef] [PubMed]
34. Kurečič, M.; Maver, T.; Virant, N.; Ojstršek, A.; Gradišnik, L.; Hribernik, S.; Kolar, M.; Maver, U.; Kleinschek, K.S. A multifunctional electrospun and dual nano-carrier biobased system for simultaneous detection of ph in the wound bed and controlled release of benzocaine. *Cellulose* **2018**, *25*, 7277–7297. [CrossRef]
35. Maver, T.; Smrke, D.; Kurečič, M.; Gradišnik, L.; Maver, U.; Kleinschek, K.S. Combining 3d printing and electrospinning for preparation of pain-relieving wound-dressing materials. *J. Sol-Gel Sci. Technol.* **2018**, *88*, 33–48. [CrossRef]
36. Shi, R.; Geng, H.; Gong, M.; Ye, J.; Wu, C.; Hu, X.; Zhang, L. Long-acting and broad-spectrum antimicrobial electrospun poly (ε-caprolactone)/gelatin micro/nanofibers for wound dressing. *J. Colloid Interface Sci.* **2018**, *509*, 275–284. [CrossRef] [PubMed]
37. Dwivedi, C.; Pandey, H.; Pandey, A.C.; Ramteke, P.W. Fabrication and assessment of gentamicin loaded electrospun nanofibrous scaffolds as a quick wound healing dressing material. *Curr. Nanosci.* **2015**, *11*, 222–228. [CrossRef]
38. Gentile, P.; Chiono, V.; Carmagnola, I.; Hatton, P. An overview of poly (lactic-co-glycolic) acid (PLGA)-based biomaterials for bone tissue engineering. *Int. J. Mol. Sci.* **2014**, *15*, 3640–3659. [CrossRef]
39. Singh, A.V.; Mehta, K.K.; Worley, K.; Dordick, J.S.; Kane, R.S.; Wan, L.Q. Carbon nanotube-induced loss of multicellular chirality on micropatterned substrate is mediated by oxidative stress. *ACS Nano* **2014**, *8*, 2196–2205. [CrossRef]
40. Singh, A.V.; Hosseinidoust, Z.; Park, B.-W.; Yasa, O.; Sitti, M. Microemulsion-based soft bacteria-driven microswimmers for active cargo delivery. *ACS Nano* **2017**, *11*, 9759–9769. [CrossRef]
41. Pandey, H.; Parashar, V.; Parashar, R.; Prakash, R.; Ramteke, P.W.; Pandey, A.C. Controlled drug release characteristics and enhanced antibacterial effect of graphene nanosheets containing gentamicin sulfate. *Nanoscale* **2011**, *3*, 4104–4108. [CrossRef] [PubMed]
42. Maver, T.; Gradišnik, L.; Smrke, D.M.; Kleinschek, K.S.; Maver, U. Systematic evaluation of a diclofenac-loaded carboxymethyl cellulose-based wound dressing and its release performance with changing ph and temperature. *AAPS PharmSciTech* **2019**, *20*, 29. [CrossRef] [PubMed]
43. Meng, Z.; Xu, X.; Zheng, W.; Zhou, H.; Li, L.; Zheng, Y.; Lou, X. Preparation and characterization of electrospun plga/gelatin nanofibers as a potential drug delivery system. *Colloids Surf. B Biointerfaces* **2011**, *84*, 97–102. [CrossRef] [PubMed]
44. Meng, Z.; Wang, Y.; Ma, C.; Zheng, W.; Li, L.; Zheng, Y. Electrospinning of plga/gelatin randomly-oriented and aligned nanofibers as potential scaffold in tissue engineering. *Mater. Sci. Eng. C* **2010**, *30*, 1204–1210. [CrossRef]
45. Pal, K.; Banthia, A.K.; Majumdar, D.K. Polyvinyl alcohol–glycine composite membranes: Preparation, characterization, drug release and cytocompatibility studies. *Biomed. Mater.* **2006**, *1*, 49. [CrossRef]
46. Murugan, R.; Ramakrishna, S. Nano-featured scaffolds for tissue engineering: A review of spinning methodologies. *Tissue Eng.* **2006**, *12*, 435–447. [CrossRef]
47. Chong, E.; Phan, T.; Lim, I.; Zhang, Y.; Bay, B.; Ramakrishna, S.; Lim, C. Evaluation of electrospun pcl/gelatin nanofibrous scaffold for wound healing and layered dermal reconstitution. *Acta Biomater.* **2007**, *3*, 321–330. [CrossRef]
48. Gander, B.; Gamazo, C.; Irache, J.M.; Prior, S. Gentamicin-loaded microspheres for treatment of experimental brucella abortus infection in mice. *J. Antimicrob. Chemother.* **2005**, *55*, 1032–1036.

49. Singh, A.V.; Baylan, S.; Park, B.W.; Richter, G.; Sitti, M. Hydrophobic pinning with copper nanowhiskers leads to bactericidal properties. *PLoS ONE* **2017**, *12*, e0175428. [CrossRef]
50. Singh, V.; Kumar, V.; Kashyap, S.; Singh, A.V.; Kishore, V.; Sitti, M.; Saxena, P.S.; Srivastava, A. Graphene oxide synergistically enhances antibiotic efficacy in vancomycin-resistant staphylococcus aureus. *ACS Appl. Bio Mater.* **2019**, *2*, 1148–1157. [CrossRef]
51. Singh, A.V.; Gemmati, D.; Kanase, A.; Pandey, I.; Misra, V.; Kishore, V.; Jahnke, T.; Bill, J. Nanobiomaterials for vascular biology and wound management: A review. *Veins Lymphat.* **2018**, *7*. [CrossRef]
52. Vikram Singh, A. Editorial (thematic issue: Recent trends in nano-biotechnology reinforcing contemporary pharmaceutical design). *Curr. Pharm. Des.* **2016**, *22*, 1415–1417. [CrossRef]

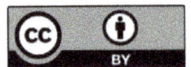

© 2019 by the authors. Licensee MDPI, Basel, Switzerland. This article is an open access article distributed under the terms and conditions of the Creative Commons Attribution (CC BY) license (http://creativecommons.org/licenses/by/4.0/).

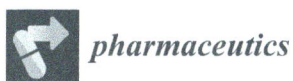

Review

Drug Delivery Applications of Core-Sheath Nanofibers Prepared by Coaxial Electrospinning: A Review

Bishweshwar Pant [1], Mira Park [2,*] and Soo-Jin Park [1,*]

1. Department of Chemistry, Inha University, 100 Inharo, Incheon 402-751, Korea
2. Department of Bioenvironmental Chemistry, College of Agriculture & Life Science, Chonbuk National University, Jeonju 561-756, Korea
* Correspondence: wonderfulmira@jbnu.ac.kr (M.P.); sjpark@inha.ac.kr (S.-J.P.)

Received: 22 May 2019; Accepted: 28 June 2019; Published: 1 July 2019

Abstract: Electrospinning has emerged as one of the potential techniques for producing nanofibers. The use of electrospun nanofibers in drug delivery has increased rapidly over recent years due to their valuable properties, which include a large surface area, high porosity, small pore size, superior mechanical properties, and ease of surface modification. A drug loaded nanofiber membrane can be prepared via electrospinning using a model drug and polymer solution; however, the release of the drug from the nanofiber membrane in a safe and controlled way is challenging as a result of the initial burst release. Employing a core-sheath design provides a promising solution for controlling the initial burst release. Numerous studies have reported on the preparation of core-sheath nanofibers by coaxial electrospinning for drug delivery applications. This paper summarizes the physical phenomena, the effects of various parameters in coaxial electrospinning, and the usefulness of core-sheath nanofibers in drug delivery. Furthermore, this report also highlights the future challenges involved in utilizing core-sheath nanofibers for drug delivery applications.

Keywords: electrospinning; coaxial spinning; core-sheath nanofibers; biomedical; drug delivery

---

1. Electrospinning

To date, several approaches, such as phase separation, self-assembly, drawing, template synthesis, and electrospinning, have been put forward for the fabrication of one-dimensional (1D) fibrous structures from various polymers [1–6]. In comparison with other methods, electrospinning is considered to be a simple, versatile, and cost-effective technique for generating continuous, nonwoven nanofiber mats from various polymeric solutions [2,7]. A variety of precursor solutions, including natural and synthetic polymers, polymer blends, polymer/metal particles, and polymer/ceramics particles, have been electrospun into fiber/nanofiber structures with diameters ranging from the nanometer to micrometer scale [1,8]. The electrospun nanofibers bear several remarkable properties such as a small diameter, large surface area, high aspect ratio, unique physiochemical properties, and flexibility [2,9,10].

The standard electrospinning setup consists of four main components: a capillary tube containing a polymer solution (or melt), a spinneret or nozzle, a collector, and a high voltage source [2,11]. The nanofibers can be obtained either from polymer melt or solution. A majority of the work has been focused on solution-based electrospinning. In the electrospinning process, a high voltage (typically 10 to 30 kV) is applied to a polymer solution in order to induce a charge on the surface of the droplet. When the intensity of the electric field is increased, the hemispherical surface of the solution elongates at the tip of the capillary and forms a Taylor cone. Upon further increasing the applied voltage, the charged jet is ejected from the Taylor cone and flows in the direction of the collector. During this process, the solvent evaporates and dry polymer fibers are randomly deposited on the collector. In electrospinning, the spinneret is the most important component, by which the multiple configurations can be implemented. Depending on the spinneret, the electrospinning process can be divided into different types such as needle-less, single, coaxial, side-by-side, and tri-axial electrospinning. The schematic of the typical electrospinning process is given in Figure 1A.

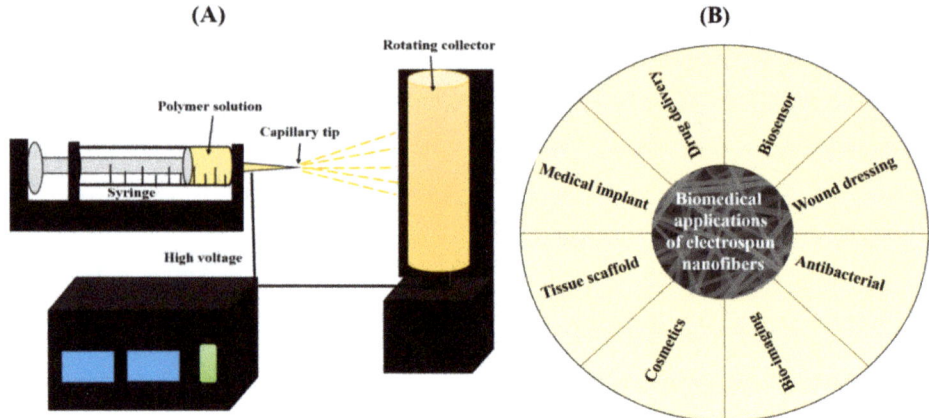

Figure 1. (A) Schematic diagram showing the electrospinning setup and (B) various biomedical applications of electrospun nanofibers.

In the electrospinning process, there are several factors that contribute to the fiber morphology [4,12]. These factors can be divided into tree category: (i) Solution parameters; (ii) process parameters; and (iii) ambient parameters [13]. The solution parameters include the type of solvent, the molecular weight of the polymer, the concentration of the solution, the viscosity of the solution, the conductivity of the solution, the surface tension, the dipole moment, and the dielectric constant. The process parameters include the applied electric field, the distance from the tip of the needle to the collector, the flow rate, etc. The relative humidity and temperature are considered as environmental factors affecting the electrospinning process. All the parameters affect the morphology of the nanofibers. It is noteworthy to mention that all the parameters affect the morphology of the nanofibers and none of them act independently during electrospinning. Therefore, the optimization of the different parameters is essential in order to design a nanofiber with the desired structure and properties. The effect of various parameters on the properties of the electrospun nanofibers is summarized in Table 1.

Table 1. Effect of various parameters on the properties of electrospun nanofibers.

Parameter	Effect	Reference
Applied voltage	High voltage generally reduces fiber diameter.	[14]
Concentration of solution	A higher concentration results in higher nanofiber diameter and the chances of bead formation are less. High concentration may clog the nozzle whereas low concentration may lead to sputtering.	[14–16]
Flow rate	Most flow rates are limited to 1 mL/h or lower. Increase in flow rate is associated with an increase in fiber diameter.	[16]
Inner diameter of needle	If large, beaded fiber may form.	[4]

Table 1. *Cont.*

Parameter	Effect	Reference
Conductivity of solution	High conductivity leads to thinner nanofibers with less chances of bead formation.	[15]
Viscosity of solution	High viscosity leads to the formation of thicker and continuous nanofibers whereas low viscosity is associated with finer and shorter nanofibers.	[17]
Tip-to-collector distance (TCD)	Longer distance results in thinner fibers. If the distance is very short, nanofibers become sticky and tend to stick to each other, resulting in the formation of a film. Diameter also increases with the decrease in TCD.	[14]
Humidity	If humidity is high, beads and pores may form on nanofibers.	[18]
Volatility of the solvent	High volatility of the solvent is associated with higher chances of porosity and increased surface area.	[15]
Temperature	Both environmental and working fluid temperatures affect the fiber formation. Generally, the diameters of the nanofibers are uniform at higher temperatures.	[9]
Type of the collector	Smooth fibers can be obtained from metal collectors. Aligned fibers can be obtained using a conductive frame, rotating drum, or a wheel-like bobblin collector.	[19]

2. Biomedical Applications of the Electrospun Nanofibers

A wide range of polymers have been electrospun to prepare nanofibers. So far, more than 200 polymers have been reported to have been made into nanofiber structures with the electrospinning technique [14]. Electrospun nanofibers possess several outstanding characteristics, for example, a large surface area to volume ratio, superior mechanical strength, flexibility, ease of surface modification, etc., which are beneficial for diverse applications including those in the biomedical sector, energy storage, and environmental remediation [1,4,20,21].

Electrospun nanofibers have already been proposed for various biomedical applications. The structure and chemical composition of the electrospun nanofibers resemble the natural fibrillary extracellular matrix (ECM) [22,23]. The interconnecting porous nature of the electrospun fibers facilitates cells attaching, migrating, and proliferating [23]. The biocompatibility and biodegradability of the nanofibers along with their suitable mechanical properties also favor their use in biomedical applications. Some potential areas of applications are given in Figure 1B. The electrospun nanofibers have been applied in various biomedical applications such as tissue engineering, wound dressing, the biosensor field, drug delivery, stent coating, implants, cosmetics, facial masks, etc. [24–26]. Many biocompatible polymers have been electrospun to generate nanofibers to be applied in the biomedical field; these polymers can either be biodegradable or non-biodegradable. Natural polymers such as collagen, chitosan, gelatin, hyaluronic acid, and silk fibroin have been electrospun into nanofiber form to form potential scaffolds for biomedical applications [27,28]. Other polymers include polycaprolactone (PCL), poly (lactic-co-glycolic acid) (PLGA), polylactic acid (PLA), poly (glycolic acid) (PGA), and poly(L-lactide-co-caprolactone) (PLCL) [27,29,30]. Currently, research is focused on three main issues: (i) Scaffold for tissue engineering; (ii) drug delivery mechanisms; and (iii) enzyme immobilization for faster reaction rates in biological reactions.

Among the various applications in the biomedical field, electrospun nanofibers use is potentially very promising in drug delivery applications. The electrospun nanofibers have been used in drug delivery applications for treating various diseases and gained popularity in the field of pharmaceutics [6,30–32]. The advantageous characteristics of nanofibers such as high surface area, high drug loading capacity, porosity, ease of functionalization and surface modification, simultaneous delivery of diverse therapies, adequate mechanical strength, and cost-effectiveness are appealing for use in drug delivery systems. Since the Kenaway group [33] prepared tetracycline loaded electrospun nanofiber mats of PLA, poly (ethylene-co-vinyl acetate) (PEVA), and their blend and studied the release of tetracycline for the first time, electrospun nanofiber for drug delivery gained significant interest among researchers. In the past few years, several research groups have prepared polymeric nanofibers in order to achieve different controlled drug release profiles. To date, various types of drugs, including DNA, RNA, protein, antibacterial, antiviral, and anticancer agents, etc., have been incorporated into electrospun nanofibers for desired applications [31,34–36]. For example, electrospun nanofibers have been applied as skin care (or facial) masks for the treatment of the skin as well as for other medical or therapeutic purposes. Different types of skin revitalizing factors can be loaded into the electrospun nanofibers and can be applied directly to the skin [37]. In recent years, drug incorporated biocompatible nanofiber membranes have been explored as a stent coating material to store and elute pharmaceutical agents to the lesion site without compromising its functional behavior [38].

3. Core-Sheath Nanofibers

The main objective of the drug delivery system is to deliver a required amount of a certain drug for a defined period of time depending on the medical condition. A drug loaded nanofiber membrane can be prepared via electrospinning by using a model drug and polymer solution; however, the initial burst release is unavoidable in such a type of blend membrane, and this is not ideal for a sustained drug release. In order to eliminate the burst release, post-treatment of the membranes such as cross-linking or chemical modifications are required. These types of post-treatment may lead to toxicity and a reduction in biocompatibility. The incorporation of the bioactive molecules or drugs into the thin fiber structure remains challenging since it should not adversely affect either the scaffold's properties or the drug's activity. The drug release rate can be tailored by tuning fiber diameter, porosity, and the drug-binding mechanism [39–43]. In recent years, many modifications have been incorporated into the electrospinning technique for producing nanofibers with enhanced performances. One such modification is the preparation of core-sheath nanofibers using coaxial electrospinning, in which one polymer nanofiber is surrounded by another, thus benefiting from the properties of both polymers [44–46]. In drug delivery systems, coating the fiber with a shell could effectively control the release profile of the drugs [47]. The specific core-shell design is helpful to incorporate the active drugs into the core part of the nanofibers, thereby providing the possibility of avoiding any damage caused to the incorporated drugs. In recent years, several core-sheath nanofibers have been fabricated to load various bioactive molecules including drugs, proteins, and genes for the sustained release of these molecules. The schematic view of the encapsulation and release procedure of drugs in core-sheath nanofibers is given in Figure 2. The advantages of core-sheath nanofibers in drug delivery applications can be summarized as follows [46–49]:

(i) It is possible to prepare nanofibers from unspinnable solutions via coaxial spinning;
(ii) It is helpful to prevent the burst release;
(iii) It enables a sustained release for a longer time;
(iv) The release kinetics of the bioactive molecules can be controlled by changing the composition or feed rate;
(v) More than one drug can be loaded in the same nanofibers and the drug release rate can be regulated;
(vi) Encapsulating the unstable bioactive molecules in mild conditions and protecting the biological activity of these molecules;
(vii) The sheath layer protects the inner ingredients, governing the release kinetics of the core which contains molecules;
(viii) It provides a better therapeutic effect and reduced toxicity;
(ix) This process eliminates the potential harm that can be caused by the post-treatment process.

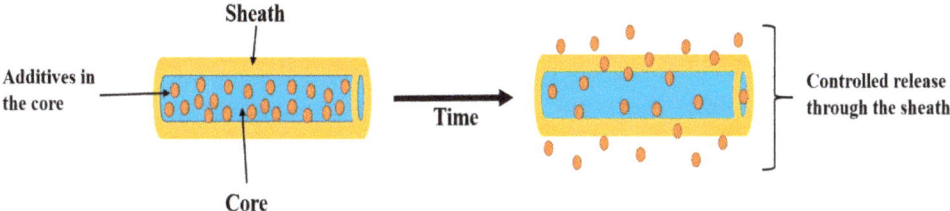

Figure 2. Schematic view showing the encapsulation and release procedure [50].

3.1. Core-Sheath Fibers from Co-Axial Electrospinning

Coaxial or triaxial electrospinning is considered to be an effective strategy to achieve sustained drug release from electrospun core-sheath nanofibers. It involves a simultaneous flow of a core and sheath solution from separate capillaries to form a fiber [51]. Coaxial electrospinning can be used to prepare core-sheath structured fibers from various core and sheath solutions to generate a fiber with different inner and outer parts: a hollow fiber, and functional fibers that may contain coatings [52]. Recently, fabrication of core-sheath fibers with triaxial electrospinning has been introduced in which the electrospun fiber contains a core, middle layer, and sheath [53,54]. By applying coaxial electrospinning, multiple drugs can be loaded into the core-sheath fibers and their release kinetics can be controlled [55]. In comparison to blend spinning, the drug loading efficiency is higher in coaxial spinning. More importantly, the initial burst release is found to be lower in core-sheath nanofibers made by coaxial spinning than that of fibers made by blend spinning. In core-sheath nanofibers, the core swells or dissolves, forming pores in the shell after the dissolutioin of hydrophilic portion in the core. While loading drugs into the core phase, the shell phase can serve as an outer protective layer. Furthermore, incompatibilities can be overcome. For instance, hydrophilic drugs in the core phase can be incorporated into the hydrophobic polymers in the shell phase. Furthermore, the shell phase can serve as a physical barrier providing sustained release kinetics, and by loading the core and shell phase, two different release patterns from one delivery system can be achieved.

3.2. General Setup and the Process of Coaxial Electrospinning

The general setup and the fiber manufacturing process is conceptually similar to that of conventional electrospinning as mentioned in Section 1. In coaxial electrospinning, the spinneret is modified by inserting a smaller capillary to fit concentrically inside the bigger capillary in order to obtain a co-axial configuration (Figure 3). The outer needle contains a sheath solution whereas the inner one contains a core solution. The inner and outer nozzles pump two different spinning solutions simultaneously, producing a core-shell droplet at the exit of the nozzle. When the polymer solutions are charged with a high voltage, the accumulation of charge takes place predominantly on the surface of the sheath solution coming out of the coaxial capillary. The pendant droplet of the sheath solution elongates and stretches as a result of the charge–charge repulsion, forming a conical shape. When the charge accumulation reaches a threshold, a jet emerges from the tip of the deformed droplet directed towards the counter electrode. Finally, a core-shell fiber is deposited on the substrate [56]. Recently, Hai et al. [57] have reported the process of Taylor cone formation in typical one-fluid electrospinning and coaxial electrospinning processes; the digital photographic observations from their study are given in Figure 4.

3.3. Effects of Various Parameters on Coaxial Electrospinning

Like in ordinary electrospinning, the fiber morphology is governed by several factors. Therefore, the selection of appropriate solution parameters and processing conditions is very important for the steady generation of the core-sheath structure in coaxial electrospinning.

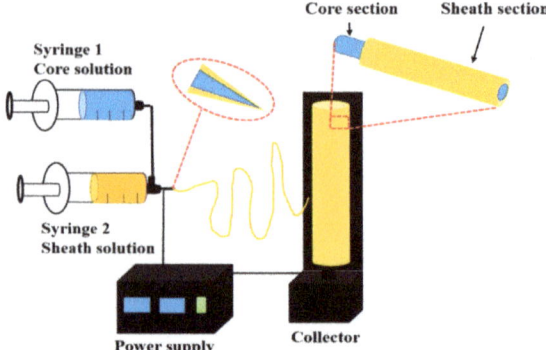

Figure 3. Schematic diagram showing the coaxial electrospinning system.

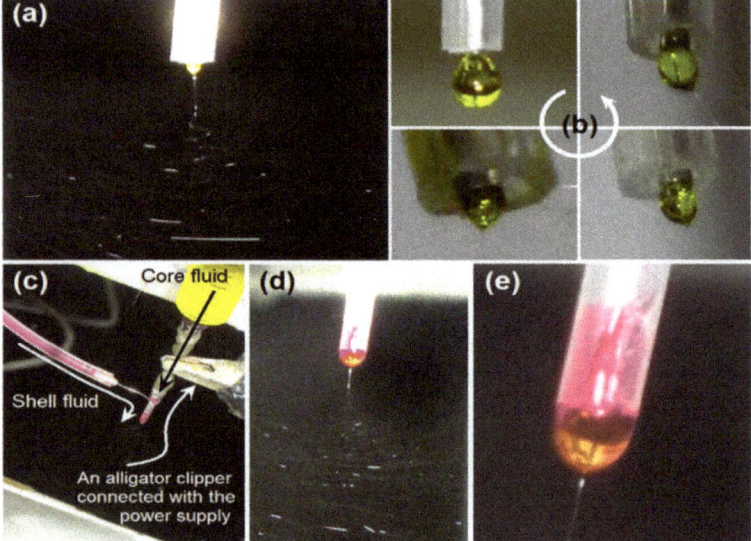

Figure 4. (**a**) Digital photographs showing a typical one-fluid electrospinning process, (**b**) formation of Taylor cone, (**c**) connection of spinneret in coaxial electrospinning, (**d**) enlarge image of the working region, and (**e**) Taylor cone with yellow core fluid encapsulate by rose-bengal shell solution [57].

3.3.1. Viscosities of the Solution

A good spinnability and sufficient viscosity of the sheath solution are required to produce enough viscous traction for the core solution. High viscosity can overcome the interfacial tension and form a stable Taylor cone. The core solution can have a lower viscosity (a minimum viscosity) to keep it intact and continuous inside the sheath fluid [55,58,59].

3.3.2. Solution Concentration

The concentration of polymer solution is a key factor in electrospinning. If the polymer concentration is increased, the viscosity also increases. An increase in the concentrations of both core and sheath solutions results in a higher core-sheath fiber diameter. The diameters of the core or sheath fibers can be tuned by controlling the concentration of the core or sheath solutions [51].

3.3.3. Solution Conductivities

In coaxial electrospinning, the sheath solution should be conductive whereas the core solution does not need to be conductive. By increasing the conductivity of the sheath solution, thinner fibers can be generated. Conversely, a highly conductive core solution can cause breakages due to the higher pulling rate in the core as compared to the sheath. A highly conductive sheath solution may affect the uniformity of the coaxial fibers due to the strong bending instability by abundant surface charges [55]. Hence, in order to obtain smooth nanofibers, the conductivity of core and sheath solutions should be maintained within an optimal range.

3.3.4. Solvent/Solution Miscibility and Incompatibility

The interaction between the inner and outer solvents determines the miscibility of the two solutions; therefore, the choice of the solvents is very important in coaxial electrospinning [51]. The solvents in the core and sheath solution should be chosen in such a way that neither of them cause the precipitation of the other. Immiscible solutions are easily spinnable into the core-sheath forms due to the phase separation during electrospinning. The core and sheath solution with the same or miscible solvents are also capable of producing core-sheath nanofibers. The use of volatile solvents can form porous nanofibers; however, a too high volatility of the solvent may cause rapid evaporation leading to the formation of clogs of the spinneret. In this case, no core-sheath fiber can be obtained.

3.3.5. Applied Voltage

For a solution, there is a small range of voltage within which a stable Taylor cone can be formed. If the applied voltage is too low, it may cause dripping of the two solutions forming a pendant drop at the exit of the nozzle. If the applied voltage is too high, it pulls the fluid jet inside the capillary and may form a clog [48,55]. Therefore, a good morphology of core-sheath nanofibers can be obtained by applying an optical range of the applied voltage.

3.3.6. Solution Flow Rates

The flow rates regulate the amount of solution which exists in the concentric tip for electrospinning. An optimal flow rate ratio for the part of polymers is required. As compared to the flow rate of the sheath solution, the flow rate of the core solution plays an important role in preparing core-sheath nanofibers in coaxial electrospinning. At a very low flow rate of the core solution, the core phase became discontinuous which leads to the breakup of the core. On the other hand, a too high flow rate can cause pendent droplets to form. Generally, the flow rate of the core solution is lower than that of the sheath solution [51].

3.3.7. Evaporation of Solvent

The solvent evaporation in coaxial electrospinning affects the Taylor cone formation and propagation and elongation of the jets. Rapid evaporation of solvents makes the solution dry at the nozzle tip before Taylor cone formation, whereas too slow evaporation causes the formation of drops [60]. The evaporation of solvents in both core and sheath solutions determines the morphology of the core and sheath structures. If the solvent in the shell solution evaporates at a higher rate than that of the core solution, the fibers collapse due to the atmospheric pressure. A high evaporation rate of the core solution also results in buckling and collapsed fibers due to the difference in pressure between the voids in the core and atmosphere.

3.3.8. Tip-to-Collector Distance (TCD)

The tip to collector distance is also one of the important parameters in electrospinning. TCD is directly related to the flight time of the fluid jet [55]. If the distance is too short, it would likely result in the formation of an interconnected fiber mesh (or film) due to the limited time for the solvent to evaporate in the air. In cases where the distance is large, there is a higher chance for the solvent to evaporate. The higher evaporation of the solvent leads to thinner nanofiber formation.

3.3.9. Nozzle Geometry

Since the nozzle geometry controls the flow rate, miscibility, and compatibility of the solutions, it has an influence on coaxial electrospinning. The diameter of the inner and outer nozzles and their geometry (length of core nozzle, the separation distance between the core and shell nozzles) may also influence the fiber morphology [60].

3.3.10. Temperature and Humidity

In addition to the above parameters, coaxial electrospinning is also affected by atmospheric conditions such as temperature and humidity, etc.; however, these parameters have shown less influence (than the aforementioned parameters) on the formation and the uniformity of the coaxial fibers.

In summary, in order to prepare uniform and steady core-sheath nanofibers, optimal solution parameters should be determined. It can be seen that the parameters affecting the coaxial electrospinning are almost the same as in traditional single-fluid electrospinning, except the nozzle geometry and core-sheath fluid flow rates and ratio. Traditional coaxial electrospinning demands spinnable sheath fluid; however, modified coaxial electrospinning can generate core-sheath fibers by using unspinnable sheath fluids such as organic solvents [61,62]. In modified coaxial electrospinning, the sheath flow must match with the drawing process of the core fluid during spinning to obtain high quality core-sheath fibers. The sheath flow must match well with the drawing process of the core fluid during the spinning process [62]. Overall, the general features for coaxial electrospinning to produce the core-sheath fibers are as follows [51,55,60,62]:

(i) The sheath solution must be electrospinnable;
(ii) The viscosity of sheath solution should be relatively high compared to the core solution;
(iii) The viscosity of the core solution is required to be above the critical value, but should not be as high as the sheath solution;
(iv) A low surface tension of core solution;
(v) Sheath solution should be conductive;
(vi) In modified coaxial electrospinning, unspinnable sheath solutions can be used; however, the sheath flow must be adjusted well to match with the flow of the core fluid.

3.4. Core-Sheath Nanofibers for Drug Delivery Applications

The advancement of materials in drug delivery should be first attributed to the biocompatibility, which is a prerequisite for biomaterials [3,22,52]. In recent years, most studies have been concerned with synthetic or natural polymers in order to fabricate core-sheath nanofibers as effective drug carrier mediums. The degradation rate of the polymer plays an important role in drug release kinetics. The degradation behavior of the polymer may depend on several characteristics such as molecular weight, wettability, crystallinity, surface roughness, and the melting temperature of the polymer [52,63] Therefore, it is important to select a biocompatible polymeric material with an appropriate degradation rate to obtain the desired drug release kinetics. Table 2 presents some examples of core-sheath nanofibers by coaxial electrospinning for drug delivery applications. Some examples of widely used polymers and recent works related to drug release form core-sheath nanofibers by coaxial electrospinning are given below.

3.4.1. Poly(vinyl alcohol) (PVA)

Water-soluble polymers offer additional advantages in electrospinning by eliminating the possible toxicity caused by solvents and represent a significant step towards clean and safe electrospinning. Among the various water-soluble polymers, poly(vinyl alcohol) (PVA), a synthetic polymer, is of great interest due to its desirable properties, such as its biocompatibility, adhesiveness, strength, swelling properties, non-carcinogenicity, film or fiber forming ability, etc. [64]. Recently, Yarin's group [65] fabricated core-sheath nanofibers with PVA containing ciprofloxacin as a core and poly(methyl methacrylate) (PMMA) as a sheath layer in order to avoid the burst release of the drug. The nanofibers were explored for use in local drug delivery systems to treat periodontal disease and skin, bone, and joint infections. The study showed that the variation of flow rate ratios between core and shell during the spinning strongly affected nanofiber morphology and drug release. A lower amount of PVA in the core was helpful to prevent the burst release. In another study, Yarin [66] developed interesting mathematic models describing drug release from nanofibers.

Tiwari et al. [67] evaluated the usefulness of core-sheath fiber to minimize the burst release. In their study, the drug (metoclopramide hydrochloride) was loaded into the core (PVA) which was surrounded by different shells of various polymers (PCL, PLGA, and PLLA). The work clearly shows the sensitivity of the observed release to various parameters, related to both the process and material.

Yan et al. [68] used two water-soluble polymers, PVA and chitosan, as the core and sheath matrix, respectively, to prepare core-sheath fibers. Doxorubicin was used as a model drug and incorporated into the core matrix. PVA–chitosan nanofibers with different feed ratios were prepared as in Figure 5. The chitosan sheath was crosslinked by treatment with glutaraldehyde vapor to restrict the swelling of the polymer. The potential of nanofibers for use as a scaffold for chemotherapy of ovary cancer was evaluated in vitro against SKOV3 cancer cells and the obtained resulted indicated that the fibers were good in prohibiting cell attachment and proliferation. They observed that the release rate of drugs can be adjusted by changing the feed ratio and by keeping the feed ratio constant. More importantly, the core-sheath nanofibers exhibited controlled release of doxorubicin (DOX), showing potential for use in the chemotherapy of ovary cancer.

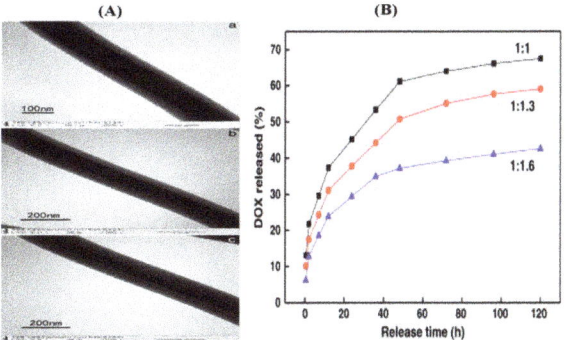

Figure 5. (**A**) TEM image of poly(vinyl alcohol)/chitosan (PVA/CS) core-sheath nanofibers with different feed ratios of (**a**) 1:1, (**b**) 1:1.3, and (**c**) 1:1.6 and (**B**) drug release profiles [68]. Reprinted with the permission from *Materials Science and Engineering: C*. Copyright Elsevier, 2014.

3.4.2. Polycaprolactone (PCL)

PCL is a biocompatible and biodegradable synthetic polymer approved by the Food and Drug Administration (FDA). It has been widely used in drug delivery systems due to its broad range of molecular weight (from 3000 to 85,000 g/mol), solubility in varieties of solvents such as acetic acid, chloroform, methanol, benzene, dichloromethane, and its non-enzymatic degradation. PCL has been extensively explored in coaxial electrospinning for drug delivery applications.

Jing et al. [69] employed coaxial electrospinning in order to incorporate and control the release of two proteins, bovine serum albumin (BSA) and lysosome, from core-sheath nanofibers with protein containing polyethylene glycol (PEG) as a core and PCL as a shell. The protein release kinetics were characterized by a slight burst release during the first day followed by a relatively steady release extending over the complete time of the analysis of 30 days. The release profile of the incorporated proteins was found to be dependent on the feeding rate of the core solution. It was noticed that a higher feeding rate resulted in rapid protein release. In another study [70], the same group prepared biodegradable core-sheath fibers with PCL or a PCL/PEG blend as shell and BSA-dextran as core by coaxial electrospinning. PEG was added to the shell in order to further finely modulate the release behavior of BSA. Their study showed that the release rate of BSA increased with the PEG content in the shell.

He et al. [71] reported the fabrication of an anti-inflammatory agent loaded guided tissue regeneration membrane (GTRM) by coaxial electrospinning. In their study, metronidazole was loaded in PCL core fibers surrounded by gelatin as a sheath layer. They suggest that the dissolving of the gelatin sheath layer could be inhibited by crosslinking, and this resulted in sustained release of metronidazole for six days. The improved hydrophilicity also resulted in better cell adhesion and proliferation without toxicity. The prepared nanofiber membrane was capable of controlled drug release and inhibited the inflammatory response during the healing process, thereby showing better results as compared to PCL fibers only.

3.4.3. Polyethylene oxide (PEO)

As a result of the solubility of hydrophilic drugs in the aqueous medium, it is challenging to maintain their prolonged release with a minimum release at the initial stage. Producing nanofibers from the blending solution of hydrophobic and hydrophilic polymers along with the drugs can reduce the burst release of hydrophilic drugs; however, the incompatibility between the drugs and hydrophilic polymers may cause the drug to migrate towards the surface of the nanofibers. In this regard, coaxial electrospinning can provide a better approach by encapsulating the drugs into the core portion of the nanofibers. The core-sheath nanofibers can be prepared by incorporating hydrophilic drugs with the polymer in the core and hydrophobic polymer as a sheath layer. Esmaeili and Haseli [72] prepared core-sheath and blend nanofibers to encapsulate tetracycline hydrochloride with PEO in the core and carboxymethyl cellulose in the sheath. As compared to the blend nanofibers, the core-sheath fibers showed a much slower and prolonged release of the drug. In the optimized core-sheath sample, the burst release was reduced from 54% to 26% and the total release was enhanced from 76% to 92% compared to the blend nanofibers. The initial burst release of the tetracycline hydrochloride in the case of the blend nanofibers might be associated with two factors: (i) The presence of the drugs on the surface of the blended nanofibers; and (ii) the hydrophilicity of the polymer which facilitates water uptake and swelling of the polymer matrix.

Recently, stimuli-responsive materials (smart materials) have gained extensive interest in controlled drug delivery applications. Various external stimuli such as light, temperature, magnetism, sound, etc., can bring change in the physical or chemical status of the smart materials. Li et al. [73] prepared a thermally switched drug delivery system, whose release can be tuned in response to a temperature change. Core-sheath fibers were prepared by coaxial electrospinning, in which drug encapsulated PEO forms a core layer, whereas a mixture of PCL and temperature stimuli-responsive nanogels form the sheath layer. The nanogels in the PCL matrix act as valves to generate a path for the diffusion of encapsulated drugs during the shrinkage and swelling above or under lower critical solution temperature (LCST) [73].

3.4.4. Polyvinylpyrrolidone (PVP)

PVP is a water-soluble polymer with an amphiphilic character. As a result of its excellent properties, such as its solubility, film or fiber forming ability, adhesion and bonding, and biocompatibility, it has been extensively investigated for various applications in the biomedical field, including drug release. Core-sheath PVP/PCL nanofibers were developed by coaxial electrospinning in which graphene oxide (GO) sheets were blended into the core (PVP) solution to adjust the release behavior of vancomycin hydrochloride (VAN) [74]. The addition of GO into the nanofibers resulted in a reduction in burst release from 73% to 60%, and it was concluded that the amount of release can be tailored by adjusting the amount of GO in the core. The molecular interactions, such as hydrogen bonds, Var der Waal's force, π–π bonds, between GO and the drugs played an important role in the typical biphasic release behavior the drug [74].

Yu et al. [75] prepared ketoprofen (KET) loaded core-sheath nanofibers by coaxial electrospinning using PVP as the sheath and ethyl cellulose (EC) as the core matrix and studied the drug release behavior. The drug was present in the polymer matrix in an amorphous state and the composite nanofibers provided a biphasic drug release profile consisting of an immediate and tunable sustained release. It was shown that the first and second phase of drug release could be tailored by adjusting the sheath flow rate and diffusion mechanism, respectively.

3.4.5. Cellulose acetate (CA)

Cellulose is the primary structural component of the cell walls of green plants. It has been a material of choice in nanotechnology due to its advantageous properties including its biocompatibility, biodegradability, and regenerative properties [76,77]. Despite its advantageous properties, preparation of electrospun nanofibers is challenging because of its limited solubility in general organic solvents and disability to melt as a result of extra inter- and intramolecular bonding [31,78]. Cellulose acetate (CA), the acetate ester of cellulose, has been widely investigated for a wide variety of applications related to electrospun membranes [31]. The electrospun CA nanofibers can be converted into cellulose fibers by deacetylation or aqueous hydrolysis [79].

Yu et al. [76] applied the electrospinning process to develop ketoprofen (KET) loaded CA nanofibers. The drug was loaded into the CA fibers via both the single and modified coaxial electrospinning process. The core fluid was prepared by dissolving CA, KET, and a mixture of solvent (acetone, dimethylacetamide (DMAc), and ethanol), whereas the same mixed solvent was taken as sheath fluid. In addition, a CA solution containing KET in the same solvent was prepared for single fluid electrospinning. The nanofibers obtained from coaxial electrospinning had a smaller diameter, narrower size distribution, and smoother surface morphologies as compared to those generated from single fluid electrospinning. It was found that the fibers obtained from coaxial electrospinning offered a better zero-order drug release profile with a smaller tailing residue than that of single nozzle electrospinning. Another study by Yu's group [80] showed a zero-order drug release profile from ketoprofen incorporated into CA nanofibers prepared via coaxial electrospinning using 2% CA solution as a sheath fluid and a mixture of CA, KET, and methylene blue in a mixed solvent system (acetone, DMAc, and ethanol) [76,80]. The obtained nanofibers provided zero-order drug release kinetics for 96 h via a diffusion mechanism.

3.4.6. Zein

Zein, a mixture of proteins with different molecular weights in corn gluten meal, is widely known for its biocompatibility, biodegradability, antioxidant activity, and electrospinnability [81,82]. In recent years, it has drawn increasing attention in various applications, particularly in the biomedical field, including drug delivery [81,83–87]. In this regard, Huang et al. [84] investigated the preparation of ibuprofen (IBU) loaded fibers using a coaxial electrospinning process, in which zein/ibuprofen dissolved in ethanol aqueous solution and N,N-dimethylformamide were used as core and sheath fluids, respectively.

Table 2. Various core-sheath nanofibers for drug delivery applications.

Core Fluid	Sheath Fluid	Name of Drug	Application	Reference
PVA	PCL, PLLA, PLGA	Metoclopramidehydrochloride	Drug delivery vehicle	[67]
PVA	PMMA	Ciprofloxacin	Periodontal disease and skin, bone, and joint infections	[65]
PVA	Chitosan	Doxorubicin	Chemotherapy against ovary cancer	[68]
Silk fibroin	PVA	Rosuvastatin	For enhancing osteogenesis of human adipose-derived stem cells	[90]
PCL	PCL	Ampicillin	Controlled release	[49]
PCL	PCL	Dipyridamole	Controlled release	[91]
PCL	Gelatin	Metronidazole	Controlled release	[71]
PCL	PEG	Salicylic acid	Studying the relationship between shell thickness and drug release rate	[42]
PCL	PCL	Ampicillin	Controlled release of a hydrophilic drug	[49]
Protein	PCL-PEG	BSA or PDGF	Controlled release of growth factor	[92]
Dextran	PCL, PLGA, PLCL	Dextran	Controlled release of proteins and drugs for tissue engineering	[70,93,94]
PEG	PCL	BSA	Controlled release	[95]
pHMGCL, PVPD	PCL	rhTGF-β1	Sustained release of growth factor	[96]
PEO	PCL & PIPAAm/AAC-nanogels	MO	Thermally switched release	[73]
PEO	Carboxymethyl cellulose	Tetracycline hydrochloride	Drug delivery study	[72]
PEO	PCL-PEG	BMP-2	Drug release for bone tissue	[97]
PEO	PCL	FGF-2	Growth factor delivery for fibroblast proliferation	[98]
PEO	Eudragit S100	Indomethacin, mebeverine hydrochloride	Site specific drug release	[99]
PEG	PLA	Salicylic acid	Effect of pores in the drug release	[43]
PEG	PBSc	Triclosan/Curcumin	Drug release	[100]
PVP	CA	Amoxicillin	Hydrophilic drug release	[101]
PVP	EC	Maraviroc and Metronidazole	Drug release	[102]
PVP/GO	PCL	Vancomycin hydrochloride	Time-programmed biphasic drug release	[74]
PVP or PCL	PVP	Quercetin or Tamoxifen citrate	Dissolution of poorly water-soluble drugs	[103]

Table 2. Cont.

Core Fluid	Sheath Fluid	Name of Drug	Application	Reference
Ethyl cellulose	PVP	Ketoprofen	Drug release profile study	[75]
Naringin-loaded PVP	poly(lactic-co-glycolic acid)	Naringin Metronidazole	Fabrication of anti-infective guided tissue regeneration mats with promoting tissue regeneration	[104]
Zein	Acetic acid	Ferulic acid	Modified coaxial spinning. The effect of acetic acid to stabilize core fibers.	[89]
Zein	Zein	Ketoprofen	Hydrophobic drug release from protein fiber	[88]
Zein	PVP	Ketoprofen	Hydrophobic drug release from protein fiber	[85]
Tetracycline hydrochloride/Ethanol	Zein, PVA-SbQ	Tetracycline hydrochloride	Drug release study	[105]
PLGA	Collagen	Fibronectin and Cadherin 11	Dual drug delivery vehicle	[106]
PLLCL	Collagen	BMP2 Dexamethasone	Dual drug delivery vehicle	[107]
PLGA-HA	Collagen	Amoxicillin	Hydrophilic drug release from hydrophilic shell	[108]
Silk/collagen blend	Polyethylene oxide	Flurbiprofen and Vancomycin	Programmable release of anti-inflammatory and anti-bacterial agents	[35]
CA	CA	Ketoprofen	Drug release study	[80]
CA	Acetone-DMAc-ethanol	Ketoprofen	Controlled release	[76]
Sodiumhyaluronate	Cellulose acetate	Naproxen	Controlled release for wound dressing	[109]
Gelatin	PLLCL	Insulin, Hydrocortisone, and Retinoic acid	Dual drug delivery system Skin regeneration	[110]
PDLLA	PHB	Dimethyl oxalylglycine	Controlled release of hygroscopic drug	[111]
PMMA	Nylon	Ampicillin	Release of hydrophilic drug in hydrophobic solvent	[112]
PolyCD	PMAA	Proprannodol hydrochloride	Controlled release of hydrophobic drug	[113]
PLA	N-isopropylacrylamide	Combretastatin A4	Thermo-sensitivity study	[114]
Shellac	Ethanol/DMF	Ferulic acid	Colon targeted drug delivery	[115]
IBU solution in HFIP	Gliadin	Ibuprofen	Drug release behavior study	[116]
Gliadin	Gliadin	Ketoprofen	Drug release study	[117]
AAm/BIS-AAm	PLCL	BSA	Protein release	[59]

Poly(vinyl)alcohol (PVA), polycaprolactone (PCL), poly (lactic-co-glycolic acid) (PLGA), poly-L-lactic acid (PLLA), polymethyl(methacrylate) (PMMA), polyethylene glycol (PEG), polyethylene oxide (PEO), polylactic acid (PLA), cellulose acetate (CA), poly(L-lactide-co-caprolactone) (PLCL), poly(L-lactic acid)-co-poly(ε-caprolactone)(PLLCL), poly-d,l-lactic acid (PDLLA), polyhydroxybutyrate (PHB), poly-cyclodextrin (polyCD), graphene oxide (GO), platelet-derived growth factor (PDGF), bovine serum albumin (BSA), bone morphogenic protein (BMP), fibroblast growth factor (FGF), acrylamide (AAm), N,N′-methylene bisacrylamide (BIS-AAm), stilbazole quaternized (SbQ), recombinant human transforming growth factor (rh TGF-β1), methyl orange (MO).

Jiang et al. [85] prepared core-sheath nanofibers from two polymers, PVP and Zein, to provide a biphasic drug release profile. Ketoprofen was exploited as the model drug in the study and was loaded into both the sheath and core fluids. Zein and PVA were selected as the core and sheath parts, respectively. Linear core-sheath nanofiber was produced with an average diameter of 730 ± 190 nm, in which the sheath part had a thickness of 90 nm. The study further showed good compatibility of the core and sheath matrix with KET due to hydrogen bonding. The dissolution tests showed an immediate release of 42.3% of the KET, followed by a sustained release over 10 h. Another study also demonstrated that the burst release can be prevented by using a blank or low concentration of zein solution in the sheath [88]. In another study, ferulic acid loaded zein was used as a core fluid and acetic acid was chosen as sheath fluid to stabilize the outer surface of the fibers [89]. The authors identified hydrogen bonding as a driving force of encapsulation of fluoric acid into the zein and the strategy of surface cross-linking was helpful for improving the release rate of the drug from the nanofibers [89].

4. Conclusions, Challenges, and Future Perspectives

In recent years, electrospinning technology has made a significant contribution in drug delivery applications. Optimization of the various parameters is important to design fibers with the desired morphology and function. Coaxial electrospinning ensures a homogeneous encapsulation of wide varieties of drugs into the core-sheath structured nanofiber along with a sustained release. Apart from drugs, several biomolecules have also been loaded into the core-sheath nanofibers via coaxial electrospinning. Additionally, some nonspinnable materials can be formed into a fiber structure due to the protection and guidance of the electrospinnable sheath layer. Easy loading of the drugs, mitigation of burst release, controlled sustained release, resemblance with the ECM, promotion of cell adhesion, and migration and proliferation are exciting features of core-sheath nanofibers which make them a suitable candidate in drug delivery applications.

It is evident from previous studies that core-sheath nanofibers are superior in terms of preserving the bioactivity of the biomolecules/drugs loaded in the fiber body and release behavior; however, there are several issues that must be addressed in order to obtain better results in drug delivery applications. To obtain the desired form of core-sheath nanofibers with satisfactory results, many experimental trails with different parameters are needed and this is complicated compared to conventional methods. The selection of core and sheath fluids is also important. The sheath layer may prevent rapid evaporation of the solvent during coaxial spinning; however, there is a chance that organic solvents will remain. To date, most reports of core-sheath fibers regarding drug delivery have focused on in vitro studies; therefore, in vivo studies with relevant preclinical studies are required for practical applications. Overall, coaxial electrospinning is an effective strategy for drug encapsulation and controlled release from nanofibers. Proper adjustment of parameters and a correct choice of core and sheath fluids are suggested to obtain good results, and further investigations and modifications are required to overcome the challenges in coaxial electrospinning.

Core-sheath devices should be further studied and advanced, in time making them more attractive for large-scale production. Furthermore, new strategies such as coaxial and tri-axial electrospinning combined with electrospraying can be adopted to prepare core-sheath fibers from spinnable and nonspinnable solutions [118,119]. In addition, designing a composite system using nanoparticles, hydrogels, and nanofibers may lead to significant advances in drug delivery applications. Recently, similar to the coaxial spinning technique, fabrication of drug loaded core-sheath nanostructures has been performed via coaxial and modified coaxial electrospraying processes [120,121]. The coaxial electrospraying method can secure drug entrapment into the core-sheath morphology, thereby giving the desired release kinetics [120]. Since both electrospinning and electrospraying are advanced nanofabrication methods that take advantage of the interactions between the working fluids and electrostatic energy, the contents and strategies reviewed in this paper as regards coaxial electrospinning and core-sheath nanofibers could also be applicable to coaxial electrospraying and core-shell nanoparticles.

Funding: This research was supported by the Traditional Culture Convergence Research Program through the National Research Foundation of Korea (NRF) funded by the Ministry of Science, ICT & Future Planning (grant number 2018M3C1B5052283) and also supported by Korea Evaluation institute of Industrial Technology (KEIT) through the Carbon Cluster Construction project (10083586, Development of petroleum based graphite fibers with ultra-high thermal conductivity) funded by the Ministry of Trade, Industry and Energy (MOTIE, Korea)

Conflicts of Interest: The authors declare no conflict of interest.

References

1. Pant, B.; Pant, H.R.; Pandeya, D.R.; Panthi, G.; Nam, K.T.; Hong, S.T.; Kim, C.S.; Kim, H.Y. Characterization and antibacterial properties of Ag NPs loaded nylon-6 nanocomposite prepared by one-step electrospinning process. *Colloids Surf. A Physicochem. Eng. Asp.* **2012**, *395*, 94–99. [CrossRef]
2. Wang, X.; Ding, B.; Sun, G.; Wang, M.; Yu, J. Electro-spinning/netting: A strategy for the fabrication of three-dimensional polymer nano-fiber/nets. *Progr. Mater. Sci.* **2013**, *58*, 1173–1243. [CrossRef]
3. Thakkar, S.; Misra, M. Electrospun polymeric nanofibers: New horizons in drug delivery. *Eur. J. Pharm. Sci.* **2017**, *107*, 148–167. [CrossRef] [PubMed]
4. Haider, A.; Haider, S.; Kang, I.-K. A comprehensive review summarizing the effect of electrospinning parameters and potential applications of nanofibers in biomedical and biotechnology. *Arabian J. Chem.* **2018**, *11*, 1165–1188. [CrossRef]
5. Peng, Y.; Dong, Y.; Fan, H.; Chen, P.; Li, Z.; Jiang, Q. Preparation of polysulfone membranes via vapor-induced phase separation and simulation of direct-contact membrane distillation by measuring hydrophobic layer thickness. *Desalination* **2013**, *316*, 53–66. [CrossRef]
6. Kamble, P.; Sadarani, B.; Majumdar, A.; Bhullar, S. Nanofiber based drug delivery systems for skin: A promising therapeutic approach. *J. Drug Deliv. Sci. Technol.* **2017**, *41*, 124–133. [CrossRef]
7. Pant, B.; Park, M.; Park, S.-J.; Kim, H.Y. High Strength Electrospun Nanofiber Mats via CNT Reinforcement: A Review. *Compos. Res.* **2016**, *29*, 186–193. [CrossRef]
8. Pant, H.R.; Kim, H.J.; Joshi, M.K.; Pant, B.; Park, C.H.; Kim, J.I.; Hui, K.S.; Kim, C.S. One-step fabrication of multifunctional composite polyurethane spider-web-like nanofibrous membrane for water purification. *J. Hazard. Mater.* **2014**, *264*, 25–33. [CrossRef] [PubMed]
9. Demir, M.M.; Yilgor, I.; Yilgor, E.; Erman, B. Electrospinning of polyurethane fibers. *Polymer* **2002**, *43*, 3303–3309. [CrossRef]
10. Schreuder-Gibson, H.L.; Gibson, P. Applications of electrospun nanofibers in current and future materials. In *Polymeric Nanofibers*; American Chemical Society: Washington, DC, USA, 2006; Volume 918, pp. 121–136.
11. Ramakrishna, S.; Fujihara, K.; Teo, W.-E.; Yong, T.; Ma, Z.; Ramaseshan, R. Electrospun nanofibers: solving global issues. *Mater. Today* **2006**, *9*, 40–50. [CrossRef]
12. Thompson, C.J.; Chase, G.G.; Yarin, A.L.; Reneker, D.H. Effects of parameters on nanofiber diameter determined from electrospinning model. *Polymer* **2007**, *48*, 6913–6922. [CrossRef]
13. Doshi, J.; Reneker, D.H. Electrospinning process and applications of electrospun fibers. *J. Electrost.* **1995**, *35*, 151–160. [CrossRef]
14. Tijing, L.D.; Yao, M.; Ren, J.; Park, C.-H.; Kim, C.S.; Shon, H.K. Nanofibers for water and wastewater treatment: Recent advances and developments. In *Water and Wastewater Treatment Technologies*; Bui, X.-T., Chiemchaisri, C., Fujioka, T., Varjani, S., Eds.; Springer: Singapore, 2019; pp. 431–468.
15. Yang, Q.; Li, Z.; Hong, Y.; Zhao, Y.; Qiu, S.; Wang, C.; Wei, Y. Influence of solvents on the formation of ultrathin uniform poly(vinyl pyrrolidone) nanofibers with electrospinning. *J. Polym. Sci. B Polym. Phys.* **2004**, *42*, 3721–3726. [CrossRef]
16. Zong, X.; Kim, K.; Fang, D.; Ran, S.; Hsiao, B.S.; Chu, B. Structure and process relationship of electrospun bioabsorbable nanofiber membranes. *Polymer* **2002**, *43*, 4403–4412. [CrossRef]
17. Shahreen, L.; Chase, G.G. Effects of electrospinning solution properties on formation of beads in Tio2 fibers with PdO particles. *J. Eng. Fibers Fabrics* **2015**, *10*, 155892501501000308. [CrossRef]
18. Casper, C.L.; Stephens, J.S.; Tassi, N.G.; Chase, D.B.; Rabolt, J.F. Controlling surface morphology of electrospun polystyrene fibers: Effect of humidity and molecular weight in the electrospinning process. *Macromolecules* **2004**, *37*, 573–578. [CrossRef]

19. Unnithan, A.R.; Arathyram, R.S.; Kim, C.S. Chapter 3—Electrospinning of polymers for tissue engineering. In *Nanotechnology Applications for Tissue Engineering*; Thomas, S., Grohens, Y., Ninan, N., Eds.; William Andrew Publishing: Oxford, UK, 2015; pp. 45–55.
20. Pant, B.; Ojha, G.P.; Kim, H.-Y.; Park, M.; Park, S.-J. Fly-ash-incorporated electrospun zinc oxide nanofibers: Potential material for environmental remediation. *Environ. Pollut.* **2019**, *245*, 163–172. [CrossRef] [PubMed]
21. Pant, B.; Park, M.; Ojha, G.P.; Park, J.; Kuk, Y.-S.; Lee, E.-J.; Kim, H.-Y.; Park, S.-J. Carbon nanofibers wrapped with zinc oxide nano-flakes as promising electrode material for supercapacitors. *J. Colloid Interface Sci.* **2018**, *522*, 40–47. [CrossRef]
22. Pant, B.; Park, M.; Ojha, G.P.; Kim, D.-U.; Kim, H.-Y.; Park, S.-J. Electrospun salicylic acid/polyurethane composite nanofibers for biomedical applications. *Int. J. Polym. Mater. Polym. Biomater.* **2018**, *67*, 739–744. [CrossRef]
23. Bhattarai, N.; Li, Z.; Gunn, J.; Leung, M.; Cooper, A.; Edmondson, D.; Veiseh, O.; Chen, M.-H.; Zhang, Y.; Ellenbogen, R.G.; et al. Natural-synthetic polyblend nanofibers for biomedical applications. *Adv. Mater.* **2009**, *21*, 2792–2797. [CrossRef]
24. Lagaron, J.M.; Solouk, A.; Castro, S.; Echegoyen, Y. 3—Biomedical applications of electrospinning, innovations, and products. In *Electrospun Materials for Tissue Engineering and Biomedical Applications*; Uyar, T., Kny, E., Eds.; Woodhead Publishing: Cambridge, UK, 2017; pp. 57–72.
25. Al-Enizi, A.M.; Zagho, M.M.; Elzatahry, A.A. Polymer-based electrospun nanofibers for biomedical applications. *Nanomaterials* **2018**, *8*, 259. [CrossRef] [PubMed]
26. Villarreal-Gómez, L.J.; Cornejo-Bravo, J.M.; Vera-Graziano, R.; Grande, D. Electrospinning as a powerful technique for biomedical applications: A critically selected survey. *J. Biomater. Sci. Polym. Ed.* **2016**, *27*, 157–176. [CrossRef] [PubMed]
27. Shahriar, S.M.S.; Mondal, J.; Hasan, M.N.; Revuri, V.; Lee, D.Y.; Lee, Y.-K. Electrospinning nanofibers for therapeutics delivery. *Nanomaterials* **2019**, *9*, 532. [CrossRef] [PubMed]
28. Chen, S.; Li, R.; Li, X.; Xie, J. Electrospinning: An enabling nanotechnology platform for drug delivery and regenerative medicine. *Adv. Drug Deliv. Rev.* **2018**, *132*, 188–213. [CrossRef] [PubMed]
29. Thenmozhi, S.; Dharmaraj, N.; Kadirvelu, K.; Kim, H.Y. Electrospun nanofibers: New generation materials for advanced applications. *Mater. Sci. Eng. B* **2017**, *217*, 36–48. [CrossRef]
30. Agrahari, V.; Agrahari, V.; Meng, J.; Mitra, A.K. Chapter 9—Electrospun nanofibers in drug delivery: Fabrication, advances, and biomedical applications. In *Emerging Nanotechnologies for Diagnostics, Drug Delivery and Medical Devices*; Mitra, A.K., Cholkar, K., Mandal, A., Eds.; Elsevier: Boston, MA, USA, 2017; pp. 189–215.
31. Khoshnevisan, K.; Maleki, H.; Samadian, H.; Shahsavari, S.; Sarrafzadeh, M.H.; Larijani, B.; Dorkoosh, F.A.; Haghpanah, V.; Khorramizadeh, M.R. Cellulose acetate electrospun nanofibers for drug delivery systems: Applications and recent advances. *Carbohydr. Polym.* **2018**, *198*, 131–141. [CrossRef] [PubMed]
32. Ghafoor, B.; Aleem, A.; Najabat Ali, M.; Mir, M. Review of the fabrication techniques and applications of polymeric electrospun nanofibers for drug delivery systems. *J. Drug Deliv. Sci. Technol.* **2018**, *48*, 82–87. [CrossRef]
33. Kenawy, E.-R.; Bowlin, G.L.; Mansfield, K.; Layman, J.; Simpson, D.G.; Sanders, E.H.; Wnek, G.E. Release of tetracycline hydrochloride from electrospun poly(ethylene-co-vinylacetate), poly(lactic acid), and a blend. *J. Controlled Release* **2002**, *81*, 57–64. [CrossRef]
34. Liu, M.; Zhang, Y.; Sun, S.; Khan, A.R.; Ji, J.; Yang, M.; Zhai, G. Recent advances in electrospun for drug delivery purpose. *J. Drug Target.* **2019**, *27*, 270–282. [CrossRef]
35. Wen, S.; Hu, Y.; Zhang, Y.; Huang, S.; Zuo, Y.; Min, Y. Dual-functional core-shell electrospun mats with precisely controlled release of anti-inflammatory and anti-bacterial agents. *Mater. Sci. Eng. C* **2019**, *100*, 514–522. [CrossRef]
36. Jin, M.; Yu, D.-G.; Wang, X.; Geraldes, C.F.G.C.; Williams, G.R.; Bligh, S.W.A. Electrospun contrast-agent-loaded fibers for colon-targeted MRI. *Adv. Healthc. Mater.* **2016**, *5*, 977–985. [CrossRef] [PubMed]
37. Fathi-Azarbayjani, A.; Qun, L.; Chan, Y.W.; Chan, S.Y. Novel vitamin and gold-loaded nanofiber facial mask for topical delivery. *AAPS PharmSciTech* **2010**, *11*, 1164–1170. [CrossRef] [PubMed]

38. Janjic, M.; Pappa, F.; Karagkiozaki, V.; Gitas, C.; Ktenidis, K.; Logothetidis, S. Surface modification of endovascular stents with rosuvastatin and heparin-loaded biodegradable nanofibers by electrospinning. *Int. J. Nanomed.* **2017**, *12*, 6343–6355. [CrossRef] [PubMed]
39. Weng, L.; Xie, J. Smart electrospun nanofibers for controlled drug release: Recent advances and new perspectives. *Curr. Pharm. Des.* **2015**, *21*, 1944–1959. [CrossRef] [PubMed]
40. Kuang, G.; Zhang, Z.; Liu, S.; Zhou, D.; Lu, X.; Jing, X.; Huang, Y. Biphasic drug release from electrospun polyblend nanofibers for optimized local cancer treatment. *Biomat. Sci.* **2018**, *6*, 324–331. [CrossRef] [PubMed]
41. Pillay, V.; Dott, C.; Choonara, Y.E.; Tyagi, C.; Tomar, L.; Kumar, P.; du Toit, L.C.; Ndesendo, V.M.K. A Review of the effect of processing variables on the fabrication of electrospun nanofibers for drug delivery applications. *J. Nanomat.* **2013**, *2013*, 22. [CrossRef]
42. Yu, H.; Jia, Y.; Yao, C.; Lu, Y. PCL/PEG core/sheath fibers with controlled drug release rate fabricated on the basis of a novel combined technique. *Int. J. Pharm.* **2014**, *469*, 17–22. [CrossRef]
43. Nguyen, T.T.T.; Ghosh, C.; Hwang, S.-G.; Chanunpanich, N.; Park, J.S. Porous core/sheath composite nanofibers fabricated by coaxial electrospinning as a potential mat for drug release system. *Int. J. Pharm.* **2012**, *439*, 296–306. [CrossRef]
44. McCann, J.T.; Li, D.; Xia, Y. Electrospinning of nanofibers with core-sheath, hollow, or porous structures. *J. Mater. Chem.* **2005**, *15*, 735–738. [CrossRef]
45. Xin, Y.; Huang, Z.; Li, W.; Jiang, Z.; Tong, Y.; Wang, C. Core–sheath functional polymer nanofibers prepared by co-electrospinning. *Eur. Polym. J.* **2008**, *44*, 1040–1045. [CrossRef]
46. Naeimirad, M.; Zadhoush, A.; Kotek, R.; Esmaeely Neisiany, R.; Nouri Khorasani, S.; Ramakrishna, S. Recent advances in core/shell bicomponent fibers and nanofibers: A review. *J. Appl. Polym. Sci.* **2018**, *135*, 46265. [CrossRef]
47. Wang, J.; Windbergs, M. Controlled dual drug release by coaxial electrospun fibers—Impact of the core fluid on drug encapsulation and release. *Int. J. Pharm.* **2019**, *556*, 363–371. [CrossRef]
48. Moghe, A.K.; Gupta, B.S. Co-axial Electrospinning for Nanofiber Structures: Preparation and Applications. *Polym. Rev.* **2008**, *48*, 353–377. [CrossRef]
49. Sultanova, Z.; Kaleli, G.; Kabay, G.; Mutlu, M. Controlled release of a hydrophilic drug from coaxially electrospun polycaprolactone nanofibers. *Int. J. Pharm.* **2016**, *505*, 133–138. [CrossRef] [PubMed]
50. Elahi, M.F.; Lu, W. Core-shell fibers for biomedical applications—A Review. *J. Bioeng. Biomed. Sci.* **2013**, *03*. [CrossRef]
51. Qin, X. 3—Coaxial electrospinning of nanofibers. In *Electrospun Nanofibers*; Afshari, M., Ed.; Woodhead Publishing: Cambridge, UK, 2017; pp. 41–71.
52. Khalf, A.; Madihally, S.V. Recent advances in multiaxial electrospinning for drug delivery. *Eur. J. Pharm. Biopharm.* **2017**, *112*, 1–17. [CrossRef] [PubMed]
53. Nagarajan, S.; Bechelany, M.; Kalkura, N.S.; Miele, P.; Bohatier, C.P.; Balme, S. Chapter 20—Electrospun nanofibers for dug delivery in regenerative medicine. In *Applications of Targeted Nano Drugs and Delivery Systems*; Mohapatra, S.S., Ranjan, S., Dasgupta, N., Mishra, R.K., Thomas, S., Eds.; Elsevier: Amsterdam, The Netherlands, 2019; pp. 595–625.
54. Yu, D.-G.; Li, X.-Y.; Wang, X.; Yang, J.-H.; Bligh, S.W.A.; Williams, G.R. Nanofibers fabricated using triaxial electrospinning as zero order drug delivery systems. *ACS Appl. Mater. Interfaces* **2015**, *7*, 18891–18897. [CrossRef] [PubMed]
55. Lu, Y.; Huang, J.; Yu, G.; Cardenas, R.; Wei, S.; Wujcik, E.K.; Guo, Z. Coaxial electrospun fibers: applications in drug delivery and tissue engineering. *Wiley Interdisciplinary Rev. Nanomed. Nanobiotechnol.* **2016**, *8*, 654–677. [CrossRef]
56. Vasita, R.G.F. Core-sheath fibers for regenerative medicine. *Nanomater. Drug Deliv. Imaging Tissue Eng.* **2013**. [CrossRef]
57. Hai, T.; Wan, X.; Yu, D.-G.; Wang, K.; Yang, Y.; Liu, Z.-P. Electrospun lipid-coated medicated nanocomposites for an improved drug sustained-release profile. *Mater. Des.* **2019**, *162*, 70–79. [CrossRef]
58. Yu, J.H.; Fridrikh, S.V.; Rutledge, G.C. Production of submicrometer Diameter fibers by two-fluid electrospinning. *Adv. Mater.* **2004**, *16*, 1562–1566. [CrossRef]
59. Nakielski, P.; Pawłowska, S.; Pierini, F.; Liwińska, W.; Hejduk, P.; Zembrzycki, K.; Zabost, E.; Kowalewski, T.A. Hydrogel nanofilaments via core-shell electrospinning. *PLoS ONE* **2015**, *10*, e0129816. [CrossRef]

60. Yoon, J.; Yang, H.-S.; Lee, B.-S.; Yu, W.-R. Recent progress in coaxial electrospinning: New parameters, various structures, and wide applications. *Adv. Mater.* **2018**, *30*, 1704765. [CrossRef]
61. Zhou, H.; Shi, Z.; Wan, X.; Fang, H.; Yu, D.-G.; Chen, X.; Liu, P. The relationships between process parameters and polymeric nanofibers fabricated using a modified coaxial electrospinning. *Nanomaterials* **2019**, *9*, 843. [CrossRef]
62. Wang, Q.; Yu, D.-G.; Zhang, L.-L.; Liu, X.-K.; Deng, Y.-C.; Zhao, M. Electrospun hypromellose-based hydrophilic composites for rapid dissolution of poorly water-soluble drug. *Carbohydr. Polym.* **2017**, *174*, 617–625. [CrossRef] [PubMed]
63. Tokiwa, Y.; Calabia, B.P.; Ugwu, C.U.; Aiba, S. Biodegradability of plastics. *Int. J. Mol. Sci.* **2009**, *10*, 3722–3742. [CrossRef] [PubMed]
64. Hassan, C.M.; Peppas, N.A. Structure and applications of poly(vinyl alcohol) hydrogels produced by conventional crosslinking or by freezing/thawing methods. In *Biopolymers PVA Hydrogels, Anionic Polymerisation Nanocomposites*; Springer: Berlin/Heidelberg, Germany, 2000; pp. 37–65.
65. Zupančič, Š.; Sinha-Ray, S.; Sinha-Ray, S.; Kristl, J.; Yarin, A.L. Controlled release of ciprofloxacin from core–shell nanofibers with monolithic or blended core. *Mol. Pharm.* **2016**, *13*, 1393–1404. [CrossRef]
66. Yarin, A.L. Coaxial electrospinning and emulsion electrospinning of core–shell fibers. *Polym. Adv. Technol.* **2011**, *22*, 310–317. [CrossRef]
67. Tiwari, S.K.; Tzezana, R.; Zussman, E.; Venkatraman, S.S. Optimizing partition-controlled drug release from electrospun core–shell fibers. *Int. J. Pharm.* **2010**, *392*, 209–217. [CrossRef]
68. Yan, E.; Fan, Y.; Sun, Z.; Gao, J.; Hao, X.; Pei, S.; Wang, C.; Sun, L.; Zhang, D. Biocompatible core–shell electrospun nanofibers as potential application for chemotherapy against ovary cancer. *Mater. Sci. Eng. C* **2014**, *41*, 217–223. [CrossRef]
69. Jiang, H.; Hu, Y.; Li, Y.; Zhao, P.; Zhu, K.; Chen, W. A facile technique to prepare biodegradable coaxial electrospun nanofibers for controlled release of bioactive agents. *J. Controlled Release* **2005**, *108*, 237–243. [CrossRef] [PubMed]
70. Jiang, H.; Hu, Y.; Zhao, P.; Li, Y.; Zhu, K. Modulation of protein release from biodegradable core–shell structured fibers prepared by coaxial electrospinning. *J. Biomed. Mater. Research B Appl. Biomater.* **2006**, *79B*, 50–57. [CrossRef] [PubMed]
71. He, M.; Xue, J.; Geng, H.; Gu, H.; Chen, D.; Shi, R.; Zhang, L. Fibrous guided tissue regeneration membrane loaded with anti-inflammatory agent prepared by coaxial electrospinning for the purpose of controlled release. *Appl. Surf. Sci.* **2015**, *335*, 121–129. [CrossRef]
72. Esmaeili, A.; Haseli, M. Electrospinning of thermoplastic carboxymethyl cellulose/poly(ethylene oxide) nanofibers for use in drug-release systems. *Mater. Sci. Eng. C* **2017**, *77*, 1117–1127. [CrossRef] [PubMed]
73. Li, L.; Yang, G.; Zhou, G.; Wang, Y.; Zheng, X.; Zhou, S. Thermally switched release from a nanogel-in-microfiber device. *Adva. Healthc. Mater.* **2015**, *4*, 1658–1663. [CrossRef] [PubMed]
74. Yu, H.; Yang, P.; Jia, Y.; Zhang, Y.; Ye, Q.; Zeng, S. Regulation of biphasic drug release behavior by graphene oxide in polyvinyl pyrrolidone/poly(ε-caprolactone) core/sheath nanofiber mats. *Colloids Surf. B Biointerfaces* **2016**, *146*, 63–69. [CrossRef] [PubMed]
75. Yu, D.G.; Wang, X.; Li, X.Y.; Chian, W.; Li, Y.; Liao, Y.Z. Electrospun biphasic drug release polyvinylpyrrolidone/ethyl cellulose core/sheath nanofibers. *Acta Biomater.* **2013**, *9*, 5665–5672. [CrossRef]
76. Yu, D.-G.; Yu, J.-H.; Chen, L.; Williams, G.R.; Wang, X. Modified coaxial electrospinning for the preparation of high-quality ketoprofen-loaded cellulose acetate nanofibers. *Carbohydr. Polym.* **2012**, *90*, 1016–1023. [CrossRef]
77. Deng, H.; Zhou, X.; Wang, X.; Zhang, C.; Ding, B.; Zhang, Q.; Du, Y. Layer-by-layer structured polysaccharides film-coated cellulose nanofibrous mats for cell culture. *Carbohydr. Polym.* **2010**, *80*, 474–479. [CrossRef]
78. Kim, C.-W.; Kim, D.-S.; Kang, S.-Y.; Marquez, M.; Joo, Y.L. Structural studies of electrospun cellulose nanofibers. *Polymer* **2006**, *47*, 5097–5107. [CrossRef]
79. Son, W.K.; Youk, J.H.; Lee, T.S.; Park, W.H. Electrospinning of ultrafine cellulose acetate fibers: Studies of a new solvent system and deacetylation of ultrafine cellulose acetate fibers. *J. Polym. Science B Polym. Phys.* **2004**, *42*, 5–11. [CrossRef]
80. Yu, D.-G.; Li, X.-Y.; Wang, X.; Chian, W.; Liao, Y.-Z.; Li, Y. Zero-order drug release cellulose acetate nanofibers prepared using coaxial electrospinning. *Cellulose* **2013**, *20*, 379–389. [CrossRef]

81. Maharjan, B.; Joshi, M.K.; Tiwari, A.P.; Park, C.H.; Kim, C.S. In-situ synthesis of AgNPs in the natural/synthetic hybrid nanofibrous scaffolds: Fabrication, characterization and antimicrobial activities. *J. Mech. Behav. Biomed. Mater.* **2017**, *65*, 66–76. [CrossRef] [PubMed]
82. Jiang, H.; Zhao, P.; Zhu, K. Fabrication and characterization of zein-based nanofibrous scaffolds by an electrospinning method. *Macromol. Biosci.* **2007**, *7*, 517–525. [CrossRef] [PubMed]
83. Karthikeyan, K.; Guhathakarta, S.; Rajaram, R.; Korrapati, P.S. Electrospun zein/eudragit nanofibers based dual drug delivery system for the simultaneous delivery of aceclofenac and pantoprazole. *Int. J. Pharm.* **2012**, *438*, 117–122. [CrossRef] [PubMed]
84. Huang, W.; Zou, T.; Li, S.; Jing, J.; Xia, X.; Liu, X. Drug-loaded zein nanofibers prepared using a modified coaxial electrospinning process. *AAPS PharmSciTech* **2013**, *14*, 675–681. [CrossRef]
85. Jiang, Y.-N.; Mo, H.-Y.; Yu, D.-G. Electrospun drug-loaded core–sheath PVP/zein nanofibers for biphasic drug release. *Int. J. Pharm.* **2012**, *438*, 232–239. [CrossRef]
86. Demir, M.; Ramos-Rivera, L.; Silva, R.; Nazhat, S.N.; Boccaccini, A.R. Zein-based composites in biomedical applications. *J. Biomed. Mater. Res. A* **2017**, *105*, 1656–1665. [CrossRef]
87. Paliwal, R.; Palakurthi, S. Zein in controlled drug delivery and tissue engineering. *J. Controlled Release* **2014**, *189*, 108–122. [CrossRef]
88. Yu, D.-G.; Chian, W.; Wang, X.; Li, X.-Y.; Li, Y.; Liao, Y.-Z. Linear drug release membrane prepared by a modified coaxial electrospinning process. *J. Membr. Sci.* **2013**, *428*, 150–156. [CrossRef]
89. Yang, J.-M.; Zha, L.-s.; Yu, D.-G.; Liu, J. Coaxial electrospinning with acetic acid for preparing ferulic acid/zein composite fibers with improved drug release profiles. *Colloids Surf. B Biointerfaces* **2013**, *102*, 737–743. [CrossRef] [PubMed]
90. Kalani, M.M.; Nourmohammadi, J.; Negahdari, B.; Rahimi, A.; Sell, S.A. Electrospun core-sheath poly(vinyl alcohol)/silk fibroin nanofibers with rosuvastatin release functionality for enhancing osteogenesis of human adipose-derived stem cells. *Mater. Sci. Eng. C* **2019**, *99*, 129–139. [CrossRef] [PubMed]
91. Repanas, A.; Glasmacher, B. Dipyridamole embedded in Polycaprolactone fibers prepared by coaxial electrospinning as a novel drug delivery system. *J. Drug Deliv. Sci. Technol.* **2015**, *29*, 132–142. [CrossRef]
92. Liao, I.; Chew, S.; Leong, K. Aligned core–shell nanofibers delivering bioactive proteins. *Nanomed.* **2006**, *1*, 465–471. [CrossRef] [PubMed]
93. Jia, X.; Zhao, C.; Li, P.; Zhang, H.; Huang, Y.; Li, H.; Fan, J.; Feng, W.; Yuan, X.; Fan, Y. Sustained release of VEGF by coaxial electrospun dextran/PLGA fibrous membranes in vascular tissue engineering. *J. Biomater. Sci. Polym. Ed.* **2011**, *22*, 1811–1827. [CrossRef] [PubMed]
94. Li, H.; Zhao, C.; Wang, Z.; Zhang, H.; Yuan, X.; Kong, D. Controlled Release of PDGF-bb by Coaxial electrospun dextran/poly(L-lactide-co-ε-caprolactone) fibers with an ultrafine core/shell structure. *J. Biomater. Sci. Polym. Ed.* **2010**, *21*, 803–819. [CrossRef]
95. Zhang, Y.Z.; Wang, X.; Feng, Y.; Li, J.; Lim, C.T.; Ramakrishna, S. Coaxial electrospinning of (fluorescein isothiocyanate-conjugated bovine serum albumin)-encapsulated poly(ε-caprolactone) nanofibers for sustained release. *Biomacromolecules* **2006**, *7*, 1049–1057. [CrossRef]
96. Man, Z.; Yin, L.; Shao, Z.; Zhang, X.; Hu, X.; Zhu, J.; Dai, L.; Huang, H.; Yuan, L.; Zhou, C.; et al. The effects of co-delivery of BMSC-affinity peptide and rhTGF-β1 from coaxial electrospun scaffolds on chondrogenic differentiation. *Biomaterials* **2014**, *35*, 5250–5260. [CrossRef]
97. Srouji, S.; Ben-David, D.; Lotan, R.; Livne, E.; Avrahami, R.; Zussman, E. Slow-release human recombinant bone morphogenetic protein-2 embedded within eectrospun scaffolds for regeneration of bone defect: In vitro and In vivo evaluation. *Tissue Eng. A* **2011**, *17*, 269–277. [CrossRef]
98. Rubert, M.; Dehli, J.; Li, Y.-F.; Taskin, M.B.; Xu, R.; Besenbacher, F.; Chen, M. Electrospun PCL/PEO coaxial fibers for basic fibroblast growth factor delivery. *J. Mater. Chem. B* **2014**, *2*, 8538–8546. [CrossRef]
99. Jia, D.; Gao, Y.; Williams, G.R. Core/shell poly(ethylene oxide)/Eudragit fibers for site-specific release. *Int. J. Pharm.* **2017**, *523*, 376–385. [CrossRef] [PubMed]
100. Llorens, E.; Ibañez, H.; del Valle, L.J.; Puiggalí, J. Biocompatibility and drug release behavior of scaffolds prepared by coaxial electrospinning of poly(butylene succinate) and polyethylene glycol. *Mater. Sci. Eng. C* **2015**, *49*, 472–484. [CrossRef] [PubMed]

101. Castillo-Ortega, M.M.; Nájera-Luna, A.; Rodríguez-Félix, D.E.; Encinas, J.C.; Rodríguez-Félix, F.; Romero, J.; Herrera-Franco, P.J. Preparation, characterization and release of amoxicillin from cellulose acetate and poly(vinyl pyrrolidone) coaxial electrospun fibrous membranes. *Mater. Sci. Eng. C* **2011**, *31*, 1772–1778. [CrossRef]
102. Ball, C.; Chou, S.-F.; Jiang, Y.; Woodrow, K.A. Coaxially electrospun fiber-based microbicides facilitate broadly tunable release of maraviroc. *Mater. Sci. Eng. C* **2016**, *63*, 117–124. [CrossRef] [PubMed]
103. Li, J.-J.; Yang, Y.-Y.; Yu, D.-G.; Du, Q.; Yang, X.-L. Fast dissolving drug delivery membrane based on the ultra-thin shell of electrospun core-shell nanofibers. *Eur. J. Pharm. Sci.* **2018**, *122*, 195–204. [CrossRef] [PubMed]
104. He, P.; Zhong, Q.; Ge, Y.; Guo, Z.; Tian, J.; Zhou, Y.; Ding, S.; Li, H.; Zhou, C. Dual drug loaded coaxial electrospun PLGA/PVP fiber for guided tissue regeneration under control of infection. *Mater. Sci. Eng. C* **2018**, *90*, 549–556. [CrossRef]
105. Cui, J.; Wang, Q.-Q.; Qiu, Y.-Y.; Wei, Q.-F. Electrospun poly(vinyl alcohol)-stilbazole quaternized/zein-tetracycline hydrochloride core-sheath nanofibers for drug release. *J. Nanosci. Nanotechnol.* **2016**, *16*, 9497–9504. [CrossRef]
106. Wang, J.; Cui, X.; Zhou, Y.; Xiang, Q. Core-shell PLGA/collagen nanofibers loaded with recombinant FN/CDHs as bone tissue engineering scaffolds. *Connect. Tissue Res.* **2014**, *55*, 292–298. [CrossRef]
107. Su, Y.; Su, Q.; Liu, W.; Lim, M.; Venugopal, J.R.; Mo, X.; Ramakrishna, S.; Al-Deyab, S.S.; El-Newehy, M. Controlled release of bone morphogenetic protein 2 and dexamethasone loaded in core–shell PLLACL–collagen fibers for use in bone tissue engineering. *Acta Biomater.* **2012**, *8*, 763–771. [CrossRef]
108. Tang, Y.; Chen, L.; Zhao, K.; Wu, Z.; Wang, Y.; Tan, Q. Fabrication of PLGA/HA (core)-collagen/amoxicillin (shell) nanofiber membranes through coaxial electrospinning for guided tissue regeneration. *Compos. Sci. Technol.* **2016**, *125*, 100–107. [CrossRef]
109. Li, Z.; Kang, H.; Che, N.; Liu, Z.; Li, P.; Li, W.; Zhang, C.; Cao, C.; Liu, R.; Huang, Y. Controlled release of liposome-encapsulated Naproxen from core-sheath electrospun nanofibers. *Carbohydr. Polym.* **2014**, *111*, 18–24. [CrossRef] [PubMed]
110. Jin, G.; Prabhakaran, M.P.; Kai, D.; Ramakrishna, S. Controlled release of multiple epidermal induction factors through core–shell nanofibers for skin regeneration. *Eur. J. Pharm. Biopharm.* **2013**, *85*, 689–698. [CrossRef] [PubMed]
111. Wang, C.; Yan, K.-W.; Lin, Y.-D.; Hsieh, P.C.H. Biodegradable core/shell fibers by coaxial electrospinning: Processing, fiber characterization, and its application in sustained drug release. *Macromolecules* **2010**, *43*, 6389–6397. [CrossRef]
112. Sohrabi, A.; Shaibani, P.M.; Etayash, H.; Kaur, K.; Thundat, T. Sustained drug release and antibacterial activity of ampicillin incorporated poly(methyl methacrylate)–nylon6 core/shell nanofibers. *Polymer* **2013**, *54*, 2699–2705. [CrossRef]
113. Oliveira, M.F.; Suarez, D.; Rocha, J.C.B.; de Carvalho Teixeira, A.V.N.; Cortés, M.E.; De Sousa, F.B.; Sinisterra, R.D. Electrospun nanofibers of polyCD/PMAA polymers and their potential application as drug delivery system. *Mater. Sci. Eng. C* **2015**, *54*, 252–261. [CrossRef]
114. Zhang, H.; Niu, Q.; Wang, N.; Nie, J.; Ma, G. Thermo-sensitive drug controlled release PLA core/PNIPAM shell fibers fabricated using a combination of electrospinning and UV photo-polymerization. *Eur. Polym. J.* **2015**, *71*, 440–450. [CrossRef]
115. Wang, X.; Yu, D.-G.; Li, X.-Y.; Bligh, S.W.A.; Williams, G.R. Electrospun medicated shellac nanofibers for colon-targeted drug delivery. *Int. J. Pharm.* **2015**, *490*, 384–390. [CrossRef]
116. Xu, Y.; Li, J.-J.; Yu, D.-G.; Williams, G.R.; Yang, J.-H.; Wang, X. Influence of the drug distribution in electrospun gliadin fibers on drug-release behavior. *Eur. J. Pharm. Sci.* **2017**, *106*, 422–430. [CrossRef]
117. Liu, X.; Shao, W.; Luo, M.; Bian, J.; Yu, D.-G. Electrospun blank nanocoating for improved sustained release profiles from medicated gliadin nanofibers. *Nanomaterials* **2018**, *8*, 184. [CrossRef]
118. Wang, K.; Wen, H.-F.; Yu, D.-G.; Yang, Y.; Zhang, D.-F. Electrosprayed hydrophilic nanocomposites coated with shellac for colon-specific delayed drug delivery. *Mater. Des.* **2018**, *143*, 248–255. [CrossRef]
119. Nguyen, D.N.; Clasen, C.; Van den Mooter, G. Encapsulating darunavir nanocrystals within Eudragit L100 using coaxial electrospraying. *Eur. J. Pharm. Biopharm.* **2017**, *113*, 50–59. [CrossRef] [PubMed]

120. Yu, D.-G.; Zheng, X.-L.; Yang, Y.; Li, X.-Y.; Williams, G.R.; Zhao, M. Immediate release of helicid from nanoparticles produced by modified coaxial electrospraying. *Appl. Surf. Sci.* **2019**, *473*, 148–155. [CrossRef]
121. Huang, W.; Hou, Y.; Lu, X.; Gong, Z.; Yang, Y.; Lu, X.-J.; Liu, X.-L.; Yu, D.-G. The process–property–performance relationship of medicated nanoparticles prepared by modified coaxial electrospraying. *Pharmaceutics* **2019**, *11*, 226. [CrossRef] [PubMed]

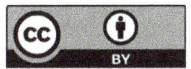

© 2019 by the authors. Licensee MDPI, Basel, Switzerland. This article is an open access article distributed under the terms and conditions of the Creative Commons Attribution (CC BY) license (http://creativecommons.org/licenses/by/4.0/).

MDPI
St. Alban-Anlage 66
4052 Basel
Switzerland
Tel. +41 61 683 77 34
Fax +41 61 302 89 18
www.mdpi.com

Pharmaceutics Editorial Office
E-mail: pharmaceutics@mdpi.com
www.mdpi.com/journal/pharmaceutics

www.ingramcontent.com/pod-product-compliance
Lightning Source LLC
LaVergne TN
LVHW071946080526
838202LV00064B/6688